T0205861

Antioxidants in Health and Disease

Antioxidants in Health and Disease

Edited by

Antonis Zampelas
Renata Micha

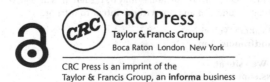

CRC Press
Taylor & Francis Group
Boca Raton London New York

CRC Press is an imprint of the
Taylor & Francis Group, an **informa** business

CRC Press
Taylor & Francis Group
6000 Broken Sound Parkway NW, Suite 300
Boca Raton, FL 33487-2742

First issued in paperback 2021

© 2015 by Taylor & Francis Group, LLC
CRC Press is an imprint of Taylor & Francis Group, an Informa business

No claim to original U.S. Government works

Version Date: 20150504

ISBN 13: 978-1-03-209858-6 (pbk)
ISBN 13: 978-1-4665-8003-9 (hbk)

Visit the Taylor & Francis Web site at
http://www.taylorandfrancis.com

and the CRC Press Web site at
http://www.crcpress.com

To our families for their love and support

and

to our students for their constant inspiration

Contents

Preface...ix
Acknowledgments.. xiii
Editors.. xv
Contributors xvii

SECTION I Interest in Antioxidants: Why and How?

Chapter 1 Reactive Oxygen Species: Production, Regulation, and Essential
Functions 3

Robert B. Rucker

Chapter 2 Major Dietary Antioxidants and Their Food Sources.......................23

Moschos Polissiou and Dimitra Daferera

SECTION II Antioxidants in Health

Chapter 3 Oxidative Stress in Pregnancy 47

Ung Lim Teo and Andrew Shennan

Chapter 4 The Role of Antioxidants in Children's Growth and Development ... 53

*Fátima Pérez de Heredia, Ligia Esperanza Díaz,
Aurora Hernández, Ana María Veses, Sonia Gómez-Martínez,
and Ascensión Marcos*

Chapter 5 Adulthood and Old Age 71

Antonios E. Koutelidakis and Maria Kapsokefalou

Chapter 6 Smoking, Oxidative Stress, and Antioxidant Intake 83

Aristea Baschali and Dimitrios Karayiannis

Chapter 7 Physical Exercise...103

*Mustafa Atalay, Jani Lappalainen, Ayhan Korkmaz,
and Chandan K. Sen*

SECTION III   Antioxidants in Various Disease States

Chapter 8   Coronary Heart Disease and Stroke.. 117

Antonis Zampelas and Ioannis Dimakopoulos

Chapter 9   Diabetes.. 151

Vaia Lambadiari, Foteini Kousathana, and George Dimitriadis

Chapter 10 Cancer 165

Eleni Andreou

Chapter 11 Antioxidants in Neurodegeneration—Truth or Myth?.................... 199

Francisco Capani, George Barreto, Eduardo Blanco Calvo, and Christopher Horst Lillig

Chapter 12 Gastrointestinal Disorders.. 215

Michael Georgoulis, Ioanna Kechribari, and Meropi D. Kontogianni

Chapter 13 Antioxidants in Obesity and Inflammation.................................... 233

Chrysi Koliaki, Alexander Kokkinos, and Nicholas Katsilambros

Chapter 14 Modulation of Immune Response by Antioxidants......................... 249

Kathrin Becker, Florian Überall, Dietmar Fuchs, and Johanna M. Gostner

Chapter 15 HIV/AIDS... 263

Heike Englert and Germaine Nkengfack

SECTION IV   Role of Herbs

Chapter 16 Role of Herbs and Spices—In Health and Longevity and in Disease 281

Krishnapura Srinivasan

Index.. 301

Preface

The present book, *Antioxidants in Health and Disease*, explores the effects of dietary antioxidants and/or antioxidant supplementation on various stages of the human life cycle, as well as on disease states, in a very balanced way.

Since the development of the "antioxidant hypothesis," which is based on the assumption that oxidation in the body has deleterious effects on health, and thus subsequent antioxidant intake may prove beneficial, numerous studies have been carried out to test this hypothesis. After decades of scientific output, this area remains controversial. This book systematically explores these controversies and provides answers to key questions.

The book aims to critically review and synthesize the latest evidence-based findings in this area, and subsequently inform health professionals, such as physicians, dietitians, nutritionists, and nurses, and additionally biochemists, policy makers, and the general audience about the true role of antioxidants in health and disease. It disentangles myths from facts associated with antioxidant intake and further provides practical advice about recommended intakes whether from diet, supplements, or both.

The book is divided into three major sections. In Section I, mechanisms of action and major food sources are given. In Section II, the role of antioxidants in different stages of the life cycle is explored. Finally, in Section III, the effect of dietary antioxidants and/or antioxidant supplementation on the prevention and the treatment of various diseases are investigated.

In Chapter 1, the way by which reactive oxygen species are formed and regulated is presented. As stated, free radicals are not always harmful, and mechanisms to maintain a balance between essential functions and potential pathologies are outlined in this chapter.

In Chapter 2, the major natural antioxidants are classified and their distribution in food sources is presented. The major antioxidants presented include phenols and polyphenols, carotenoids, and essential oils, while major food sources are fruits, grapes and wine, vegetables, herbs, olive, and olive oil.

In Chapter 3, the implications of oxidative stress in pregnancy are explored. This chapter also reviews the most recent evidence available regarding the clinical potential of antioxidants in preventing some common and serious conditions in pregnancy.

Chapter 4 initially explores the effects of oxidative stress on children's health. Then, a very balanced overview of the effects of antioxidants on various conditions during childhood is given, such as their effects on growth, physical and cognitive performance, treatment of deficiencies, and asthma and allergies.

Chapter 5 explores the needs of adults and the elderly in antioxidants. Owing to population aging, especially in westernized societies, and more people reaching the ages of 70, 80, or even 90 years, the possible effects of antioxidants on diseases such as cataract and Alzheimer's are of great interest.

Chapter 6 explores the mechanisms involved in the increased oxidative stress in people who smoke. It also gives an overview on the prevention and treatment of diseases caused by smoking, relying on a combined application of antioxidants, substitution of important factors for human oxidant defense, and metal-detoxifying agents.

Chapter 7 discusses the role of endogenous and exogenous antioxidants on physical exercise and human performance. More specifically, it focuses on the need for, as well as the advantages and disadvantages of, antioxidant supplements for the physically active population and gives a special emphasis on thiol antioxidants, which play a key role in cellular redox regulation.

Chapter 8 initially gives a brief overview of the potential relationship between oxidation and the development of cardiovascular diseases, namely coronary heart disease and stroke. Then, data on the effects of antioxidants on risk factors and on end points of the diseases are presented.

Diabetes is a disease where increased oxidative stress is present. Chapter 9 explores mechanisms that contribute to increased oxidative stress in diabetic patients, and it also gives an overview of the antioxidant effects on the disease and the controversies related to antioxidant supplements.

Chapter 10 initially gives an overview of the effects of free radicals on cancer development. Then it gives, in extensive detail, the impact and the controversies of antioxidant intake through dietary sources or supplementation on cancer prevention and on the treatment of some types of cancer.

Chapter 11 explores the influence of antioxidants on neurodegenerative diseases. It explores mechanisms and gives data from interventions with more specific focus on the thioredoxin protein family (Trxs).

Chapter 12 provides an overview on the role of oxidative stress in the pathogenesis of inflammation-based gastrointestinal tract diseases, namely celiac disease and inflammatory bowel diseases, as well as the potential role of antioxidants in their prevention and treatment.

Oxidative stress is one of the unifying mechanisms underlying the development of obesity-related comorbidities, mainly type 2 diabetes and cardiovascular diseases. Chapter 13 explores the multiple contributing factors that may promote increased oxidative stress in obesity, including hyperglycemia, hyperleptinemia, increased tissue lipid availability that leads to lipotoxicity, inadequate antioxidant capacity, and chronic subclinical inflammation. It also gives a very balanced overview of the effects of antioxidants on oxidative stress in obese patients.

During immune response, activated immunocompetent cells produce large amounts of reactive oxygen species and reactive nitrogen species as a defense strategy. Chapter 14 focuses on the interference of antioxidants with the immune response, and discusses the possible consequences of unconsidered high-dose antioxidant supplementation.

Chapter 15 discusses controversies regarding antioxidant supplementation on HIV/AIDS patients.

Finally, Chapter 16 explores the role of herbs. The chapter argues that although spices are typically consumed at relatively low levels, some data indicate that spices are in fact a very concentrated source of antioxidants and may provide a meaningful level of antioxidant activity if consumed at higher levels.

We hope that this book will provide all the valuable information to unravel current myths and straighten out facts associated with antioxidant intake, and that any reader will enjoy reading it.

Antonis Zampelas
Renata Micha

Acknowledgments

It was some years ago when Ira Wolinsky approached me and enquired whether I would be interested in editing a book on antioxidants. It is obvious that this field remains highly controversial, and I thus accepted this challenge with great enthusiasm. I would really like to thank him for this opportunity, and I look forward to future collaborations.

We, as coeditors, would also like to acknowledge the hard work of all the staff at CRC Press and thank them for their professional conduct and their efficient collaboration. Namely, we would like to thank Randy Brehm, Amor Nanas, and Jill Jurgensen who accommodated our deadline misses and editing requests, and effectively made this book possible. We couldn't have done this without them.

Special thanks are due to Nantia Mavrommataki, who provided administrative support, for her constant dedication.

Finally, we would like to sincerely thank all the authors for their scientific input to this book and for ensuring its accuracy and practicality. Its success is primarily due to their commitment and to their high-level scientific knowledge, which they transferred to the book's text outstandingly. Thank you!

Antonis Zampelas
Renata Micha

Editors

Antonis Zampelas earned his BSc in Food Science and Technology from the Agricultural University of Athens, Greece. He holds an MSc degree in food science from the University of Reading, UK, and a PhD in Human Nutrition from the University of Surrey, UK. Professor Zampelas worked in the University of Surrey, as research fellow and also in the UK Ministry of Agriculture, Fisheries and Food, as a senior scientific officer. In Greece, and before joining the Agricultural University of Athens in 2006, he worked as an assistant professor of human nutrition and director of the professional training year in the Department of Nutrition and Dietetics at Harokopio University, Athens. He also served as president of the Hellenic Food Authority (2008–2010). He has been involved in numerous trials and projects related to the effects of diet on parameters influencing the development of cardiovascular diseases. Professor Zampelas' research interest also includes the development of nutritional educational programs for Greek school children to prevent childhood obesity. He is also the principal investigator of the Hellenic Nutrition and Health Examination Survey. Professor Zampelas served as chair of the Department of Food Science and Human Nutrition, at the Agricultural University of Athens (2011–2014), and as a member of its senate; as president of the Hellenic Society of Lipidology, Atherosclerosis and Vascular Diseases; vice chairman of the Committee of National Drug Administration for the approval of Nutritional Supplements (2005–2007); member of the National Committee of Nutritional Policy; and member of the Executive Committee of the European Atherosclerosis Society (2005–2008). He is now vice president of the Hellenic Society of Medical Nutrition and associate editor of the international journal *Atherosclerosis*. Professor Zampelas currently works at the Department of Nutrition and Health of the United Arab Emirates University, at the Department of Food Science and Human Nutrition of the Agricultural University of Athens, and he is also a visiting professor at the Department of Nutrition of the University of Nicosia, Cyprus. Professor Zampelas is editor-in-chief of two nutrition textbooks, coeditor of two others, coauthor of 20 textbook chapters, and contributed to 120 peer-reviewed publications in international scientific journals.

Renata Micha is a clinical dietician, public health nutritionist, and epidemiologist who specializes in nutritional and cardiovascular epidemiology, with a focus on global diet and chronic disease and population strategies to improve diet. Dr. Micha earned her degree in nutrition and dietetics from Harokopio University of Athens, Greece (2004), and her PhD in public health nutrition from King's College London, UK (2008). She subsequently did her 3-year (2008–2011) postdoctoral training in nutritional and cardiovascular epidemiology at the Department of Epidemiology, Harvard School of Public Health, Boston, United States. During her postdoc, she mainly focused on leading the work of the 2010 Global Burden of Diseases (GBD) Nutrition and Chronic Diseases Expert Group (NutriCoDE), a global WHO project funded by the Bill and Melinda Gates Foundation. In November 2011, she was appointed research associate (junior faculty) at the Department of Epidemiology, Harvard School of Public Health, and in July 2014 she was appointed research assistant professor at Friedman School of Nutrition Science and Policy, Tufts University. In this role, she is involved in cutting-edge international research, including expanding the 2010 GBD NutriCoDE work and evaluating the comparative effectiveness of population strategies and policies to improve diet and reduce cardiovascular disease. Furthermore, in Greece, she was instrumental in the design, development, and funding of the 1st Hellenic National Health and Nutrition Examination Survey (H-NHANES), the largest national surveillance survey of its kind to ever take place in Greece. Dr. Micha currently serves as the director of the H-NHANES; in this role, she directs a team of more than 100 people of various backgrounds, with aims of evaluating dietary and lifestyle habits and related health indicators and risk factors in a nationally representative sample of the Greek population. In addition to her research, Dr. Micha has extensive teaching experience. She has developed and led teaching for one undergraduate and three graduate courses in the field of nutritional science, including in nutritional epidemiology, public health nutrition, and advanced research methods. She has designed and contributed to multiple epidemiological studies (clinical and observational) relating to the investigation of the effect of diet on the development of chronic diseases, particularly cardiometabolic diseases. Dr. Micha has received several awards and honors, and she is an *ad hoc* manuscript reviewer in international journals, including the *New England Journal of Medicine*. She has contributed to more than 35 peer-reviewed publications in international high-impact scientific journals such as *New England Journal of Medicine, Lancet, British Medical Journal, Circulation*, and *PLoS Medicine*; presented more than 40 abstracts in international scientific meetings; is a coauthor of three international books; and is a coeditor of one book.

Contributors

Eleni Andreou
Life and Health Sciences
University of Nicosia
Nicosia, Cyprus

Mustafa Atalay
Institute of Biomedicine, Physiology
University of Eastern Finland
Kuopio, Finland

George Barreto
Department of Nutrition and
    Biochemistry Faculty of Sciences
Pontificia Universidad Javeriana
Bogotá, D.C., Colombia

Aristea Baschali
Department of Clinical Nutrition
Evaggelismos Hospital
Athens, Greece

Kathrin Becker
Division of Biological Chemistry,
    Biocenter
Innsbruck Medical University
Innsbruck, Austria

Eduardo Blanco Calvo
Institute of Biomedical Research
    (IBIMA)
Regional Hospital of Málaga
Málaga, Spain

Francisco Capani
Laboratory of Cytoarchitecture and
    Neuronal Plasticity
Institute of Cardiological Research
    "Prof. Dr. Alberto C. Taquini"
    (ININCA)
Buenos Aires University and CONICET
and
Department of Biology
Universidad Argentina John F. Kennedy
Buenos Aires, Argentina

Dimitra Daferera
Laboratory of General Chemistry
Department of Food Science and
    Human Nutrition
Agricultural University of Athens
Athens, Greece

Fátima Pérez de Heredia
School of Natural Sciences and
    Psychology
Liverpool John Moores University
Liverpool, United Kingdom

Ligia Esperanza Díaz
Immunonutrition Research Group
Department of Metabolism and
    Nutrition
Institute of Food Science and
    Technology and Nutrition (ICTAN)
Spanish National Research Council
    (CSIC)
Madrid, Spain

Ioannis Dimakopoulos
Agricultural University of Athens
Athens, Greece

George Dimitriadis
Second Department of Internal
    Medicine
Research Unit and Diabetes Centre
Athens University Medical School
Attikon General Hospital
Athens, Greece

Heike Englert
University of Applied Sciences
    Muenster
Muenster, Germany

Dietmar Fuchs
Division of Biological Chemistry,
    Biocenter
Innsbruck Medical University
Innsbruck, Austria

Michael Georgoulis
Department of Nutrition and Dietetics
Harokopio University
Athens, Greece

Sonia Gómez-Martínez
Immunonutrition Research Group
Department of Metabolism and
    Nutrition
Institute of Food Science and
    Technology and Nutrition (ICTAN)
Spanish National Research Council
    (CSIC)
Madrid, Spain

Johanna M. Gostner
Division of Medical Biochemistry,
    Biocenter
Innsbruck Medical University
Innsbruck, Austria

Aurora Hernández
Immunonutrition Research Group
Department of Metabolism and
    Nutrition
Institute of Food Science and
    Technology and Nutrition (ICTAN)
Spanish National Research Council
    (CSIC)
Madrid, Spain

Maria Kapsokefalou
Unit of Human Nutrition
Department of Food Science and
    Human Nutrition
Agricultural University of Athens
Athens, Greece

Dimitrios Karayiannis
Department of Clinical Nutrition
Evaggelismos Hospital
Athens, Greece

Nicholas Katsilambros
First Department of Propaedeutic
    Medicine
Athens University Medical School
Laiko General Hospital
Athens, Greece

Ioanna Kechribari
Department of Nutrition and Dietetics
Harokopio University
Athens, Greece

Alexander Kokkinos
First Department of Propaedeutic
    Medicine
Athens University Medical School
Laiko General Hospital
Athens, Greece

Chrysi Koliaki
Institute for Clinical Diabetology
German Diabetes Center
Leibniz Center for Diabetes Research
Heinrich Heine University
Düsseldorf, Germany

Meropi D. Kontogianni
Department of Nutrition and Dietetics
Harokopio University
Athens, Greece

Ayhan Korkmaz
Institute of Biomedicine, Physiology
University of Eastern Finland
Kuopio, Finland

Foteini Kousathana
Second Department of Internal
    Medicine
Research Unit and Diabetes Centre
Athens University Medical School
Attikon General Hospital
Athens, Greece

Antonios E. Koutelidakis
Unit of Human Nutrition
Department of Food Science and
    Human Nutrition
Agricultural University of Athens
Athens, Greece

Vaia Lambadiari
Second Department of Internal
    Medicine
Research Unit and Diabetes Centre
Athens University Medical School
Attikon General Hospital
Athens, Greece

Jani Lappalainen
Institute of Biomedicine, Physiology
University of Eastern Finland
Kuopio, Finland

Christopher Horst Lillig
Institute for Medical Biochemistry and
    Molecular Biology
Universitätsmedizin Greifswald Ernst-
    Moritz Arndt-Universitat Greifswald
Greifswald, Germany

Ascensión Marcos
Immunonutrition Research Group
Department of Metabolism and
    Nutrition
Institute of Food Science and
    Technology and Nutrition (ICTAN)
Spanish National Research Council
    (CSIC)
Madrid, Spain

Germaine Nkengfack
Department of Nutrition
University of Applied Sciences
Muenster, Germany

and

Department of Biomedical Sciences
University of Dschang
Dschang, Cameroon

Moschos Polissiou
Laboratory of General Chemistry
Department of Food Science and
    Human Nutrition
Agricultural University of Athens
Athens, Greece

Robert B. Rucker
Nutrition Department
University of California, Davis
Davis, California

Chandan K. Sen
Department of Surgery
College of Medicine
Center for Regenerative Medicine and
    Cell-Based Therapies
OSU Comprehensive Wound Center
The Ohio State University Wexner
    Medical Center
Columbus, Ohio

Andrew Shennan
Womens Health Academic Centre
Kings College London
London, United Kingdom

Krishnapura Srinivasan
Department of Biochemistry and
   Nutrition
CSIR—Central Food Technological
   Research Institute
Mysore, India

Ung Lim Teo
Maternity Unit
St Thomas' Hospital
London, United Kingdom

Florian Überall
Division of Medical Biochemistry,
   Biocenter
Innsbruck Medical University
Innsbruck, Austria

Ana María Veses
Immunonutrition Research Group
Department of Metabolism and
   Nutrition
Institute of Food Science and
   Technology and Nutrition (ICTAN)
Spanish National Research Council
   (CSIC)
Madrid, Spain

Section I

Interest in Antioxidants:
Why and How?

1 Reactive Oxygen Species
Production, Regulation, and Essential Functions

Robert B. Rucker

CONTENTS

Introduction 3
Some Oxygen Chemistry Basics 4
Production and Types of O_2-Derived ROS 7
    ROS Production 7
    Types of O_2-Derived ROS 10
        Hydrogen Peroxide 10
        Hydroxyl Radicals 12
        Peroxynitrite 13
        Hypochlorous Acid (HOCl) and Myeloperoxidase 14
        Singlet Oxygen and Ozone 15
        Oxidative Stress 16
    Common Targets of the Damaging Effects of ROS 19
Final Perspectives 20
References 20

INTRODUCTION

This chapter provides basic information and background to set the stage for the subsequent chapters that address health or disease conditions in which reactive oxygen species (ROS) and oxidant stress play important roles. The major forms of ROS are described along with mechanisms that account for their production. Strictly defined, ROS include chemically reactive oxygen ions and peroxides. Abnormally high levels of ROS initiate reactions that structurally alter important molecules, such as DNA, RNA, proteins, and lipids, particularly lipids comprising cellular membranes [1,2]. Such events contribute to a number of pathological conditions. Ischemic muscle damage, desynchronies in growth due to excessive apoptosis, necrosis, inflammation, and insulin resistance are examples.

Despite their destructive potential, however, ROS also play essential roles in cell turnover and replacement (e.g., apoptosis or programmed cell death), as secondary messengers in a variety of cellular processes and as catalyst in the modulation of protein structure, host defense mechanisms, wound repair, chemotaxis, and the mobilization of cellular transport systems [2,3]. Whether ROS serve as healthful biological agents or initiate oxidative damage depends on the delicate equilibrium between ROS production and their scavenging.

A free radical is an atom or molecule that contains unpaired electrons and maintains an independent existence. Free radicals can have positive, negative, or neutral charges. In most instances, free radicals initiate a change in other atoms or molecules by abstracting a hydrogen atom from C–H, N–H, or O–H bonds within biomolecules or an electron from a metal or metal complex capable of catalyzing oxidation/reduction (redox) reactions [2]. In simple reactions, there may be only a change in a given redox state of the targeted molecule. However, if the free radical does not reattach to the redox molecule or another molecule that can act as a free radical acceptor (e.g., an antioxidant), such reactions can become potentially harmful. The descriptions that follow outline the mechanisms important to maintaining the balance between essential functions and potential pathologies.

SOME OXYGEN CHEMISTRY BASICS

Oxygen is the third most abundant element in the universe and constitutes 20.8% of the volume of air [4,5]. In most compounds containing oxygen, the oxidation state of oxygen is −2. An oxidation state of −1 is found in peroxides. From an evolutionary perspective, the dominant forms of early life on Earth were anaerobic organisms until oxygen began to accumulate in the atmosphere. The accumulation of atmospheric oxygen started about 2.5 billion years ago, and the first aerobic organisms followed about a billion years later [5].

Oxygen is an unusual element in several ways. For example, at temperatures compatible with life, molecular oxygen exists in a triplet state, whereas almost all molecules encountered in daily life exist in a singlet state. Triplet oxygen (not to be confused with the oxygen allotrope ozone, O_3) is the ground state for dioxygen, O_2. Oxygen in the triplet state needs to transition into a singlet state before chemical reactions can more easily occur (Figure 1.1). The need for such transitions makes the vast bulk of atmospheric oxygen kinetically nonreactive on a relative scale despite being a strong oxidant from a thermodynamic perspective. For example, although dioxygen is not a highly reactive molecule, its two unpaired electrons give it free radical character. There are also other allotropic states of oxygen ranging from molecular oxygen (O_2), the most familiar form, to highly reactive ozone (O_3) and oxygen in several solid states [1–5].

The electron configuration of ground-state oxygen has two unpaired electrons occupying two degenerate molecular orbitals, i.e., orbitals that have different quantum states but the same energy level [2,4]. Degenerate orbitals are antibonding, which prevents molecular oxygen from reacting directly or readily with other molecules.

Ground-state oxygen (O_2): common representations of electron distributions

$$\sigma 1s \mid \sigma°1s \mid \sigma 2s \mid \sigma°2s \mid \sigma 2p \mid \pi 2p \mid \pi°2p$$

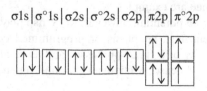

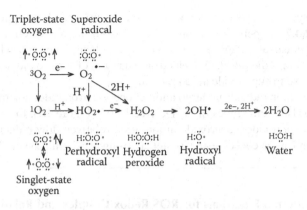

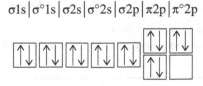

FIGURE 1.1 ROS are generated as by-products and intermediates from many types of oxidation reactions. Some relationships between oxygen in the triplet state and major forms of ROS are given. Triplet oxygen ($^3O_2$) has two unpaired electrons occupying two degenerate molecular orbitals, which are antibonding. However, triplet oxygen can be transformed into several forms of singlet oxygen, which contains paired electrons, and with the addition of an electron, the superoxide anion radical. Singlet oxygen is more reactive than triplet oxygen. Various ROS may then be formed from singlet oxygen and superoxide in steps involving one electron and/or one or two H^+ transfers. In the Lewis structures corresponding to a given form of oxygen, the electrons that have "free radical" potential are designated with small open circles (o) and arrows represent potential spin states.

To iterate, O_2 in its ground state can absorb energy and be transformed into the more reactive singlet oxygen (Figure 1.1). This achieves the goal of producing a molecule in which there is the same number of electrons but with a pair of outer electrons that have antiparallel spin. When this occurs, one of the electrons can potentially jump to an empty orbital, creating an unpaired electron. Singlet oxygen is not a radical, but is more reactive than dioxygen, because it can react with atoms with outer shell electrons in either spin direction. In this regard, singlet oxygen violates Hund's rule, which states that every orbital in an atom's subshell is singly occupied with one electron before any one orbital is doubly occupied, and all electrons in singly occupied orbitals have the same spin. Singlet oxygen has eight outer electrons existing in pairs, leaving one orbital of the same energy level empty [2,5].

In nature, singlet oxygen is formed from water during photosynthesis, using the energy of sunlight [5,6]. It can also be produced in the troposphere by the photolysis of ozone $\left(O_3 + \text{ultraviolet light} \rightarrow O_2^* + O\right)$, and in mammalian systems by reactions that occur in cells of the immune system (also cf. comments related to HOCl in "Types of O_2-Derived ROS").

Singlet oxygen: common representations of electron distributions

$$\sigma 1s \mid \sigma°1s \mid \sigma 2s \mid \sigma°2s \mid \sigma 2p \mid \pi 2p \mid \pi°2p$$

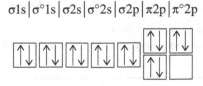

Another oxygen species that can be formed from ground-state oxygen is superoxide anion [1,2,4,7]. Superoxide anion is formed from the one-electron reduction of dioxygen and exists as a negatively charged free radical of oxygen. The systematic name of the anion is dioxide^{-1}. One electron reduction of the ground-state molecular oxygen gives rise to superoxide anion radical $\left(O_2^{\cdot-}\right)$.

Superoxide anion radicals undergo another one-electron reduction to yield hydrogen peroxide (H_2O_2, cf. "Types of O_2-Derived ROS"; Figure 1.1). In spite of its designation as a *super*oxide, superoxide anion has a relatively low reduction potential (Table 1.1), and as a consequence is not a strong oxidizing agent. Nevertheless,

TABLE 1.1
Standard Reduction Potentials for ROS Redox Couples and Relative Rate Constants for Selected ROS

Redox Couple	Standard Reduction Potential (E) and pH 7.0 in MV
OH$^{\cdot}$, H$^+$/H$_2$O	+2310
Lipid-LO$^{\cdot}$, H$^+$/LOH	+1600
HOO$^{\cdot}$, H$^+$/H$_2$O$_2$	+1060
Lipid-LOO$^{\cdot}$, H$^+$/LOOH	+800–1400
GS$^-$/GSH	+920
PUFA[–C$^{\cdot}$], H$^+$/PUFA–H	+600
H$_2$O$_2$, H$^+$/H$_2$O, OH$^{\cdot}$	+320
Ascorbate$^{-\cdot}$, H$^+$/ascorbate	+282
CoQH$^{\cdot}$, H$^+$/CoQH$_2$ (ubiquinol)	+200
Cu^{2+}/Cu^{1+}	+150
Fe^{3+}/Fe^{2+} (aqueous)	+110
CoQ (ubiquinone), H$^+$/CoQH$^{\cdot}$	−40
Dehydroascorbate/dehydroascorbate$^{-\cdot}$	−170
Fe^{3+} [ferritin]/Fe^{2+} [ferritin]	−190
NAD$^+$, H$^+$/NADH	−320
O$_2$/O$_2^{\cdot-}$	−330
O$_2$, H$^+$/HOO$^{\cdot}$	−460
H$_2$O/hydrated electron $\left(e_{aq}^-\right)$	−2870

Relative Half-Lives of Reactive Oxygen Species	
Hydroxyl radical	10^{-9} seconds (s)
Alkoxyl radical	10^{-6} s
Singlet oxygen	10^{-5} s
Peroxyl radical	1–10 s
Nitric oxide radical	1–10 s
Semiquinones	Days
Hydrogen peroxide (aqueous solutions, pH ~7)	Minutes to days
Superoxide anion radical	Seconds to minutes

Source: Sies, H., *Eur. J. Biochem.*, 215, 213, 1993.

Note: The half-lives of ROS markedly differ, which underscores the need for different types of defense mechanisms.

because of its ability to reduce transition metals capable of reduction, such as iron and copper, and act as a precursor to compounds, such as H_2O_2, it is clearly a major facilitator of free radical reactions (cf. "Production and Types of O_2-Derived ROS").

Superoxide anion radical: common representations of electron distributions representations

$$\sigma1s \,|\, \sigma°1s \,|\, \sigma2s \,|\, \sigma°2s \,|\, \sigma2p \,|\, \pi2p \,|\, \pi°2p$$

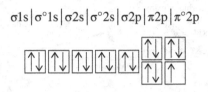

PRODUCTION AND TYPES OF O_2-DERIVED ROS

ROS PRODUCTION

ROS are not an entity, but a group of compounds, each with distinct features. Accordingly, ROS can be produced by multiple chemical, physical, and biological mechanisms. Numerous examples are developed in subsequent chapters that range from pollutants, tobacco smoke, excessive drug or xenobiotic exposure, to radiation exposure. With respect to cellular metabolism, from 2% to 4% of the total oxygen during both rest and exercise can be potentially converted to some type of ROS (Refs. [1–4]; also cf. Chapters 4, 5, and 7). This amounts to ~0.44–0.9 mol of ROS equivalents generated per day for a person weighing ~70 kg and consuming 500 liters of O_2, i.e., equivalent to an energy expenditure of ~2500 kcal or ~10.5 MJ/day [8]. ROS production is particularly associated with metabolic processes that take place within mitochondria, peroxisomes, and the endoplasmic reticulum (ER) (Figure 1.2):

- In mitochondria, high rates of ATP production are often associated with increased levels of ROS as a result of the superoxide radical generation associated with the increase in oxygen flux through the mitochondrial respiratory complex [9,10]—an increase that can be dissipated in part by uncoupling electron transport from ATP synthesis. Uncoupling proteins (UCPs), located in the mitochondrial inner membrane, dissipate mitochondrial proton gradients before they can be used to provide the energy for oxidative phosphorylation leading to ATP generation [10]. Although the major function of UCPs is heat regulation, UCPs also help modulate mitochondrial ROS levels (Figure 1.3).
- In peroxisomes, an organelle designed for branched and long-chain fatty acid and D-amino acid oxidations, ROS are produced predominantly by the actions of various oxidases. As an example, the first step in the oxidation of fatty acids is catalyzed by the enzyme acyl-CoA oxidase, which results in H_2O_2 and a dehydroacyl moiety:

$$\text{Acyl-CoA} + O_2 \rightarrow \textit{trans}\text{-2,3-dehydroacyl-CoA} + H_2O_2$$

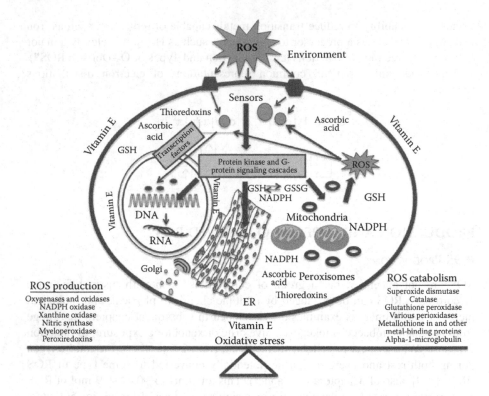

FIGURE 1.2 ROS generation and regulation. Oxidative stress is the balance between events that are important to the control of ROS synthesis versus catabolism. Cellular regulation of ROS is organized at several levels and involves expression of enzymes and proteins involved in both ROS generation and catabolism. The reactions occur predominantly in the ER, mitochondria, and peroxisomes. Many small molecules are also involved in acting as antioxidants and reductants (e.g., ascorbic acid, reduced glutathione, NADPH, thioredoxins, vitamin E, and carotenoids). Apolar antioxidants, such as vitamin E or carotenoids, are localized in cellular and organelle membranes. External factors, such as chemical and ultraviolet radiation, can also be important to ROS generation. Not shown is the contribution of dietary antioxidants, which can serve as an important defense to excessive generation of ROS. The need for a balance relates in large degree to the important roles ROS play in cellular signaling and defenses that require strong oxidants (e.g., inflammation caused by foreign substances). Cellular signaling involves recognition by receptors that are linked to pathways important to generating protein kinase cascades or expression of transcription factors that control the enzymes involved in ROS production (synthesis/catabolism).

- In the ER, particularly the smooth ER, numerous reactions occur that involve oxidases and oxygenases. The smooth ER is important to the synthesis, catabolism, or modification of complex lipids, phospholipids, and steroids not metabolized directly by peroxisomes or mitochondria. The smooth ER is also essential for detoxification and the modification of xenobiotics (foreign chemical substances found within an organism that are not normally produced by the organism, e.g., drugs and food-derived pigments). Families of enzymes localized in the smooth ER (the cytochrome P450 mono- and

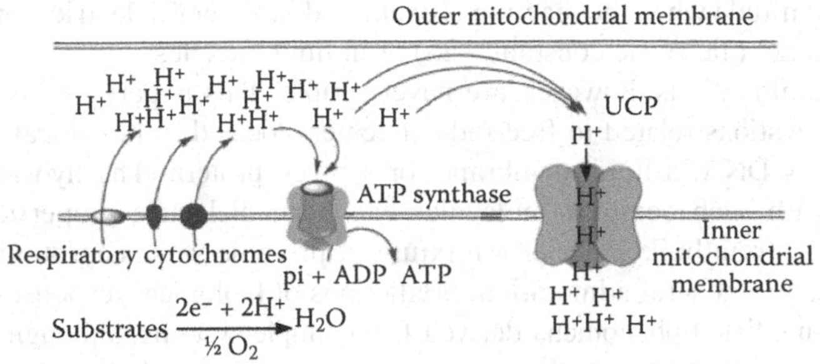

Outer mitochondrial membrane

FIGURE 1.3 Relationships between H$^+$ flux, ATP synthase, and uncoupling protein complexes in mitochondria. In mitochondria, there is balance between the respiratory system, ATP synthase (for work-related functions), and the UCP complexes (for control of heat regulation). In part, this is achieved by regulating the H$^+$ concentrations in the compartments defined by the outer and inner mitochondrial membranes. The presence of protons in the intermembrane space together with the difference in membrane potential between this space and the mitochondrial matrix is a driving force for the conversion of ADP to ATP. Furthermore, an increase in ATP levels can slow mitochondrial respiration, owing to the ability of ATP to regulate the phosphorylation of ADP by ATP synthase. In this regard, uncoupling the proton flux is an adaptive way to avoid excessive inhibition of mitochondrial respiration. Uncoupling the proton flux from ATP synthase also helps buffer ROS production by controlling the rate of respiration. As an additional control, when the rates of respiration and substrate oxidation are high, O$_2^{\cdot-}$ production increases. The increase in O$_2^{\cdot-}$ levels activates UCPs. This is another important control in that it occurs when the dismutation of O$_2^{\cdot-}$ is insufficient to avoid ROS-related damage to mitochondria. (From Ricquier, D, *Proc. Nutr. Soc.*, 64, 47, 2005.)

[D]ioxygenases, Cyt P450) modify toxins and useful secondary metabolites to facilitate their partitioning into pathways for further transport or eventual elimination [11]. Oxygen is a co-substrate for many of the reactions carried out by such enzymes. Superoxide radicals are produced when the flow of electrons from the respective substrates for a given Cyt P450 to the reaction intermediates to the final products is compromised. Moreover, reduced glutathione (GSH) is used as a co-substrate for some of the modifications in the smooth ER. In situations where glutathione is used faster than it can be resynthesized, one result is reduced levels of GSH for antioxidant enzymes, such as glutathione peroxidase that use GSH as a reductant [12].

As an additional point, regardless of the process involved, changes in pH, temperature, the presence of sequestrants or inhibitors, and the polarity of the environment are noteworthy as factors important to free radical formation and stability. For example, the dielectric constant of the cellular environment can have a significant influence on the rates of free radical reactions [12]. The dielectric constant is a measure of solvent polarity and its ability to reduce the field strength of an electric field surrounding a charged particle. Solvents most often encountered in biology have dielectric constants >15; at <15, a solvent is usually defined as nonpolar. For perspective, superoxide radical generated from redox cycling systems (e.g., the repetitive coupling of a given reduction and subsequent oxidation reactions) can vary several orders of magnitude when the reaction is examined in water (dielectric constant, ~70) versus in alcohol (dielectric constant, ~25) or in lipid micelles.

Such medium effects, however, are never simple. This is particularly true when addressing questions related to free radical centers located in biological macromolecules such as DNA, a lipid membrane, or a given protein. The hydration sheath associated with such complex molecules can have dielectric properties that are quite different from bulk water or a mixture of protonic versus aprotonic solvents. Accordingly, as a general admonition, predictions of biological responses related to free radical–mediated phenomena derived from simple systems, although helpful for hypothesis generation, may not be universal or straightforward.

TYPES OF O_2-DERIVED ROS

Hydrogen Peroxide

H_2O_2 is not a free radical and is freely permeable across cell membranes. Analogous to its precursor, superoxide anion radical, in its radical form, it is also less reactive than other ROS and compounds capable of oxidation or initiation of free radical cascades (Table 1.1, Ref. [13]):

$$O_2^{-\bullet} + e + 2H^+ \rightarrow H_2O_2 \rightarrow HOO^\bullet + H^+$$

From a chemical and biological perspective, this has some advantages. It is well appreciated that within cellular membranes, carbon chains associated with membrane lipids are major sites of oxidative damage. In lipids containing unsaturated, nonconjugated carbon chains, the hydrogen associated with the carbon not involved in π-bonding ($-CH=CH-C[H_2]-CH=CH-$) is more easily abstracted than hydrogens associated with π-bonded carbons in conjugated carbon chains or completely saturated carbon chains. The resulting radical ($-CH=CH-CH^\bullet-CH=CH-$) is highly reactive and can lead to the formation of other radicals or cause isomerization and polymerization. In the presence of O_2, a likely free radical product of a nonconjugated lipid is lipid peroxide:

$$-CH=CH-CH^\bullet-CH=CH- + O_2 \rightarrow -CH=CH-CHOO^\bullet-CH=CH-$$

Reactions initiated by ROS that result in free radicals as products are called chain reactions because the product may also serve as reactant, thereby creating a chain of events that only stops when the reagents are used up or blocked by antioxidants. In this regard, as a consequence of being a slower-reacting free radical, lipid peroxides are more easily controlled and quenched in the presence of antioxidants. O_2 may even be viewed as an important free radical modulator in this context.

Whether H_2O_2 is going to act as a potentially useful versus destructive chemical often depends on its concentration in a given tissue. All aerobic organisms studied to date from prokaryotes to humans appear to tightly regulate their intracellular H_2O_2 concentrations at relatively similar levels. H_2O_2 concentrations range from ~0.001 μM to as high as ~0.1 μM during peak periods of H_2O_2 generation. In mitochondria, it is estimated that the steady-state level of H_2O_2 is ~0.04 μM [14,15].

At controlled and low concentrations, H_2O_2 is involved in oxidative reactions important to (i) the regulation of protein function by altering structure via the modification of critical amino acid residues, (ii) cell signaling, (iii) thyroxin production, and a number of cellular and organismal defense systems [14,15]. Examples related to important protein modifications include the oxidation of cysteinyl residues to form sulfenic (–SOH), sulfinic (–SO$_2$H), sulfonic (–SO$_3$H), or S-glutathionylated (–SSG) derivatives. Such reactions can result in protein dimerization or modification of Fe–S moieties or other metal complexes at the active sites of certain enzymes [16,17]. As noted, thyroxin formation (particularly iodination of tyrosyl residues in thyroglobulin) also requires H_2O_2 generation. Moreover, H_2O_2 is required for the oxidation of tyrosine residues, and, in some proteins, is essential for their cross-linking to form active dimers, oligomers, and even polymers.

Hydrogen peroxide is also important to cell signaling. A number of kinase-driven pathways important to cell proliferation, migration, survival, and autophagy depend on H_2O_2, which aids in catalyzing changes in the redox state of given kinases [13–15]. H_2O_2 is also essential in phagocytic processes by cells such as neutrophils, monocytes, macrophages, dendritic cells, and mast cells, i.e., cells that are critical in fighting infections, as well as removing dead and dying cells that have reached the end of their lifespan [13–15]. Compounds with well-defined roles are usually highly regulated either through control of synthesis and catabolism (Figure 1.2); H_2O_2 is no exception.

With regard to synthesis, H_2O_2 is generated from the spontaneous or enzyme-catalyzed dismutation (simultaneous oxidation and reduction) of superoxide anion or enzymes that catalyze the electron reduction of molecular oxygen (e.g., xanthine oxidase; Refs. [1–4]). Furthermore, as noted previously, inefficient metabolism by cytochrome P450 enzymes in the smooth ER or oxidases associated with peroxisomes is often associated with the production of superoxide radical or excessive amounts of hydrogen peroxide [1–4]. Other cellular sources of hydrogen peroxide are NADPH oxidase [1–4,18], which is found in all major classes of phagocytic cells. A general scheme for the NADPH oxidase reaction is

$$NADPH + 2O_2 \leftrightarrow NADP^+ + 2O_2^{\cdot-} + H^+$$

The production of superoxide anion by NADPH (nicotinamide adenine dinucleotide phosphate) oxidase and the eventual production of hydrogen peroxide by superoxide dismutase (SOD) serve as good examples of the complexity of H_2O_2 regulation [18]. NADPH oxidase is a membrane-bound enzyme complex found in the cellular plasma membrane as well as in the membranes of phagosomes used by neutrophils. The production of superoxide anion by NADPH oxidase is commonly referred to as the oxidative or respiratory burst reaction. There is first rapid generation of superoxide anion. Next, in the presence of the enzyme SOD, which is found in high concentrations in both the cytosol and mitochondria of cells, superoxide anion is converted to hydrogen peroxide [1–4]:

$$M^{n+} - SOD + O_2^{\cdot-} + 2H^+ \rightarrow M^{(n+1)+} - SOD + H_2O_2$$

where M = Cu ($n = 1$), Mn ($n = 2$), Fe ($n = 2$), and Ni ($n = 2$).

Owing to the need for a high level of control, both the activities of SOD and NADPH oxidase are controlled by a number of regulatory strategies at the cellular and organismal levels. As examples, NADPH oxidase activity is controlled both by the transcriptional regulation of NADPH oxidase complex components as well as factors that control their rates of assembly [18]. Moreover, depending on the metabolic need or function, the number of agents may stimulate assembly or act as activators, such as growth factors and cytokines (platelet-activating factor, interleukin [IL]-8), various physical stimuli, ATP, and N-formylated peptides. This suggests that H_2O_2 production is linked to processes that use a number of differing cellular signals depending on the metabolic function that is needed. There are also a number of well-controlled events that extend from the activation of the NADPH oxidase complex at the cell surface. For example, NADPH oxidase activation is followed by the hydrolysis of membrane-associated phosphatidylinositol bisphosphate, which results in an increase in the levels of inositol trisphosphate (inositol 1,4,5-trisphosphate) and diacylglycerol [18]. These molecules, in turn, promote the opening of calcium channels, and the combination of diacylglycerol and calcium causes the activation of protein kinase C. Many other cell signaling factors are also involved, such as Rac, a transcription factor associated with the Rho family of "G-protein" GTPases. G proteins act as molecular switches and play roles in cellular events ranging from organelle development, cytoskeletal dynamics, and cell movement.

Regarding SOD, there are three major families of SOD, each requiring specific metal cofactors: (i) Cu/Zn (the cytosolic form); (ii) Fe and Mn types (the mitochondrial form); and (iii) the Ni type, which is found mostly in prokaryotes [19]. SOD overcomes the potentially damaging reactions of superoxide by catalyzing its dismutation. Dietary deficiencies of dietary copper and manganese can influence SOD activity [19]. SOD activity is lower and superoxide anion concentrations are higher in Cu-deficient animal models, which can be accompanied by malformations and ROS-related developmental defects. In mitochondria, SOD upregulation has been associated with the extension of lifespan, using invertebrates and arthropods as experimental models [19]. In this regard, whenever there is complex cellular regulation of molecules, the reasons often center on maintaining plasticity. Owing to the both healthful and potentially deleterious effects of oxidants, regulation must have features that address both specificity and safety, particularly when there are opportunities for nonspecific or deleterious modifications to normal cell signaling function.

Hydroxyl Radicals

Hydroxyl radicals are produced from the decomposition of hydrogen peroxides (often as the result of Fenton-type reactions or photolysis) or water (as a result of radiolysis). In the Fenton reaction, transition elements are usually used as catalysts [1–4,20] if they are capable of engaging in redox cycling reactions. For example, the addition of metals such as iron and copper (most often encountered in biology) to a solution containing hydrogen peroxide can result in the following reactions with hydroxyl radical and peroxyl radical as products:

$$M^n + H_2O_2 \rightarrow M^{n+1} + HO^\bullet + OH^-$$

$$M^{n+1} + H_2O_2 \rightarrow M^n + HOO^{\bullet} + H^+$$

In cells, these reactions are modulated by the presence of proteins such as ferritin (binds iron) and metallothionein (binds Cu, Zn, and Cd). An important observation is that metal-binding proteins keep the concentrations of many redox transition metals (e.g., Cu or Fe) at extremely low levels. For example, it has been calculated that the concentration of free copper in cells is maintained at less than one atom per cell [21], thereby assuring that the probability of nonspecific interactions with OH$^{\bullet}$ remains low.

Exposure of H_2O_2 to ultraviolet light can also cause the homolytic cleavage of hydrogen peroxide to yield hydroxyl radicals; in particular, ultraviolet light as a form of electromagnetic radiation (i.e., between 400 and 10 nm, corresponding to photon energies from 3 to 124 eV). In a homolytic cleavage of a chemical bond, each fragment retains one of the original electrons involved in bonding; that is, the exposed electrons are distributed equally within the two resulting fragments [1–4,20]:

$$H_2O_2 \rightarrow HO^{\bullet} + HO^{\bullet}$$

Water, in the presence of alpha radiation, dissociates into hydrogen and hydroxyl radicals:

$$H_2O \rightarrow H^{\bullet} + HO^{\bullet}$$

Regardless of the process, the hydroxyl radicals that are produced have high reduction potentials and rapid rates of reaction (Table 1.1). In this regard, the rates of reactions are very near the diffusion limit; that is, the reactions take place at sites where hydroxyl radicals are generated. Hydroxyl radicals also react nonselectively and are probably the most responsible for the injury induced by ionizing radiation or when tissues are exposed to excessive levels of H_2O_2. Furthermore, unlike superoxide, which can be detoxified by SOD, the hydroxyl radical cannot be eliminated by an enzymatic reaction [20]. Accordingly, hydroxyl radicals are the most reactive of the known ROS.

Peroxynitrite

The free radical nitric oxide (NO) is an essential endothelial-derived relaxing factor and powerful vasodilator [22]. Low nanomolar concentrations of NO activate guanylyl cyclase to produce cGMP. The production of NO is derived from arginine by a reaction that is controlled by NO synthetase (NOS). NO and citrulline are products of this reaction.

There are several forms of NOS. The endothelial isoform (eNOS) is the primary signal generator of NO in the control of vascular tone. It is also involved in the regulation of insulin secretion, cardiac function, and angiogenesis. The neuronal isoform (nNOS) is involved in the regulation and development of the nervous system. There is also an inducible isoform (iNOS) that is capable of producing large amounts of NO. NO is synthesized in response to inflammatory cytokines in phagocytic cells (monocytes, macrophages, and neutrophils) and is important to defense against parasites, infections, and even tumor growth. At high levels of NO (usually the result of iNOS activation), there is reduced mitochondrial activity [22]. As a consequence, there can be an increase in tissue oxygen saturation, followed by increases in superoxide anion radical, hydrogen peroxide, and NO levels [22].

Such conditions can lead to the formation of peroxynitrite via a reaction in which superoxide reacts rapidly with NO to form peroxynitrite anion ($ONOO^-$):

$$^\bullet NO + O_2^{\bullet -} \rightarrow ONOO^- \text{ (rate constant, } k \sim 10^{10})$$

Peroxynitrite is a very strong oxidizing and nitrating agent. Although not a free radical, peroxynitrite is much more reactive than superoxide and NO; accordingly, peroxynitrite can damage a wide array of molecules in cells. Peroxynitrite can react with CO_2 to form nitrosoperoxycarbonate $\left(ONOOCO_2^-\right)$. Potentially damaging effects in cells may result from the decomposition to $ONOOCO_2^-$, which yields carbonate $\left(CO_3^{\bullet -}\right)$ and nitrogen dioxide radicals $\left(^\bullet N^+ O_2^-\right)$. Such radicals can react with tyrosine to form phenoxy radical intermediates that can initiate free radical chain reactions.

Hypochlorous Acid (HOCl) and Myeloperoxidase

HOCl is synthesized largely by the action of myeloperoxidase in phagocytic cells (e.g., mostly neutrophils) using H_2O_2 and chloride anion as substrates [23]. Myeloperoxidase is expressed as a part of the respiratory burst reaction. Myeloperoxidase can also oxidize tyrosine to tyrosyl radical using hydrogen peroxide as an oxidizing agent:

$$H_2O_2 + Cl^- \rightarrow HOCl + OH^-$$

The reaction of HOCl with superoxide radical produces hydroxyl radical (A) and with H_2O_2 produces singlet oxygen (B):

$$(A) \quad HOCl + O_2^{\bullet -} \rightarrow O_2 + Cl^- + HO^\bullet$$

$$(B) \quad HOCl + H_2O_2 \rightarrow O_2^1 + H_2O + HCl$$

In addition, hypochlorous acid can be the precursor of potent oxidizing species that react with proteins, lipids, nucleic acids, and carbohydrates and even foreign substances (e.g., inhaled particles, molds, and dust). In this regard, HOCl plays an integral part in the innate or nonspecific immune defense system designed to kill microorganisms or destroy substances that may lead to more serious cell and tissue injury [23]. However, as with other oxidants, when in excess, HOCl can be toxic. Moreover, the amount of HOCl required for toxicity is markedly lower than the concentrations of H_2O_2 needed to destroy otherwise healthy cells. HOCl can cause an irreversible loss of intracellular GSH, an essential reductant in cells, and is more likely to oxidize thiol groups in proteins than H_2O_2 [24]. Glutathione is only replaced by resynthesis.

Singlet Oxygen and Ozone

The reaction of ozone with a number of biological molecules produces singlet oxygen in high yield. In turn, singlet oxygen is an important intermediate in the biochemical damage attributed to ozone exposure. Both can be produced *in vivo* by reactions and processes associated with inflammation and, analogous to the other ROS, play both healthful and potentially damaging effects in biological systems. A number of consequences of the interactions between ROS and inflammation are described in the chapters focusing on gastrointestinal disorders (cf. Chapters 12 through 15).

Singlet Oxygen

In plants, singlet oxygen is produced during the process of photosynthesis [6]. In animals, singlet oxygen is often associated with lipoprotein oxidation and skin photosensitivity. Singlet oxygen reacts with many kinds of biological molecules, particularly reactions that often involve carbon–carbon double bonds. Singlet oxygen is a powerful electrophile. Schenck-ene reactions and Diels–Alder reactions are examples [25]. The addition of singlet oxygen to an *ene*-containing molecule, such as a polyunsaturated fatty acid, often results in a peroxide adduct, which can result in bond cleavage, rearrangements, and aldehyde-containing products (R-CHO).

Ozone

In nature, atmospheric ozone is formed from dioxygen by the action of ultraviolet light and electrical discharges. Typical ozone concentrations found in the natural atmosphere range from 0.001 to 0.125 ppm. The levels of concentration vary with altitude, atmospheric conditions, and locale [1–4,26].

In animals, compounds with the chemical signatures of ozone are produced as a product of innate immune reactions; more specifically, the intrinsic ability of antibodies to generate hydrogen peroxide from singlet oxygen via the so-called antibody-catalyzed water oxidation pathway [27,28]. The process is independent of antigenic specificity and is triggered upon binding of $^1O_2$ to conserved (specific) binding sites within the antibody's structure:

$$x O_2^1 + H_2O \rightarrow H_2O_2 + (x-1)3 O_2$$

Like other ROS, ozone also can play a role in combating foreign substances and bacteria [27,28]. For example, exposure to ozone triggers responses, such as secretion of various cytokines, tumor necrosis factor, and γ-interferon. Given that ozone is highly reactive, it would be expected that at higher than normal levels, ozone's interaction with biologically important molecules may lead to premature cell death and inflammation.

Epithelial cells lining the respiratory tract are the main target of ozone and its products. Moreover, epithelial cells in response to ozone exposure release a number of inflammatory mediators that may initiate events leading to pathologies related to small airway obstruction and decreased integrity of the airway epithelium (e.g., prostaglandin E2, IL-6 and IL-8, granulocyte-macrophage colony-stimulating factor, monocyte chemotactic protein-1, chemokine [ligand 5], which is also known as RANTES or "regulated on activation, normal T-cell expressed and secreted" protein [27,28]).

Regarding levels of ozone that are considered a hazard, the allowable limit in many countries (United States, United Kingdom, Japan, France, Netherlands, and Germany) is 0.1 ppm or less. In many industrial cities, levels of 0.15–0.51 ppm are often observed. High ozone levels usually occur in summer months and reach their peak in mid to late afternoon because of an increase in exhaust fumes from morning traffic and industrial activities. Exposures of 0.4-ppm ozone are often used in experimental animal studies to induce lung pathology. A 3-h exposure at 12 ppm is usually lethal for guinea pigs. Those exposed to 5–9 ppm ozone concentrations plus other air pollutants may be subject to major lung damage [26].

Oxidative Stress

The term "oxidative stress" is used to characterize an imbalance between the ROS concentration and the ability to detoxify excesses of ROS (production via synthesis and/or catabolic processes) and their reactive intermediates, or to facilitate the repair of ROS-mediated damage (Figure 1.2). Accordingly, cellular protection against the deleterious effects of ROS is organized at several levels (prevention, interception, and repair) [29–31]. Regulation involves both small molecules that act as antioxidants and enzymatic strategies to control either the rate of synthesis or catabolism of potential oxidants or oxygen utilization.

As examples, H_2O_2 is catabolized by catalase ($2H_2O_2 \rightarrow 2H_2O + O_2$) and various hydrogen peroxidases [32]. Catalase is found in most organisms exposed to oxygen. In particular, catalase has high catalytic capacity or turnover number, the maximum number of molecules of substrate that an enzyme can convert to product per catalytic site per unit of time. The value for catalase is 40 million s^{-1}. However, the biological significance of catalase is not straightforward. For example, mice genetically engineered without catalase remain phenotypically normal. In addition to catalase, thiol and selenol peroxidases are also important to H_2O_2 regulation. There are two main subfamilies: peroxiredoxins (Prx) and glutathione peroxidases.

The Prx are antioxidant enzymes that have thiol groups at their active centers and control peroxide levels that are mediated mostly by changes in cytokine levels [33]. Prx are regenerated by thioredoxins (Trx), small molecular weight redox proteins known to be present in all organisms [34]:

$$Prx(reduced) + H_2O_2 \rightarrow Prx(oxidized) + 2H_2O$$

$$Prx(oxidized) + Trx(reduced) \rightarrow Prx(reduced) + Trx(oxidized)$$

As a consequence, Prx are often important to cell signaling involving oxidant-related processes and are relatively abundant in cells in which oxygen tension is high. Mammalian cells express six known Prx isoforms. The oxidized active-site cysteine in Prx can be reduced by cellular thiols, such as one of the Trx. Regulation of Prx can also occur through phosphorylation by kinases that respond to extracellular cytokines and related cellular signals. Of additional importance, the oxidation state of the active-site cysteine of Prx can be transferred to other proteins that cannot effectively sense changes in peroxide concentrations.

Glutathione peroxidase is a selenium-containing enzyme [35]. Glutathione peroxidases are novel because instead of sulfhydryl moieties, they employ seleno moieties at their active centers (R–SeH [red] or R–Se–Se–R [ox]). Glutathione peroxidase also catalyze both H_2O_2 and lipid peroxides to water or lipid alcohols, respectively:

$$2GSH + H_2O_2 \rightarrow GS-SG + 2H_2O$$

where GSH represents reduced glutathione as substrate and G–S–S–G oxidized glutathione as product. With regard to importance, similar to catalase knockout mice, mice genetically engineered to lack various isoforms of glutathione peroxidase or Prx only demonstrate modest phenotypic changes; however, they are more sensitive to certain exogenous sources of oxidative stress, such as hyperoxia.

Table 1.2 includes other proteins, enzymes, and examples of other molecules found in tissues that are involved in the control of ROS levels and related metabolites. Although a discussion of each of the molecules that act as reductants or antioxidants is beyond the scope of this chapter, it is important to appreciate that many of the enzymes involved in ROS regulation utilize these molecules as reductants [1–4]. As examples:

1. Ascorbic acid is important in maintaining iron and copper in reduced states at the active sites of many oxidases and peroxidases [36].
2. GSH, a tripeptide containing cysteine, is the principal reductant for glutathione peroxidase [35].
3. NADPH is essential as a cofactor for GSH regeneration from oxidized glutathione ($2GSH \leftarrow\rightarrow GS-SG$) via glutathione reductase, and for oxygenases and oxidases associated with the ER [35].
4. Vitamin E and carotenoids are often referred to as the first lines of defense in cellular membranes and act to sequester $HOO^\bullet$ radicals and retard reactions involving singlet oxygen [37].

Also listed in Table 1.2 are a number of dietary antioxidants that putatively counter ROS damage by scavenging free radicals (Refs. [4,29–31,38–40]; also cf. Chapter 2).

TABLE 1.2
Substances and Compounds with Antioxidant Activity

Substance or Compound	ROS Target or Function
Essential Compounds (Vitamins) and Related Derivatives	
A-, β-, γ-, and δ-Tocopherols	Lipid peroxide–initiated chain reaction breakers
β-Carotenes	Singlet oxygen quencher
Lycopene	Singlet oxygen quencher
Ubiquinol (CoQ-10)	Radical scavenger
Ascorbic acid	Reductant
Glutathione	Reductant
Urate	Radical scavenger
Bilirubin	Radical scavenger
Proteins and Enzymes (Primary)	
Superoxide dismutase	Dismutation of superoxide anions
GSH peroxidases	Reduce lipid hydroperoxides to their corresponding alcohols and reduce free hydrogen peroxide to water
Myeloperoxidase	Controls hypochlorous acid production from hydrogen peroxide and chloride anion
Hydrogen peroxidases	Converts hydrogen peroxide to water
Catalase	Catalyzes the decomposition of hydrogen peroxide to water and oxygen
Alpha-1-microglobulin	Degrades heme and is a radical scavenger as well as a reductase
Proteins and Enzymes (Secondary)	
Metal-binding proteins (e.g., metallothionein, chaperones, ceruloplasmin)	Sequestration, transport, and regulation of transition metals capable of redox
Cytochrome P450s	Catalyzes phase 1 metabolism, most often characterized by the addition of –OH groups to nonpolar and/or aromatic compounds to facilitate transport or elimination
Conjugation enzymes (e.g., glutathione-*S*- and UDP-glucuronosyl-transferases)	Conjugate phase 1 Cyt P450 products to more polar compounds (phase II reactions) to facilitate transport, delivery, or elimination
NADPH quinone oxidoreductases	Two electron reductions
GSSG reductase	GSH regeneration
NADPH-generating enzymes	NADPH production
DNA repair enzymes	DNA repair
Protein repair enzymes	Catalyze oxidized and denatured protein turnover or degradation

(Continued)

TABLE 1.2 (CONTINUED)
Substances and Compounds with Antioxidant Activity

Substance or Compound	ROS Target or Function
Diet-Derived Antioxidants/Nutraceuticals	
Polyphenol antioxidants (e.g., flavonoids, various flavones, flavanols such as catechins or epicatechins, flavanones, flavanols, isoflavone phytoestrogens such as daidzein and genistein, quercetin, rutin, resveratrol, pyrroloquinoline quinone, and hydroxytyrosol)	More than 4000 distinct species: many have antioxidant activity; others affect cell-to-cell signaling, receptor sensitivity, inflammatory enzyme activity, or gene regulation
Phenolic acids (e.g., cinnamic acid, caffeic acid, salicylic acid, and vanillin)	Redox cycling, general antioxidant activity
Carotenoid (e.g., lutein, zeaxanthin, carotenes)	More than 600 known carotenoids in two classes: xanthophylls (which contain oxygen) and carotenes (which are hydrocarbons, and contain no oxygen); quench singlet oxygen
Lipoic acid	Reducing agent, free radical scavenger
Selenium	Co-factor for glutathione peroxidase

COMMON TARGETS OF THE DAMAGING EFFECTS OF ROS

Carbohydrates, lipids, proteins, and nucleic acids (RNA and DNA) are all targets of ROS and their derived products [4]. Carbohydrates and lipids can be oxidized to carbonyl compounds. Such oxidation reactions can lead to the formation of the advanced glycation or lipoxidation end products (often abbreviated as AGEs/ALEs), rearrangement of double bonds, changes in conformation, and carbon chain cleavage leading to end products such as malondialdehyde [41]. When glucose is involved, the initial products are Schiff base products followed by Amadori rearrangements. A good example of an AGE is glycated hemoglobin (hemoglobin A1c), which correlates with blood glucose levels [41].

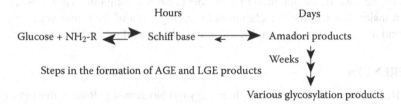

Steps in the formation of AGE and LGE products

When proteins interact with ROS, additional responses may include (i) oxidative attack of the polypeptide backbone; (ii) peptide cleavage due to ROS attack of glutamyl, aspartyl, and prolyl side chains; (iii) oxidation of amino acid side chains; or (iv) cross-linking or N-terminal modifications due to reactions with carbohydrate or lipid-derived carbonyls such as malondialdehyde. In this setting, the accumulation of damaged protein is dependent on the balance between prooxidant, antioxidant, and associated proteolytic activities [1–4,16,17,20,41]. When ROS interact with DNA, oxidation usually occurs at guanine residues due to the high oxidation potential of this base relative to cytosine, thymine, and adenine. DNA stand breaks occur with 8-oxoguanine (8-hydroxyguanine) as a measurable product in blood and urine [20]. Moreover, ROS can also randomly damage RNAs. Oxidation of mRNAs *in vitro* and *in vivo* can result in lower rates of mRNA translation efficiency and aberrant protein products [20].

FINAL PERSPECTIVES

Many compounds have gained acceptance as antioxidant supplements independent of their original dietary source (i.e., as nutraceuticals). Indeed, currently, one of the most active areas of nutrition-related research focuses on foods or food-derived compounds with putative antioxidant potential (Refs. [38–43], cf. Table 1.2). Moreover, an additional dimension includes the products derived from such compounds and their potential interactions with the intestinal microbiota [44].

Although under most conditions, combinations of conventional nutrients with antioxidant or reducing potential in addition to endogenous enzymes and their corresponding co-factors appear sufficient to regulate of ROS levels, additional secondary metabolites and compounds, particularly those found in fruits and vegetables, are now viewed by many as not only having complimentary but also potentially independent roles in oxidant defense [42]. Nevertheless, important caveats are in order when making claims about dietary antioxidants [43–47]. As examples, some claims are based on assays *in vitro* that measure antioxidant chemical potential and may have little relevance *in vivo* [47]. Furthermore, experimental studies using more diverse sets of experimental end points, rather than single end points, and clinical studies using larger pools of subjects, tend to demonstrate less benefit related to supplements than that proposed in many of the earlier preliminary studies (cf., Refs. [45,46]). It is also becoming increasingly apparent that ingestion of a complex food may set into motion dozens of cell signaling strategies and feedback loops that are likely not to occur with a single dietary supplement [38,39]. Moreover, many compounds (particularly polyphenols) with antioxidant potential at low concentrations can catalyze redox cycling and may cause free radical generation at higher concentrations [47,48]. With that said, however, the antioxidant potential of a number of natural compounds in foods remains to be a major factor in the correlation between ingestion of fruit- and vegetable-rich diets and the a reduction in pathological events that are influenced by free radicals.

REFERENCES

1. Hermes-Lima, M. 2004. Oxygen in biology and biochemistry: Role of free radicals. In *Functional Metabolism: Regulation and Adaptation*, ed. K.B. Storey, 12:319–366. John Wiley & Sons Inc, Hoboken, NJ.
2. Li, Y.R. 2011. Free radicals and related reactive species. In *Free Radical Biomedicine: Principles, Clinical Correlations, and Methodologies*, Chapter 2:10–39. Bentham Science Publishers, Sharjah, United Arab Emirates.
3. Ray, P.D., Huang, B.W., Tsuji, Y. 2012. Reactive oxygen species (ROS) homeostasis and redox regulation in cellular signaling. *Cell Signal.* 24:981–990.

4. Kalyanaraman, B. 2013. Teaching the basics of redox biology to medical and graduate students: Oxidants, antioxidants and disease mechanisms. *Redox Biol.* 1:244–257.
5. Canfield, D.E. 2014. *Oxygen: A Four Billion Year History*, 1–189. Princeton University Press, Princeton, NJ.
6. Ogilby, P.R. 2010. Singlet oxygen: There is indeed something new under the sun. *Chem. Soc. Rev.* 39:3181–3209.
7. Hayes, P., Knaus, U.G. 2013. Balancing reactive oxygen species in the epigenome: NADPH oxidases as target and perpetrator. *Antioxid. Redox Signal.* 18:1937–1945.
8. Beckman, K.B., Ames, B.N. 1998. The free radical theory of aging matures. *Physiol. Rev.* 78:547–581.
9. Shigenaga, M.K., Hagen, T.M., Ames, B.N. 1994. Oxidative damage and mitochondrial decay in aging. *Proc. Natl. Acad. Sci. U. S. A.* 91:10771–10778.
10. Ricquier, D. 2005. Respiration uncoupling and metabolism in the control of energy expenditure. *Proc. Nutr. Soc.* 64:47–52.
11. Costas Ioannides, C., Lewis, D.F.V. 2004. Cytochromes P450 in the bioactivation of chemicals. *Curr. Top. Med. Chem.* 4:1767–1788.
12. Litwinienko, G., Beckwith, A.L., Ingold, K.U. 2011. The frequently overlooked importance of solvent in free radical syntheses. *Chem. Soc. Rev.* 40:2157–2163.
13. Gough, D.R., Cotter, T.G. 2011. Hydrogen peroxide: A Jekyll and Hyde signalling molecule. *Cell Death Dis.* 2:e213.
14. Bindoli, A., Rigobello, M.P. 2013. Principles in redox signaling: From chemistry to functional significance. *Antioxid. Redox Signal.* 18:1557–1593.
15. Stone, J.R., Yang, S. 2006. Hydrogen peroxide: A signaling messenger. *Antioxid. Redox Signal.* 8:243–270.
16. Stadtman, E.R. 2001. Protein oxidation in aging and age-related diseases. *Ann. N. Y. Acad. Sci.* 928:22–38.
17. Berlett, B.S., Stadtman, E.R. 1997. Protein oxidation in aging, disease, and oxidative stress. *J. Biol. Chem.* 272:20313–20316.
18. Katsuyama, M., Matsuno, K., Yabe-Nishimura, C. 2012. Physiological roles of NOX/NADPH oxidase, the superoxide-generating enzyme. *J. Clin. Biochem. Nutr.* 50:9–22.
19. Landis, G.N., Tower, J. 2005. Superoxide dismutase evolution and life span regulation. *Mech. Ageing Dev.* 126:365–379.
20. Imlay, J.A., Linn, S. 1988. DNA damage and oxygen radical toxicity. *Science* 240:1302–1309.
21. Rae, T.D., Schmidt, P.J., Pufahl, R.A., Culotta, V.C., O'Halloran, T.V. 1999. Undetectable intracellular free copper: The requirement of a copper chaperone for superoxide dismutase. *Science* 284:805–808.
22. Pacher, P., Beckman, J.S., Liaudet, L. 2007. Nitric oxide and peroxynitrite in health and disease. *Physiol. Rev.* 87:315–424.
23. Klebanoff, S.J. 2005. Myeloperoxidase: Friend and foe. *J. Leukoc. Biol.* 77:598–625.
24. Pullar, J.M., Vissers, M.C., Winterbourn, C.C. 2001. Glutathione oxidation by hypochlorous acid in endothelial cells produces glutathione sulfonamide as a major product but not glutathione disulfide. *J. Biol. Chem.* 276:22120–22125.
25. Zhang, W., Sun, M., Salomon, R.G. 2006. Preparative singlet oxygenation of linoleate provides doubly allylic dihydroperoxides: Putative intermediates in the generation of biologically active aldehydes *in vivo. J. Org. Chem.* 71:5607–5615.
26. Apte, M.G., Buchanan, I.S., Mendell, M.J. 2008. Outdoor ozone and building-related symptoms in the BASE Study. *Indoor Air* 18:156–170.
27. Wentworth, P. Jr., Wentworth, A.D., Zhu, X. et al. 2003. Evidence for the production of trioxygen species during antibody-catalyzed chemical modification of antigens. *Proc. Natl. Acad. Sci. U. S. A.* 100:1490–1493.

28. Wentworth, P. Jr., McDunn, J.E., Wentworth, A.D. et al. 2002. Evidence for antibody-catalyzed ozone formation in bacterial killing and inflammation. *Science* 298:2195–2199.
29. Sies, H. 1993. Strategies for antioxidant defense. *Eur. J. Biochem.* 215:213–219.
30. Hollman, P.C., Cassidy, A., Comte, B. et al. 2011. The biological relevance of direct antioxidant effects of polyphenols for cardiovascular health in humans is not established. *J. Nutr.* 141:989S–1009S.
31. Sies, H. 2010. Polyphenols and health: Update and perspectives. *Arch. Biochem. Biophys.* 501:2–5.
32. Chelikani, P., Fita, I., Loewen, P.C. 2004. Diversity of structures and properties among catalases. *Cell. Mol. Life Sci.* 61:192–208.
33. Rhee, S.G., Woo, H.A., Kil, I.S., Bae, S.H. 2012. Peroxiredoxin functions as a peroxidase and a regulator and sensor of local peroxides. *J. Biol. Chem.* 287:4403–4410.
34. Stefankova, P., Kollarova, M., Barak, I. 2005. Thioredoxin—Structural and functional complexity. *Gen. Physiol. Biophys.* 24:3–11.
35. Xin, G.L., Wen-Hsing, C., McClung, J.P. 2007. Metabolic regulation and function of glutathione peroxidase-1. *Annu. Rev. Nutr.* 27:41–61.
36. Johnson, C., Steinberg, F., Rucker, R.B. 2013. Ascorbic acid, Chapter 14. In *Handbook of Vitamins*, 5th Edition, eds. J. Zempleni, J. Suttie, J.F. Gregory III, P.J. Stover, 515–549. CRC Press, Boca Raton, FL.
37. Mustacich, D.J., Bruno, R.S., Traber, M.G. 2007. Vitamin E. *Vitam. Horm.* 76:1–21.
38. Chowanadisai, W., Shenoy, S.F., Sharman, E., Keen, C.L., Liu, J.K., Rucker, R.B. 2011. Nutritionally important biofactors in foods (Part 1—Factors important to mitochondriogenesis and their importance to health). *Calif. Agric.* 65:136–140.
39. Shenoy, S.F., Chowanadisai, W., Sharman, E., Keen, C.L., Liu, J.K., Rucker, R.B. 2011. Important biofactors in foods (Part 2—Specific food components as cellular signals for mitochondriogenesis). *Calif. Agric.* 65:141–147.
40. Sies, H., Stahl, W., Sevanian, A. 2005. Nutritional, dietary and postprandial oxidative stress. *J. Nutr.* 135:969–972.
41. Kellow, N.J., Savige, G.S. 2013. Dietary advanced glycation end-product restriction for the attenuation of insulin resistance, oxidative stress and endothelial dysfunction: A systematic review. *Eur. J. Clin. Nutr.* 67:239–248.
42. Ames, B.N. 2004. A role for supplements in optimizing health: The metabolic tune-up. *Arch. Biochem. Biophys.* 423:227–234.
43. Bjelakovic, G., Nikolova, D., Gluud, C. 2014. Antioxidant supplements and mortality. *Curr. Opin. Clin. Nutr. Metab. Care* 17:40–44.
44. Devkota, S., Chang, E.B. 2013. Nutrition, microbiomes, and intestinal inflammation. *Curr. Opin. Gastroenterol.* 29:603–607.
45. Bjelakovic, G., Nikolova, D., Gluud, C. 2013. Meta-regression analyses, meta-analyses, and trial sequential analyses of the effects of supplementation with beta-carotene, vitamin A, and vitamin E singly or in different combinations on all-cause mortality: Do we have evidence for lack of harm? *PLoS One* 8:e74558.
46. Peternelj, T.T., Coombes, J.S. 2011. Antioxidant supplementation during exercise training: Beneficial or detrimental? *Sports Med.* 41:1043–1069.
47. Fraga, C.G., Oteiza, P.I., Galleano, M. 2014. *In vitro* measurements and interpretation of total antioxidant capacity. *Biochim. Biophys. Acta* 1840:931–934.
48. Carocho, M., Ferreira, I.C. 2013. A review on antioxidants, prooxidants and related controversy: Natural and synthetic compounds, screening and analysis methodologies and future perspectives. *Food Chem. Toxicol.* 51:15–25.

2 Major Dietary Antioxidants and Their Food Sources

Moschos Polissiou and Dimitra Daferera

CONTENTS

Introduction...23
Classification of Natural Antioxidants 24
   Phenols and Polyphenols...24
      Simple Phenols...24
      Phenolic Acids..24
      Flavonoids 26
      Other Polyphenols 28
   Carotenoids 28
   Essential Oils..30
Distribution of Natural Antioxidants in Selected Food Sources 30
   Fruits 30
   Grapes and Wine 34
   Vegetables 35
   Herbs 36
   Olive and Olive Oil 39
References..40

INTRODUCTION

The plant kingdom boasts of a great number of species consumed by humans in various ways: fresh, dry, cooked, processed, or as decoctions. These are fruits, vegetables, herbs and spices, olive and olive oil, grapes and wines, and juices and beverages, which contain in their chemical composition more or less antioxidant compounds classified to structurally different categories. The quality and quantity of these naturally occurring compounds depend on a number of parameters, such as the plant material, plant part, development stage, seasonal variation, environmental conditions, geographic origin, genetic factors and evolution, dehydration procedure, storage conditions, cooking method, isolation techniques, and analytical methods used for their identification (Kivilompolo et al. 2007, Figueiredo et al. 2008, Palermo et al. 2013).

An antioxidant has been defined as "any substance that, when present at low concentrations compared to those of an oxidizable substrate, significantly delays or prevents oxidation of that substrate" (Halliwell and Gutteridge 1995). Plant secondary metabolites have been the subject of research for many decades in order for their chemical structure to be characterized and their possible antioxidant effect to be attributed to this structure. In this chapter, the classification of these phytochemicals and their distribution in food sources is presented.

CLASSIFICATION OF NATURAL ANTIOXIDANTS

PHENOLS AND POLYPHENOLS

Phenols and polyphenols constitute one of the most numerous and widely distributed group of secondary metabolites in the plant kingdom. This group of compounds is characterized by the presence of at least one phenolic ring to their chemical structure, and is divided into subgroups that may differ significantly in stability, bioavailability, and physiological functions in relation to human health (Tsao 2010). More than 8000 phenolic structures have been identified from various sources; among them, fruits, grains, vegetables, spices, herbs, wine, and decoctions are important (Boskou 2006, Tsao 2010).

Simple Phenols

The most common simple phenols are thymol, carvacrol, and eugenol. The first two compounds are found in high amounts in the essential oils of many Lamiaceae species belonging to the genus *Origanum*, *Thymus*, and *Satureja*, which display various biological activities. Tyrosol, hydroxytyrosol, and oleuropein are natural phenolics occurring in olive and olive oil. Along with tocopherols, other natural antioxidants contribute to the high nutritional value of olive oil. Tocopherols consist of a chroman ring and a long, saturated phytyl chain, and are found in nature in four homologs, namely α-, β-, γ-, and δ-tocopherol (Figure 2.2). They are lipophilic compounds and are present in all oilseeds.

Phenolic Acids

Phenolic acids are usually found in plant tissues in the form of ester, salt, or glycosides, constituting the aglycone part of the compound. The aglycone part can be liberated by acid or alkaline hydrolysis, or by enzymes. Free phenolic acids can be found in fruits and vegetables; however, in other plant tissues such as grains, seeds, and in herbs, they are usually present in bound form (Tsao 2010, Hossain et al. 2010). Phenolic acids can be divided into two main categories, namely benzoic and cinnamic acid derivatives (Figure 2.1). The known representatives of benzoic acid derivatives in plants are *p*-hydroxybenzoic, vanillic, syringic, protocatechic, gallic, and salicylic acids. Among the cinnamic acid derivatives, also known as phenylpropanoids, ferulic, caffeic, *p*-coumaric, chlorogenic, and sinapic acids have been reported. Rosmarinic acid, an ester of caffeic acid and 3,4-dihydroxyphenylacetic acid, is an important naturally occurring phenolic bioactive compound found in important quantities in plants of the Lamiaceae family (Saltas et al. 2013).

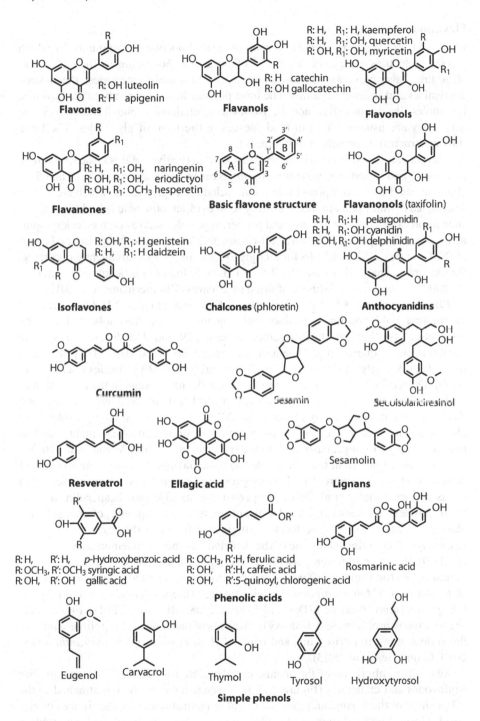

FIGURE 2.1 Molecular structures of characteristic phenols and polyphenols found in natural sources.

Flavonoids

Flavonoids are the most abundant group of natural phenolic compounds for which >4000 molecules have been identified (Tsao 2010). According to their chemical structure, flavonoids can be distinguished into two main categories: the flavone derivatives and the anthocyanins. The most popular flavone derivatives are flavones, flavonoles, flavanones, flavanonols, isoflavones, chalcones, and flavanols (Figure 2.1). They are usually found in food sources in the form of glycosides. The basic flavone structure is presented in Figure 2.1.

Flavones are considered to be the hydroxylated derivatives of this basic structure at positions 5 and 7, and one, two or three hydroxyls can be found at positions 3′, 4′, and 5′. A characteristic flavone compound is luteolin, including its glycosides, which are widely distributed in many plant families. Dietary sources of luteolin include herbs and spices such as oregano, rosemary, thyme, and pepper; vegetables such as carrots, celery, spinach, lettuce, and parsley; and olive oil (Justesen 2000, Boskou 2006, Lopez-Lazaro 2009, Cecchi et al. 2013). Luteolin 7-O-glycosides are the most frequently occurring; for example, cynaroside or luteolin 7-O-glucoside is found in artichoke (Lattanzio et al. 2009) and in aqueous infusion of dried sage leaves (Zimmermann et al. 2011).

Flavonols are the 3-hydroxy derivatives of flavones (Figure 2.1). Quercetin and kaempferol hold prominent positions among the studied flavonols, followed by myricetin. The literature has presented at least 279 and 348 different glycosidic combinations of quercetin and kaempferol, respectively (Tsao 2010). They are found in fruits as 3-O-glycosides mainly, and more rarely as 7-O-glycosides (Belitz et al. 2009). Quercetin-3-O-glucoside is found in significant amounts in the berry skin of grapes and in the wine made from them, constituting 42.6% and 39.4% of the total flavonol content, respectively (Nisco et al. 2013). Quercetin and its glycosides have also been found in dill, cress, tarragon, and in several Lamiaceae plants such as rosemary, oregano, sage, basil, and thyme (Hossain et al. 2010, Miron et al. 2011).

Flavanones contain in their molecule the basic flavone structure with the lack of double bond at C3 (Figure 2.1). This subgroup of flavonoids is mainly presented in citrus species (Ghafar et al. 2010). Hesperetin and its glycoside hesperidin (hesp-7-O-rutinoside) have been considered as the characteristic compounds of orange fruits. Naringenin and its glycosidic form, naringin, are found in the bark of grapefruit. Eriodictyol-7-O-rutinoside is one of the detected flavanones in lemon bark (Belitz et al. 2009). However, in fewer cases, the above-mentioned aglycones, alone or in combination with the same or different sugar moieties, contribute to the phenolic content of lemon balm (*Melissa officinalis*), wild thyme (*Thymus serpyllum*), and oregano (*Origanum vulgare*) extracts (Dastmalchi et al. 2008, Miron et al. 2011). Flavanonols or dihydroflavonols are the 3-hydroxy derivatives of flavanones. Taxifolin is a famous flavanonol found in citrus fruits and fruits of *Rosa canina* and *R. micrantha* (Tsao 2010, Guimarães et al. 2013).

Two other subgroups of flavonoids, closely related to the flavone structure, are isoflavones and chalcones (Figure 2.1). Isoflavones have the B ring attached to the C3 position of the C ring, and they are found in natural sources either in free or glycosidic form. The food sources of isoflavones are mainly plants of the Leguminosae family, such as beans and soya (Tsao 2010). Studies presented daidzein, genistein, and their β-glucosides conjugates as being >80% of the total determined isoflavones in soya milk (Toro-Funes et al. 2014). In chalcones, rings A and B are joined together by an unsaturated carbonyl system. They play an important role in the biosynthesis of flavonoids, as chalcone is enzymatically isomerized to a flavanone intermediate where all classes of flavonoids branch out (Tsao 2010). They have an intense yellow color and are mainly present in fruits. Phloretin is a characteristic dihydrochalcone found in the free form, and in varying glycosidic structures in apples, apple pomaces, and juices (Ramirez-Ambrosi et al. 2013).

Flavanols or flavan-3-ols are noncolor flavonoids widely distributed in all common fruits, while among herbs, black and green tea are rich sources. Flavan-3-ols are also known as catechins, and they exhibit a strong antioxidant activity. Tea polyphenols are already used in the food industry as natural antioxidants (He et al. 2009). They are structurally differentiated from the other flavonoids because they do not contain carbonyl at C4, or the double bond between C2 and C3 of the C ring (Figure 2.1). The well-known flavan-3-ols are catechin, catechin gallate, gallocatechin, gallocatechin gallate, and their corresponding isomers, namely epicatechin, epicatechin gallate, epigallocatechin, and epigallocatechin gallate. In the biosynthesis of flavonoids, it is possible to form dimeric or oligomeric compounds of flavan-3-ols, which are called proanthocyanidins or condensed tannins. Proanthocyanidins are the noncolor precursors of anthocyanins, and they usually coexist with flavanols in plant tissues.

Four catechins and six catechin gallates have been identified in the fresh young shoots of tea (*Camellia sinensis*) grown in Australia, with epigallocatechin gallate constituting up to 116 mg/g on a dry basis (Yao et al. 2004). In aqueous extracts of Chinese green tea, the total catechin content was determined to be 93.6% (w/w) of infusions, with the catechin gallates accounting for >82% (w/w) of the tea extract (He et al. 2009). Other good sources of flavanols and proanthocyanidins are plants of the genus *Cistus* (Danne et al. 1993, Barrajón-Catalan et al. 2011), which nowadays are a part of several natural mixtures used as decoctions. Other food sources of flavanols are the fruits of plants from the Ericaceae and Rosaceae families, orange juice, chocolate, red wine, and beans (Boskou 2006, Guimarães et al. 2013).

The anthocyanins are a famous flavonoid group that causes the red to violet and blue color of flowers and fruits. They exist in plants as glycosides, mainly at the C3 position, and their aglycone parts, known as anthocyanidins, are produced by acid hydrolysis. The most important anthocyanidins are pelargonidin, cyanidin, and delphinidin. Especially the last two, together with their ether derivatives, peonidin, petunidin, and malvidin, are responsible for the color of grapes, red currants, morellos, cherries, and various berries such as blackberry, blueberry, and raspberry, making them a valuable source of anthocyanins (Pantelidis et al. 2007, Nisco et al. 2013, Carrieri et al. 2013). The anthocyanin contents in black and red grapes are estimated at 70% and 23% of their total phenols, respectively (Carrieri et al. 2013). Vegetables are another food source of anthocyanins. A delphinidin glycoside was found in eggplant, two pelargonidin derivatives in radish, a cyanidin derivative in red cabbage, and a cyanidin glycoside with peonidin-3-arabinoside in red onion peel (Belitz et al. 2009). Artichoke heads were found to contain several cyanidin glycosides mainly, but two peonidin and one delphinidin derivatives are also referred (Lattanzio et al. 2009).

Other Polyphenols

In food, there are also other polyphenols, besides the simple phenols, phenolic acids, and flavonoids, that are of great biological interest.

Resveratrol (*trans*-3,4′,5-trihydroxystilbene) belongs to the stilbenes, and is a natural antioxidant mainly found in berries, leaves, and canes of grapes, as well as in red wine and lesser in white wines. Hydrolyzable tannins are another group of polyphenols found mainly in the wood and bark of oak and chestnut tree. They are divided into simple hydrolyzable tannins, which are esters of gallic acid or its glycosides or its esters with glucose, and ellagitannins, which contain in their structure a glycoside of glucose and ellagic acid (a gallic acid dimer) (Figure 2.1). Ellagitannins have been found in aqueous extracts of many *Cistus* species of the subgenus *Leucocistus* and *Halimioides* in quantities ranging from 0.63 to 15.79 mg/mL; however, they are mostly absent from plants of the subgenus *Cistus* (Barrajón-Catalan et al. 2011). Punicalin, punicalagin, and punicalagin gallate are common ellagitannins found in *Cistus salvifolius*, *C. ladanifer*, and *C. monspeliensis*. It is believed that they contribute substantially to the antioxidant properties of the crude aqueous leaf extracts of *Cistus* spp. (Saracini et al. 2005, Barrajón-Catalan et al. 2011).

Lignans are phytoestrogens present in seeds, cereals, legumes, fruits, and vegetables. Their consumption is believed to have positive effects on human health (Gerstenmeyer et al. 2013). Sesame and flax seeds are good sources of lignans, which are also found in rye grains and rye products in lesser amounts. Secoisolariciresinol and its diglycoside isolariciresinol; lariciresinol and its monoglycoside 7-hydroxymatairesinol; syringaresinol; pinoresinol with mono-, di-, and triglycosides; sesaminol with di- and triglucosides; and sesamolinol and its diglucoside have been detected in the extracts of the above-mentioned sources (Gerstenmeyer et al. 2013). Sesame seeds and oil also contain sesamin and sesamolin, which are considered antioxidant compounds (Rangkadilok et al. 2010). The sesamin and sesamolin contents in sesame range between 0 and 7.23 mg/g seed and between 0 and 2.25 mg/g seed, respectively, strongly depending on of the sesame type and origin (Rangkadilok et al. 2010).

CAROTENOIDS

Carotenoids are a group of tetraterpenes widely distributed in nature, giving fruits and vegetables from a light yellow to a dark red color. They are divided into carotenes, which are unsaturated hydrocarbons, and to xanthophylls, which are their oxygenated derivatives. Typical representatives of this group are β-carotene, α-carotene, lycopene, zeaxanthin, and lutein (Figure 2.2). Carotenoids are the precursors of vitamin A. Food sources of carotenoids are fruits like citrus, peaches, apricots, watermelon, and melon, and vegetables including all yellow ones, corn, carrots, tomatoes, red pepper, etc. Carotenoids constitute the major pigment in carrots. Apocarotenoids are natural polyenes with a shortened carbon skeleton structurally related to carotenoids. Such apocarotenoids are present in the red dark stigmas of *Crocus sativus* flowers, whose dried form is the famous and expensive spice saffron, and are known as crocins. Crocins are very water-soluble colorings, mainly found as *all-trans*- and 13-*cis*-glycosyl esters of crocetin (Tarantilis et al. 1995). Crocins are mainly composed of digentiobiosyl crocetin (Figure 2.2). Saffron, especially in powder form, is

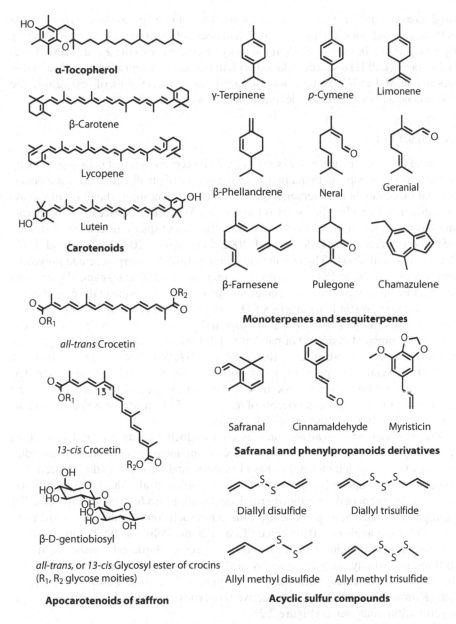

FIGURE 2.2 Molecular structures of characteristic essential oil compounds, carotenoids, and α-tocopherol found in natural food sources.

often confused and adulterated with curcumin, which is a diphenylheptanoid compound extracted from turmeric rhizome and used in the food industry as a coloring with strong antioxidant properties (Figure 2.1). The antioxidant potential of carotenoids has been reported in the literature and may play an important role in human health, protecting cells and tissues from the damaging effects of free radicals and singlet oxygen. β-Carotene can act as an antioxidant or as prooxidant, depending on both its concentration and the low or high concentration of oxygen (Lee et al. 2004). By studying the *in vitro* antioxidant activity of crocins with the 2,2-diphenyl-1-pic-rylhydrazyl (DPPH) test, a correlation with the crocin concentration was observed—crocins showed an IC_{50} value of 44 ± 1 μg/mL; at a concentration of >50 μg/mL, the antioxidant activity started to decrease (Kanakis et al. 2009).

ESSENTIAL OILS

Essential oils (EO) are natural mixtures of volatile compounds that belong principally to the terpenes group and found in a special category of plants called aromatic plants. A great variability of monoterpenes and sesquiterpenes constitute the EO composition of plants of different families, such as Lamiaceae, Asteraceae, Apiaceae, Verbenaceae, and Cistaceae, whose aerial parts are used as herbs and spices, or consumed in their fresh form as vegetables (Daferera et al. 2002, Candan et al. 2003, Güllüce et al. 2003, Petropoulos et al. 2004). Thymol and carvacrol, primarily, γ-terpinene and *p*-cymene secondarily, are basic EO compounds in oregano, thyme, marjoram, dittany, and savory. Limonene is a common monoterpene predominantly found in the peel of citrus fruits, and also present in lemongrass EO. α-Pinene is one of the main components in the EO of rosemary, mountain tea, and sage (Aligiannis et al. 2001). β-Phellandrene is a basic compound in the EO of parsley and dill leaves. Eucalyptol and camphor are characteristic compounds in sage, rosemary, and *Achillea*. Pulegone predominates in the EO composition of pennyroyal. Monoterpene alcohols such as α-terpineol, ter-pinen-4-ol, and borneol are found in *Achillea*, marjoram, and rosemary. Neral and geranial are the principal components of lemongrass EO. Farnesene and chamazulene are parts of the EO composition of chamomile.

Phenylpropanoid derivatives, such as cinnamaldehyde, eugenol, and myristicin, frequently constitute the EO composition. Cinnamaldehyde is the predominant cin-namon EO compound; eugenol is found in clove and basil oil; and myristicin is a characteristic compound in parsley EO (Petropoulos et al. 2004). In some cases, the volatile compounds are the thermal degradation products of carotenoids. For example, safranal and isophorone are considered such compounds, and are the prin-cipal EO compounds in saffron spice (Tarantilis and Polissiou 1997). Organosulfur compounds are common among the *Allium* species. Garlic oil consists of diallyl sulfides, methyl allyl sulfides, and vinyl dithiins, in quantities that vary according to the extraction technique, extraction temperature, and the solvent used for their isola-tion (Kimbaris et al. 2006). The bioactive properties of garlic oil are attributed to its acyclic sulfur compounds (Figure 2.2).

DISTRIBUTION OF NATURAL ANTIOXIDANTS IN SELECTED FOOD SOURCES

FRUITS

Fruits are very good sources of various phenolic compounds and carotenoids (Belitz et al. 2009). The content of carotenoids among different fruits varies widely, from

0.3 mg/kg of fresh weight (fw) in pears to 27 mg/kg (fw) in peaches (Belitz et al. 2009). Oranges, pears, peaches, and sweet melons contain relatively high amounts of β-carotene, cryptoxanthin, and zeaxanthin. Peaches are also rich in lycopene, phytoene, phytofluene, and ζ-carotene. Moreover, in the carotenoid composition of oranges, the epoxy carotenoids arc found in significant amounts. Fruits like pineapples, bananas, figs, and grapes are poor in β-carotene, lutein, and neoxanthine (Belitz et al. 2009).

The total phenol content in fruits shows fluctuations. Apples and grapes contain 0.1–1.0 g/100 g (fw), plums contain 0.2–1.4 g/100 g (fw), whereas peaches contain 0.03–0.14 g/100 g (fw). Cinnamic acid derivatives are the most popular phenolic compounds in fruits, mainly found as esters of p-coumaric, ferulic, and caffeic acids with quinic acid and often with D-glucose. Chlorogenic acid (syn. 5-caffeoylquinic acid) is the predominant compound in apples and pears. The major cinnamic acid derivatives found in cherries, morellos, plums, peaches, and apricots are neochlorogenic (syn. 3-caffeoylquinic) and chlorogenic acids. Cherries and morellos also contain 3-p-coumaroylquinic acid in significant amounts. In the case of strawberries and various types of berries such as blackberries, a diversity of cinnamic acid derivatives exist. Chlorogenic acid is the major one in blackberries, while the most commonly occurring, regardless of its quantity, is p-coumaroylglucose. Benzoic acid derivatives are found in strawberries, grapes, and citrus fruits. Salicylic acid is the most widespread, followed by gentisic acid. In strawberries, p-hydroxybenzoic, gallic, ellagic, protocatechic, and vanillic acids are also found. The content of phenolic acids in fruits depends of the fruit variety, degree of maturation, and storage period.

L-Ascorbic acid (a form of vitamin C) also exists in fruits, influencing their total antioxidant capacity. Small fruits of various blackberries, raspberries, gooseberries, red currants, and cherries contain variable amounts of phenols, among them anthocyanins. The anthocyanin content ranged from 1.3 to 223.0 mg cyanidin-3-glucoside equivalents per 100 g (fw), and the total phenol content from 657 to 2611 mg gallic acid equivalents per 100 g dry weight (dw) (Pantelidis et al. 2007). The largest amount of anthocyanins was found in a native Cornelian cherry population with red color, while the highest total phenol content was found in a raspberry × blackberry cultivar (sunberry). The anthocyanin content in three sweet cherry varieties was estimated to be between 2 and 24 mg cyanidin 3-O-rutinoside equivalent/100 g (Pappas et al. 2011). The ascorbic acid content in such fruits ranged from 14 to 103 mg/100 g (fw); however, it was negatively correlated with ferric reducing antioxidant power (FRAP) values, leading the authors to hypothesize that no direct correlation can be established between ascorbic acid content and total antioxidant capacity (Pantelidis et al. 2007). Literature reports show that ascorbic acid can act as an antioxidant or prooxidant depending on certain conditions (Lee et al. 2004). The major anthocyanins found in common fruits such as apples, pears, peaches, plums, figs, oranges, morellos, cherries, and blackberries are glycosides of cyanidin; those in strawberries are glycosides of pelargonin; and those in bananas are glycosides of petunidin (Belitz et al. 2009). Cyanidin 3-O-glucoside and cyanidin 3-O-rutinoside are predominant compounds in plums, sweet cherries (*Prunus avium* L.), and blackberries, although variations among different varieties were observed. The above-mentioned common fruits also contain flavonols and flavan-3-ols, with major representatives being quercetin 3-O-glucoside and epicatechin, respectively.

TABLE 2.1
Distribution of Natural Antioxidants in Selected Food Sources

Food Source	Natural Antioxidant Group	References
Fruits and Fruit Products		
Pears, peaches	Carotenoids, phenolic acids, flavonols, flavanols	Belitz et al. 2009
Apricots	Phenolic acids, flavonols, flavanols	Belitz et al. 2009
Cherries	Anthocyanins, flavanols, phenolic acids, flavonols	Belitz et al. 2009, Pappas et al. 2011
Blackberries, raspberries, gooseberries, red currant	Anthocyanins, phenols	Pantelidis et al. 2007
Strawberry tree	Anthocyanins, flavanols, flavonols, galloyl derivatives, proanthocyanidins	Guimarães et al. 2013
Blackthorn	Phenolic acids, flavones, flavonols, anthocyanins	Guimarães et al. 2013
Wild roses, dog roses	Flavononols, flavanones, anthocyanins, flavanols, flavonols, proanthocyanidins	Guimarães et al. 2013
Apples, cider apples, pomace, juice	Anthocyanins, proanthocyanidins, phenolic acids, dihydrochalkones, flavonols, flavanols	Ramirez-Ambrosi et al. 2013, Belitz et al. 2009
Citrus, citrus juice	Flavanones, carotenoids	Ghafar et al. 2009
Mandarin peel	Polymethoxylated flavones, flavanones, chalcones	Zhang et al. 2012
Grapes	Anthocyanins, phenolic acids, stilbenes, flavonols, flavanols, proanthocyanidin	Teixeira et al. 2013, Nisco et al. 2013, Carrieri et al. 2013, Cantos et al. 2002
Olive oil	Phenolic alcohols, phenolic acids, secoiridoids, lignans, flavones, flavonols, anthocyanins, carotenoids, tocopherols	Tripoli et al. 2005, Boskou 2006, Christophoridou and Dais 2009
Seeds		
Sesame, flax, rye grains	Lignans	Gerstenmeyer et al. 2013
Vegetables		
Artichoke	Cinnamic acid derivatives, flavones, flavanones, flavonols, anthocyanins	Lattanzio et al. 2009, Palermo et al. 2013
Eggplant, red cabbage, radish, red onion	Anthocyanins	Belitz et al. 2009
Spinach	Flavonoids, p-coumaric acid	Boskou 2006
Garlic/onion	Volatile sulfur compounds	Kimbaris 2006, Belitz et al. 2009
Dill	Essential oil, flavonols	Justesen 2000
Parsley	Essential oil, flavones	Petropoulos et al. 2004, Justesen 2000

(Continued)

TABLE 2.1 (CONTINUED)
Distribution of Natural Antioxidants in Selected Food Sources

Food Source	Natural Antioxidant Group	References
Herbs		
Oregano, sage, rosemary	Essential oils, phenolic acids, flavones, flavonols, phenolic triterpenes	Miron et al. 2011, Zimmermann et al. 2011, Hossain et al. 2010
Thyme, basil	Essential oils, phenolic acids, flavones, flavonols	Hossain et al. 2010
Lemon balm	Essential oil, phenolic acids, flavones, flavanones	Dastmalchi et al. 2008
Tarragon	Phenolic acids, caftaric acid, flavonols	Miron et al. 2011
Herbal Infusions		
Oregano, pennyroyal	Flavanols, essential oil compounds, phenolic acids, triterpenic acids	Kogiannou et al. 2013
Marjoram, savory, mountain tea, chamomile	Flavanols, essential oil compounds, phenolic acids	Kogiannou et al. 2013
Tea	Flavanols	Yao et al. 2004, He et al. 2009
Cistus	Flavanols, proanthocyanidins, ellagitannins	Barrajón-Catalan et al. 2011, Danne et al. 1993, Saracini et al. 2005

Strawberry tree (*Arbutus unedo*), blackthorn (*Prunus spinosa*), dog rose (*Rosa canina*), and wild rose (*Rosa micrantha*) fruits, consumed fresh or as jams, liqueurs, or decoctions, are good sources of phenolic acids and flavonoids (Guimarães et al. 2013) (Table 2.1). Blackthorn fruits presented the highest amounts of anthocyanins (100.40 mg/100 g), flavones/flavonols (57.48 mg/100 g), and phenolic acids (29.78 mg/100 g) compared with strawberry tree and wild roses. Strawberry tree contained the largest quantity of flavan-3-ol (36.30 mg/100 g), followed by wild rose (32.62 mg/100 g) and dog rose (19.90 mg/100 g), while it was not detected in blackthorn. Among the identified phenolic acids, 3-*O*-caffeoylquinic acid was the most abundant, quercetin 3-*O*-rutinoside was the most detected flavonol, and (+)-catechin was the predominant flavan-3-ol. Cyanidin 3-*O*-glucoside was detected in all samples to be the major anthocyanin, with the exception of blackthorn where cyanidin 3-*O*-rutinoside and peonidin 3-*O*-rutinoside predominated.

Nowadays, modern analytical techniques are applied in food analysis, which allows the identification of more compounds not previously reported. Nineteen new compounds were characterized in the case of cider apples (two flavanols, four dihydrochalcones, nine hydroxycinnamic acids, and four flavonols), while in apple pomace and juice, five new compounds were identified (two dihydrochalcones and three flavonols) (Ramirez-Ambrosi et al. 2013).

The flavonoid composition of citrus fruits is characterized by the presence of flavanones, which naturally occur in glycosidic form and are responsible for the bitter taste in those fruits. The intensity of the bitterness depends on the type of substituents in the basic aglycone part of the glycosides. Hesperidin is the characteristic flavanone of sweet oranges, also found in lemon peel, which has a neutral taste. The bitter taste of some orange cultivars is attributed to the compound neohesperidin. Naringin is the bitter compound of grapefruits (Belitz et al. 2009). Mandarin peel was found to contain polymethoxylated flavones, flavanones, and chalcones. It was mentioned that polymethoxylated flavonoids have high oral bioavailability, showing, among others, antioxidant activity (Zhang et al. 2012). Citrus juices are a good source of phenolic compounds whose quantity range between 105 and 490 mg of gallic acid equivalent/100 mL juice, depending on the citrus species. Their flavonoid content in different lime species and in oranges was determined to be from 2.99 to 22.25 mg of hesperidin equivalent/100 mL juice (Ghafar et al. 2010).

GRAPES AND WINE

Table and wine grapes are a special category of fruits constituting a major source of phenolic compounds. Phenolics in grapes are responsible for the color, flavor, and stringency of wine, contributing to its antioxidant properties. Phenolics in table and wine grape cultivars present qualitative similarities; however, quantitative differences were observed. The anthocyanin content in grapes fluctuates depending on the cultivar. In four red table cultivars, it was estimated to be from 69 to 151 mg/kg (fw) (Cantos et al. 2002). The berry skin and wine of the grape cultivar *Vitis vinifera* L. (cv. Aglianico), grown in southern Italy, was characterized to be a valuable source of anthocyanins, with an amount of 9996.1 mg/kg (fw) and 716.3 mg/L, respectively (Nisco et al. 2013). Malvidin and petunidin glycosides constitute the majority of the anthocyanin composition, with malvidin-3-glucoside being the predominant compound (Nisco et al. 2013). In three black table grapes, malvidin was found to be the predominant anthocyanin, while in four red ones petunidin was distinguished to be predominant (Carrieri et al. 2013). The major anthocyanin in red table grapes is peonidin-3-glucoside, while in wine grapes it was reported to be malvidin-3-glucoside (Cantos et al. 2002, Nisco et al. 2013).

Red grape cultivars contain higher amounts of phenolic compounds relative to white grapes, owing to the presence of anthocyanins in their composition (Cantos et al. 2002). However, the average total phenolic content in black, red, and white table grapes was determined to be 297 ± 70, 138 ± 15, and 196 ± 103 mg/kg (fw), respectively, indicating that, in the some white cultivars, exceptions exist (Carrieri et al. 2013). The relatively high amount of total phenolics in some white grape cultivars was attributed to the presence of flavonols and flavan-3-ols, occurring in higher quantities and contributing to the higher percentages to the total phenolic content (Cantos et al. 2002, Carrieri et al. 2013). Quercetin 3-glucuronide, quercetin 3-glucoside, and quercetin 3-rutinoside have been determined as the main flavonols in all table grapes (Cantos et al. 2002). Studies on the relation between antithrombotic activity and the polyphenolic profile of 12 table grapes showed that quercetin and cyanidin displayed a positive correlation, suggesting that the greater their concentration, the stronger the inhibition of tissue factor synthesis (Carrieri et al. 2013). Cinnamic acid derivatives were also found in grapes, constituting about 4–13% of the total phenol content.

Caffeoyltartaric acid and *p*-coumaroyltartaric acid are the most common (Cantos et al. 2002). The *trans-* and *cis*-isomers of resveratrol are both present in grapes, although the *trans*-isomers exist in larger quantities. In berry skin and wine from the Aglianico cultivar, *trans*-resveratrol was determined at 444.41 mg/kg (fw) and 3.79 mg/L respectively, while the corresponding detected levels for the *cis*-isomer was 2.7% and 1.8% lower (Nisco et al. 2013). Resveratrol is present in the skin and seeds of berry grapes but not in the flesh (Teixeira et al. 2013). The groups of phenolic compounds and their distribution in tissues of mature grape berry are presented in Table 2.1.

VEGETABLES

Vegetables are consumed by humans daily as fresh, cooked, or processed (e.g., canned). As with other food sources, their contents of natural, possible antioxidant compounds vary both qualitatively and quantitatively. Besides fruits, vegetables are also rich sources of phenolic compounds, mainly benzoic and cinnamic acid derivatives, flavones, and flavanols. Vegetables with red, violet, and blue color also contain anthocyanins. Eggplant has a delphinidin glycoside; radish contains two pelargonidin glycosides; red cabbage has a cyanidin derivative; and onions with red peel contain cyanidin and a peonidin glycoside in its anthocyanin composition (Belitz et al. 2009). Some plant species are considered vegetables, despite their content of EO or other volatile compounds, such as parsley, dill, onion, and garlic. α-Phellandrene is the main component of dill leaves EO. In aqueous methanol extract of dill, the flavonols isorhamnetin, kaempferol, and quercetin were detected as glucuronyl conjugates. Quercetin–rhamnoglucoside was also detected as a minor component of dill (Justesen 2000). β-Phellandrene was determined as the predominant compound in the EO composition of three types of parsley, namely plain, curly, and turnip-rooted. Fluctuations were observed in the relative percentages of their EO compounds, strongly depending on the sowing date, growth stage, and plant part (Petropoulos et al. 2004). Myristicin was present in notable percentages in all types of parsley; however, the highest values were observed in curly parsley. The aqueous methanol extract of parsley was found to contain a flavone fraction, consisting of apigenin-7-apiosylglucoside (apiin), apigenin-acetyl-apiosylglucoside, diosmetin-apiosylglucoside, and diosmetin-acetyl-apioglucoside (Justesen 2000).

Alliin (*S*-allyl-L-cysteine sulfoxide) is considered the precursor of the aromatic compounds of onion and garlic, and is present in fresh tissues. When garlic is chopped or crushed, the enzyme allinase is activated and acts on alliin, producing allicin (diallyl thiosulfinate). Under certain conditions, allicin is converted directly to acyclic sulfur compounds or, via thioacrolein, produces vinyl dithiins isomers, which can further decompose to acyclic sulfides with heating. Garlic EO consists mainly of acyclic polysulfides and vinyl dithiin isomers (Figure 2.2). These two groups have different properties, and their content in garlic EO is related to the applied temperature during the isolation process, as well as the time that affects the heating. Thus, the relative percentage of polysulfides decreased from 77.4% to 8.7%, whereas that of vinyl dithiin isomers increased from 4.7% to 70.8%, when the isolation techniques changed from harsh thermal (simultaneous distillation extraction, 2 h) to short time thermal (microwave-assisted hydrodistillation extraction, 30 min) and room temperature isolation (ultrasound-assisted extraction) (Kimbaris et al. 2006).

Among other vegetables, reference will be made to artichoke (*Cynara cardunculus* subsp. *solymus*), a native plant in Mediterranean countries that contains large amounts of polyphenols with high antioxidant activity and display high bioavailability (Lattanzio et al. 2009). The edible part of artichoke is the immature inflorescence, called head; however, its by-products, leaves, external bracts, and stems, also contain bioactive polyphenols and could be used as an antioxidant source. The total phenol content in artichoke heads, external bracts, and leaves was determined to be 2.32, 1.67, and 1.01 g gallic acid equivalent per 100 g of dry weight, respectively (Palermo et al. 2013). The principal phenolic group found in artichoke heads and leaves are the phenolic acids. There is a wide range of caffeoylquinic derivatives, with chlorogenic acid (5-*O*-caffeoylquinic acid) being the most abundant. In artichoke extracts, cryptochlorogenic (4-*O*-caffeoylquinic acid), neochlorogenic (3-*O*-caffeoylquinic acid), 1-*O*-caffeoylquinic, 1,3-*O*-dicaffeoylquinic (cynarin), 3,4-*O*-dicaffeoylquinic, 1,5-*O*-dicaffeoylquinic, and many other dicaffeoylquinin acids are also found. Their content in artichoke tissues is related to the physiological stage of the tissue, ranging from 8% (dw) in young to 1% (dw) in senescent tissues (Lattanzio et al. 2009). Flavonoids represent <10% of the total phenol content in artichoke. Luteolin and apigenin are the major flavones, found both as 7-*O*-glucoside and 7-*O*-rutinoside. Luteolin-7-*O*-glucoside is also known as cynaroside. Recent studies also report the presence of flavanones, mainly found as naringenin and eriodictyol glycosides, and flavonols that are represented by many quercetin and two myricetin glycosides (Palermo et al. 2013). Anthocyanins are present only in artichoke heads and consist of cyanidin, peonidin, and delphinidin glycosides. The most abundant are the cyanidin glycosides with the cyanidin 3,5-diglucoside and cyanidin 3-*O*-β-glucoside being among the principal ones (Lattanzio et al. 2009). The cooking method is one factor that affects the total phenol content and the percentage composition of the various phenolic compounds. Compared with the raw material, cooked artichoke contained reduced relative percentages of chlorogenic acid but increased percentages of cryptochloregenic acid and 4,5-*O*-dicaffeoylquinic acid, while steamed artichoke showed a higher phenolic content than the microwaved ones (Palermo et al. 2013). The antioxidant activity of artichoke extracts is related to its total phenol content, and probably to cynarin and caffeic acid, as they both present antioxidative properties. These compounds coexist in artichoke extracts with other bioactive compounds such as luteolin and cynaroside, indicating a possible additive or synergistic effect (Lattanzio et al. 2009).

HERBS

Herbs are used in food as flavorings and spices, but also for making various decoctions such as sage, chamomile, mountain tea, black and green tea, etc. The flora of the Mediterranean region includes many aromatic taxa, most of them endemic. Traditionally, people living in this region have introduced these herbs into their daily diet.

Herbs contain a variable amount of EO, which is constituted by numerous compounds in different qualitative and quantitative combinations (Aligiannis et al. 2001, Daferera et al. 2002, Güllüce et al. 2003, Candan et al. 2003, Petropoulos et al. 2004,

Tepe et al. 2004). Eucalyptol, camphor, and α-terpineol are the major components in *Achillea millefolium* EO (oil yield 0.6% v/w), as well as in many other *Achillea* species (Candan et al. 2003). Bisabolol oxides are also found in considerable percentages (total 7.1%) in *Achillea* EO. The EO of *A. millefolium* displayed a strong antioxidant effect on the *in vitro* free radical (IC_{50} = 1.56 µg/mL in DPPH, IC_{50} = 2.70 µg/mL in hydroxyl), and lipid peroxidation generation (IC_{50} = 13.50 µg/mL), compared with the corresponding values of ascorbic acid, curcumin, and butylated hydroxy toluene (BHT) (Candan et al. 2003). α-Pinene, eucalyptol, camphor, camphene, and borneol are found as basic compounds in *Salvia cryptantha* and *S. multicaulis* plants (oil yield 0.37–0.42% v/w). The EO of both *Salvia* species had greater antioxidant activity relative to the controls in DPPH and hydroxyl radicals, while their methanolic extracts were efficient only in the DPPH test (Tepe et al. 2004).

Carvacrol, thymol, γ-terpinene, and *p*-cymene are characteristic compounds of many *Origanum*, *Thymus*, and *Satureja* species (Daferera et al. 2002, Güllüce et al. 2003). *Satureja hortensis* (savory) EO displayed a lesser ability to act as a donor for hydrogen atom or electron (IC_{50} = 350 µg/mL) compared with the water subfraction of the methanol extract (IC_{50} = 30.89 µg/mL) in the DPPH test, although it inhibited 95% of the linoleic acid oxidation. The methanol extract of *S. hortensis* callus culture also showed a strong effect in the DPPH test (IC_{50} = 23.76 µg/mL) and it was comparable to the BHT effect (IC_{50} = 19.8 µg/mL) (Güllüce et al. 2003). The strong antioxidant capacity of the water/methanol extracts of *S. hortensis* can be attributed to the presence of phenolic acids, mainly rosmarinic acid, which are widespread in plants of the Lamiaceae family. Moreover, the rosmarinic acid content of 11 Lamiaceae samples of lemon balm (*M. officinalis*), sage (*Salvia officinalis*), oregano (*O. vulgare* ssp. *hirtum*), rosemary (*Rosemary officinalis*), basil (*Ocimum basilicum*), thyme (*Thymys vulgaris*), hyssop (*Hyssopus officinalis*), and savory, was determined. The rosmarinic acid content fluctuated from 81 ± 4 mg/g (in lemon balm) to 12 ± 3 mg/g (in hyssop) of dried plant material, while its quantity in savory was estimated at 56 ± 6 mg/g (dw) (Saltas et al. 2013).

Aqueous methanol extracts of rosemary, sage, oregano, basil, and thyme included various phenolic compounds belonging to the phenolic acids, flavones, phenolic terpenes, and flavonols (Hossain et al. 2010). A variety of phenolic acids was observed in all samples, among them gallic, caffeic, syringic, vanillic, protocatechuic, chlorogenic, *p*-coumaric, and rosmarinic acids. Luteolin and apigenin (in free or glycosidic form), quercetin, and quercetin-3-*O*-hexoside were also present. Carnosol and carnosic acid were present in oregano, rosemary, and sage extracts. Similar qualitative results have been observed in the aqueous and aqueous/ethanol extracts of Romanian oregano and wild thyme (*T. serpyllum*), apart from the phenolic triterpenes (Miron et al. 2011). Oregano water extract presented high content of total phenols (184.9 mg gallic acid eq./g, dw) showing important antioxidant activity (EC_{50} = 6.98 µg/mL) (Miron et al. 2011). The corresponding extracts of tarragon (*Artemisia dracunculus*) was found to contain 3-*O*-caffeoylquinic acid (neochloregenic), 4-*O*-caffeoylquinic acid (cryptochlorogenic), caftaric acid, various dicaffeoylquinic acid isomers, isorhamnetin, and quercetin (Miron et al. 2011). The aqueous ethanol extract of lemon balm leaves (*M. officinalis*) contain a phenolic fraction estimated at 268.9 ± 21.3 mg gallic acid eq./g (dw), which contained rosmarinic acid, caffeic acid, *m*-coumaric acid, eriodictyol-7-*O*-glucoside, naringin, naringenin, hespiridin, and hesperetin (Dastmalchi et al. 2008). Rosmarinic acid was the major constituent and was quantified at 96.45 ± 0.13 mg/g (dw). Lemon balm extracts possess strong antioxidant activity that can be explained by its phenolic composition (Dastmalchi et al. 2008). In the literature, qualitative and quantitative differences may be observed in the phenolic profile of the same herbs owing to the differences in plant origin, isolation method, extracting solvent system, and analytical technique (Kivilompolo et al. 2007, Dastmalchi et al. 2008, Miron et al. 2011).

The antioxidant properties, by the oxidation of *trans*-2-hexenal into the corresponding carboxylic acid, of 14 individual EOs from black and white pepper (*Piper nigrum* L.), cardamom (*Elettaria cardamomum* L.), nutmeg (*Myristica fragrans* Houtt.), mace (*Myristica fragrans* Houtt), juniper berry (*Juniperus communis* L.), fennel seed (*Foeniculum vulgare* Mill., var. *dulce* Thelling), caraway (*Carvum carvi* L.), dry cinnamon leaves (*Cinnamomum zeylanicum* Bl.), marjoram (*Origanum majorana* L.), laurel (*Laurus nobilis* L.), ginger (*Zingiber officinalis* L.), garlic (*Allium sativum* L.), and clove bud (*Caryophyllus aromaticus* L.) have been examined (Misharina et al. 2009). The EOs of garlic, clove bud, ginger, and leaves of cinnamon showed maximal efficiency, inhibiting hexenal oxidation at 80–93%, while black pepper oil showed minimal efficiency (49%). Garlic oil was the most effective. The antioxidant activity of an EO is attributed mainly to its major components; however, the synergistic or antagonistic effect of one compound present in the mixture in a minor percentage is also considered (Misharina et al. 2009, Amorati et al. 2013).

The total phenol contents in infusions of some Greek herbs, namely oregano (*O. vulgare*), Cretan marjoram (*O. microphyllum*), pink savory (*Satureja thymbra*), mountain tea (*Sideritis syriaca*), pennyroyal (*Mentha pulegium*), and chamomile (*Matricaria chamomilla*), have been determined (Kogiannou et al. 2013). The concentration of the total phenols in the herbal infusions was determined at high levels, ranging from 30.9 to 109.1 mg gallic acid equivalent per cup (200 mL). The flavanol content, also measured in these infusions, ranged between 8.3 and 40.0 mg rutin per cup. Oregano infusion was the most abundant both in total phenol and flavanol content, followed by pink savory. Pennyroyal infusion contains a high amount of phenols (82.9 mg gallic acid equivalent per cup); however, its flavanol content was estimated at only 13.2 mg/cup. On the contrary, the flavanol content in chamomile infusion (25.2 mg/cup) was high, >50% of the total phenol content (46.4 mg gallic acid equivalent per cup). The antioxidant capacity of the herbal infusion measured by the DPPH and FRAP methods showed the following sequence: oregano > pennyroyal > pink savory > chamomile > mountain tea and Cretan marjoram. The highest antioxidant activity of oregano infusion is attributed to its carvacrol, thymol, and caffeic acid contents. Carvacrol was detected in all herbal infusions, although higher amounts were measured in oregano. The herbal infusions were also rich in phenolic acids displaying a varied qualitative profile (Kogiannou et al. 2013). Protocatechic acid was the major one in oregano, mountain tea, and chamomile infusions. Syringic acid was primarily found in pink savory and Cretan marjoram infusions, while vanillic acid was the basic content in pennyroyal infusion. Among the detected cinnamic acid derivatives, caffeic acid was predominant in all cases, ranging from 73.57 µg/cup in mountain tea to 895.19 µg/cup in oregano infusion. Catechin and epicatechin were found in all herbal infusions, while kaempferol, quercetin, genistein, and naringenin were detected in specified plant cases (Kogiannou et al. 2013). Ursolic acid, a triterpenic acid, was quantified in the oregano and pennyroyal infusions, and it positively correlated with antiradical activity and FRAP, indicating that the antioxidant activity of herbal infusions can also be attributed to the presence of nonphenolic compounds (Kogiannou et al. 2013).

Another study on herbal infusions used 70 commercial medicinal plants from a local market, and their total phenol content correlated with the antioxidant capacity of the infusions (Katalinic et al. 2006). The total phenol concentration in all plant infusions varied between 9.0 and 2218.0 mg catechin equivalents (CE) per liter of infusion. The total phenol content for Thymi herba, Serpylli herba, *Mentha piperita* folium, *S. officinalis* folium, Basilici herba, Hyperici herba, Majoranae folium, *Tiliae officinalis* flos, Satureja herba, Chamomillae flos, Lauri folium, and Rormarini folium, was estimated to be between 136 and 876 mg CE/L infusion. The highest value was determined in *Melissa folium* infusion (2218.0 mg CE/L), which showed the strongest antioxidant property. In the DPPH test, *M. folium* infusion showed a similar behavior to catechin, but not as good as quercetin; however, it was more efficient as a free ABTS radical scavenger, compared with trolox and vitamin C (Katalinic et al. 2006). In infusions of different samples of dried sage leaves, rosmarinic acid and luteolin-7-*O*-glucoside were the predominant compounds with values ranging between 12.2 and 296 mg/L and between 37.9 and 166 mg/L, respectively. The phenolic triterpene carnosic acid was another compound found in significant amounts (9.1–32.9 mg/L). Moreover, the phenolic composition of sage infusion include caffeic acid, chlorogenic acid, salvianolic acid I and isomers, carnosol, rosmanol, apigenin glycosides, and other luteolin glycosides (Zimmermann et al. 2011).

OLIVE AND OLIVE OIL

Table olives and virgin olive oil are valuable food for people of all countries around the Mediterranean basin. Greece, Turkey, Spain, and Italy are the most important producer countries. Phenolics are responsible for the stability of olive against oxidation and contribute to its nutritional properties, including its antioxidant effect. The polyphenol content differ among the produced olive oils, depending on the olive cultivar, geographical origin, ripening degree, extraction procedure, and storage (Tripoli et al. 2005, Cecchi et al. 2013). The major phenols found in virgin olive oil are hydroxytyrosol and oleuropein, which are responsible for its bitter and pungent taste (Tripoli et al. 2005). Other phenolics that can be found in olive oil are caffeic acid, *p*-coumaric acid, *p*-hydroxybenzoic acid, ferulic acid, cinnamic acid, 2,3-dihydroxybenzoic acid, homovanillic acid, vanillic acid, vanillin, syringic acid, apigenin, luteolin, quercetin, 1-acetoxy-pinoresinol, pinoresinol, oleuropein, ligstroside, sinapic acid, and tyrosol derivatives (Tripoli et al. 2005, Boskou 2006, Christophoridou and Dais 2009). The lignans 1-acetoxy-pinoresinol and pinoresinol are present in extra virgin olive oil (Christophoridou and Dais 2009). Tocopherols are included in the lipophilic phenolic fraction of olive oil.

Oleuropein is found in significant amounts in olive fruit and becomes reduced with the maturation of the fruit. The oleuropein content is higher in the first stages of fruit maturation, and in green cultivars compared with black ones, while the amounts of hydroxytyrosol and tyrosol increase as the fruits ripen (Tripoli et al. 2005). Olive ripening is a crucial factor affecting the quality of the produced oil and its total phenolic content (Cecchi et al. 2013). The basic phenolic fraction in the ethanolic extracts (80%, v/v) of olive pastes of different cultivars and harvesting times was oleuropein (mean value, 139.6 ± 12.0 mg/kg on dry material [dm]) and isomers of oleuropein aglycone (sum of mean values, 667.4 mg/kg, dm), followed by verbascoside (mean value, 241.9 ± 8.9 mg/kg, dm). The hydroxytyrosol content was estimated at 35.7 ± 8.5 mg/kg, dm (Cecchi et al. 2013).

Nuclear magnetic resonance analysis of the phenolic extracts received from extra virgin olive oils using a mixture of ethanol–water (80:20, v/v) led to the qualification and quantification of hydroxytyrosol (34.03–64.37 μmol/100 g of oil), tyrosol (25.06–61.26 μmol/100 g), oleuropein, ligstroside and their aglycones (sum 22.62–61.74 μmol/100 g), pinoresinol (1.25–1.61 μmol/100 g), 1-acetoxy-pinoresinol (2.01–2.87 μmol/100 g), *p*-coumaric acid, vanillin, vanillic acid, homovanillyl alcohol, luteolin, apigenin, and syringaresinol (Christophoridou and Dais 2009). Although all examined samples showed the same qualitative pattern, quantitative differences among the individual components were observed, because of the different cultivars and locations. The largest quantitative differences were observed between olive oils of the same cultivar from the same prefecture but different locations (Christophoridou and Dais 2009).

In this chapter, the components of natural sources used in human nutrition were described. The literature reports several *in vitro* or *in vivo* biological activities, including antioxidant activity, for these compounds. The evaluation of such activities is not easy, as various components exist simultaneously and can act synergistically or antagonistically (Amorati et al. 2013). In addition, it is not necessary for a natural antioxidant to exist in high concentration in the food source to present a positive result, as each compound displays different bioavailabilities in humans (Pantelidis 2007).

REFERENCES

Aligiannis, N., Kalpoutzakis, E., Chinou, I.B., Mitakou, S., Gikas, E., Tsarbopoulos, A. 2001. Composition and antimicrobial activity of the essential oils of five taxa of *Sideritis* from Greece. *J. Agric. Food Chem.* 49: 811–815.

Amorati, R., Foti, M.C., Valgimigli, L. 2013. Antioxidant activity of essential oils. *J. Agric. Food Chem.* 61: 10835–10847.

Barrajón-Catalàn, E., Fernández-Arroyo, S., Roldán, C., Guillén, E., Saura, D., Segura-Carretero, A., Micol, V. 2011. A systematic study of the polyphenolic composition of aqueous extracts deriving from several *Cistus* genus species: Evolutionary relationship. *Phytochem. Anal.* 22: 303–312.

Belitz, H.D., Grosch, W., Schieberle, P. 2009. *Food Chemistry*. Berlin: Springer Verlag.

Boskou, D. 2006. Sources of natural phenolic antioxidants. *Trends Food Sci. Technol.* 17: 505–512.

Candan, F., Unlu, M., Tepe, B., Daferera, D., Polissiou, M., Sökmen, A., Akpulat, A. 2003. Antioxidant and antimicrobial activity of the essential oil and methanol extracts of *Achillea millefolium* subsp. *millefolium* Afan. (Asteraceae). *J. Ethnopharmacol.* 87: 215–220.

Cantos, E., Espín, J.C., Tomás-Barbefn, F.A. 2002. Varietal differences among the polyphenol profiles of seven table grape cultivars studied by LC–DAD–MS–MS. *J. Agric. Food Chem.* 50: 5691–5696.

Carrieri, C., Milella, R.A., Incampo, F., Crupi, P., Antonacci, D., Semeraro, N., Colucci, M. 2013. Antithrombotic activity of 12 table grape varieties. Relationship with polyphenolic profile. *Food Chem.* 140: 647–653.

Cecchi, L., Migliorini, M., Cherubini, C., Giusti, M., Zanoni, B., Innocenti, M., Mulinacci, N. 2013. Phenolic profiles, oil amount and sugar content during olive ripening of three typical Tuscan cultivars to detect the best harvesting time for oil production. *Food Res. Int.* 54: 1876–1884.

Christophoridou, S., Dais, P. 2009. Detection and quantification of phenolic compounds in olive oil by high resolution ^{1}H nuclear magnetic resonance spectroscopy. *Anal. Chim. Acta* 633: 283–292.

Daferera, D.J., Tarantilis, P.A., Polissiou, M.G. 2002. Characterization of essential oils from Lamiaceae species by Fourier transform Raman spectroscopy. *J. Agric. Food Chem.* 50: 5503–5507.

Danne, A., Petereit, F., Nahrstedt, A. 1993. Proanthocyanidins from *Cistus incanus*. *Phytochemistry* 34 (4): 1129–1133.

Dastmalchi, K., Dorman, D., Oinonen, P., Darwis, Y., Laakso, I., Hiltunena, R. 2008. Chemical composition and *in vitro* antioxidative activity of a lemon balm (*Melissa officinalis* L.) extract. *LWT Food Sci Technol* 41: 391–400.

Figueiredo, A.C., Barroso, J.G., Pedro, L.G., Scheffe, J.J.C. 2008. Factors affecting secondary metabolite production in plants: Volatile components and essential oils. *Flavour Fragr. J.* 23: 213–226.

Gerstenmeyer, E., Reimer, S., Berghofer, E., Schwartz, H., Sontag, G. 2013. Effect of thermal heating on some lignans in flax seeds, sesame seeds and rye. *Food Chem.* 138: 1847–1855.

Ghafar, F.A.M., Prasad, N.K., Weng, K., Ismail, A. 2010. Flavonoid, hesperidine, total phenolic contents and antioxidant activities from *Citrus* species. *Afr. J. Biotechnol.* 9 (3): 326–330.

Guimarães, R., Barros, L., Dueñas, M., Carvalho, A.-M., Queiroz, M.J., Santos-Buelga, C., Ferreira, I. 2013. Characterisation of phenolic compounds in wild fruits from Northeastern Portugal. *Food Chem.* 141: 3721–3730.

Güllüce, M., Sökmen, M., Daferera, D., Ağar, G., Özkan, H., Kartal, N., Polissiou, M., Sökmen, A., Şahin, F. 2003. *In vitro* antibacterial, antifungal, and antioxidant activities of the essential oil and methanol extracts of herbal parts and callus cultures of *Satureja hortensis* L. *J. Agric. Food Chem.* 51: 3958–3965.

Halliwell, B., Gutteridge, J.M. 1995. The definition and measurement of antioxidants in biological systems. *Free Radic. Biol. Med.* 18: 125–126.

He, Q., Yao, K., Jia, D., Fan, H., Liao, X., Shi, B. 2009. Determination of total catechins in tea extracts by HPLC and spectrophotometry. *Nat. Prod. Res.* 23 (1): 93–100.

Hossain, M.B., Rai, D.K., Brunton, N.P., Martin-Diana, A.B., Barry-Ryan, C. 2010. Characterization of phenolic composition in Lamiaceae species by LC–ESI–MS/MS. *J. Agric. Food Chem.* 58: 10576–10581.

Justesen, U. 2000. Negative atmospheric pressure chemical ionization low-energy collision activation mass spectrometry for the characterization of flavonoids in extracts of fresh herbs. *J. Chromatogr. A.* 902: 369–379.

Kanakis, C.D., Tarantilis, P.A., Pappas, C., Bariyanga, J., Tajmir-Riahi, H.A., Polissiou, M.G. 2009. An overview of structural features of DNA and RNA complexes with saffron compounds: Models and antioxidant activity. *J. Photochem. Photobiol. B Biol.* 95: 204–212.

Katalinic, V., Milos, M., Kulisic, T., Jukic, M. 2006. Screening of 70 medicinal plant extracts for antioxidant capacity and total phenols. *Food Chem.* 94: 550–557.

Kimbaris, A.C., Siatis, N.G., Daferera, D.J., Tarantilis, P.A., Pappas, C.S., Polissiou, M.G. 2006. Comparison of distillation and ultrasound-assisted extraction methods for the isolation of sensitive aroma compounds from garlic (*Allium sativum*). *Ultrason. Sonochem.* 13: 54–60.

Kivilompolo, M., Obůrka, V., Hyötyläinen, T. 2007. Comparison of GC–MS and LC–MS methods for the analysis of antioxidant phenolic acids in herbs. *Anal. Bioanal. Chem.* 388: 881–887.

Kogiannou, D., Kalogeropoulos, N., Kefalas, P., Polissiou, M., Kaliora, A. 2013. Herbal infusions: Their phenolic profile, antioxidant and anti-inflammatory effects in HT29 and PC3 cells. *Food Chem. Toxicol.* 61: 152–159.

Lattanzio, V., Kroon, P.A., Linsalata, V., Cardinali, A. 2009. Globe artichoke: A functional food and source of nutraceutical ingredients. *J. Funct. Foods* 1: 131–144.

Lee, J., Koo, N., Min, D.B. 2004. Reactive oxygen species, aging, and antioxidative nutraceuticals. *Compr. Rev. Food Sci. Food Saf.* 3: 21–33.

Lopez-Lazaro, M. 2009. Distribution and biological activities of the flavonoid luteolin. *Mini-Rev. Med. Chem.* 9: 31–59.

Miron, T.L., Plaza, M., Bahrima, G., Ibãnez, E., Herrero, M. 2011. Chemical composition of bioactive pressurized extracts of Romanian aromatic plants. *J. Chromatogr. A* 1218: 4918–4927.

Misharina, T.A., Terenina, M.B., Krikunova, N.I. 2009. Antioxidant properties of essential oils. *Appl. Biochem. Microbiol.* 45 (6): 642–647.

Nisco, M., Manfra, M., Bolognese, A., Sofo, A., Scopa, A., Tenore, G., Pagano, F., Milite, C., Russo, M.T. 2013. Nutraceutical properties and polyphenolic profile of berry skin and wine of *Vitis vinifera* L. (cv. Aglianico). *Food Chem.* 140: 623–629.

Palermo, M., Colla, G., Barbieri, G., Fogliano, V. 2013. Polyphenol metabolite profile of artichoke is modulated by agronomical practices and cooking method. *J. Agric. Food Chem.* 61: 7960–7968.

Pantelidis, G.E., Vasilakakis, M., Manganaris, G.A., Diamantidis, Gr. 2007. Antioxidant capacity, phenol, anthocyanin and ascorbic acid contents in raspberries, blackberries, red currants, gooseberries and Cornelian cherries. *Food Chem.* 102: 777–783.

Pappas, C.S., Takidelli, C., Tsantili, E., Tarantilis, P.A., Polissiou, M.G. 2011. Quantitative determination of anthocyanins in three sweet cherry varieties using diffuse reflectance infrared Fourier transform spectroscopy. *J. Food Compos. Anal.* 24: 17–21.

Petropoulos, S.A., Daferera, D., Akoumianakis, C.A., Passam, H.C., Polissiou, M.G. 2004. The effect of sowing date and growth stage on the essential oil composition of three types of parsley (*Petroselinum crispum*). *J. Sci. Food Agric.* 84: 1606–1610.

Ramirez-Ambrosi, M., Abad-Garcia, B., Viloria-Bernal, M., Garmon-Lobato, S., Berrueta, L.A., Gallo, B. 2013. A new ultrahigh performance liquid chromatography with diode array detection coupled to electrospray ionization and quadrupole time-of-flight mass spectrometry analytical strategy for fast analysis and improved characterization of phenolic compounds in apple products. *J. Chromatogr. A* 1316: 78–91.

Rangkadilok, N., Pholphana, N., Mahidol, C., Wongyai, W., Saengsooksree, K., Nookabkaew, S., Satayavivad, J. 2010. Variation of sesamin, sesamolin and tocopherols in sesame (*Sesamum indicum* L.) seeds and oil products in Thailand. *Food Chem.* 122: 724–730.

Saltas, D., Pappas, C., Daferera, D., Tarantilis, P., Polissiou, M. 2013. Direct determination of rosmarinic acid in Lamiaceae herbs using diffuse reflectance infrared Fourier transform spectroscopy (DRIFTS) and chemometrics. *J. Agric. Food Chem.* 61: 3235–3241.

Saracini, E., Tattini, M., Traversi, M.L., Vincieri, F.F., Pinelli, P. 2005. Simultaneous LC–DAD and LC–MS determination of ellagitannins, flavonoid glycosides, and acyl-glycosyl flavonoids in *Cistus salvifolius* L. leaves. *Chromatographia* 62: 245–249.

Tarantilis, P.A., Polissiou, M.G. 1997. Isolation and identification of the aroma components from saffron (*Crocus sativus*). *J. Agric. Food Chem.* 45: 459–462.

Tarantilis, P.A., Tsoupras, G., Polissiou, M. 1995. Determination of saffron (*Crocus sativus* L.) components in crude plant extracts using high-performance liquid chromatography–UV–visible photodiode–array detection–mass spectrometry. *J. Chromatogr. A* 699: 107–118.

Teixeira, A., Eiras-Dias, J., Castellarin, S.D., Gerós, H. 2013. Review. Berry phenolics of grapevine under challenging environments. *Int. J. Mol. Sci.* 14: 18711–18739.

Tepe, B., Donmez, E., Unlu, M., Candan, F., Daferera, D., Vardar-Unlu, G., Polissiou, M., Sokmen, A. 2004. Antimicrobial and antioxidative activities of the essential oils and methanol extracts of *Salvia cryptantha* (Montbret et Aucher ex Benth.) and *Salvia multicaulis* (Vahl). *Food Chem.* 84: 519–525.

Toro-Funes, N., Bosch-Fusté, J., Veciana-Nogués, M.T., Vidal-Carou, M.C. 2014. Effect of ultra high pressure homogenization treatment on the bioactive compounds of soya milk. *Food Chem.* 152: 597–602.

Tripoli, E., Giammanco, M., Tabacchi, G., Di Majo, D., Giammanco, S., La Guardia, M. 2005. The phenolic compounds of olive oil: Structure, biological activity and beneficial effects on human health. *Nutr. Res. Rev.* 18: 98–112.

Tsao, R. 2010. Chemistry and biochemistry of dietary polyphenols. *Nutrients* 2: 1231–1246.

Yao, L., Jiang, Y., Datta, N., Singanusong, R., Liu, X., Duan, J., Raymont, K., Lisle, A., Xu, Y. 2004. HPLC analyses of flavanols and phenolic acids in the fresh young shoots of tea (*Camellia sinensis*) grown in Australia. *Food Chem.* 84: 253–263.

Zhang, J.-Y., Zhang, Q., Zhang, H.-X., Ma, Q., Lu, J.-Q., Qiao, Y.-J. 2012. Characterization of Polymethoxylated flavonoids (PMFs) in the peels of 'Shatangju' mandarin (*Citrus reticulata* Blanco) by online high-performance liquid chromatography coupled to photodiode array detection and electrospray tandem mass spectrometry. *J. Agric. Food Chem.* 60: 9023–9034.

Zimmermann, B.F., Walch, S.G., Tinzoh, L.N., Stohlinger, W., Lanchenmeier, D.W. 2011. Rapid UHPLC determination of polyphenols in aqueous infusions of *Salvia officinalis* L. (sage tea). *J. Chromatogr. B.* 879: 2459–2464.

Section II

Antioxidants in Health

3 Oxidative Stress in Pregnancy

Ung Lim Teo and Andrew Shennan

CONTENTS

Introduction 47
Fertility 47
Miscarriage 48
Preeclampsia 48
Intrauterine Growth Restriction 49
Preterm Labor 49
Preterm Premature Rupture of Membrane 50
Gestational Diabetes Mellitus 50
Conclusion 51
References 51

INTRODUCTION

The role of antioxidants in pregnancy is promising as we move toward disease prevention rather than cure, and recent findings that oxidative stress may be linked to some maternal–fetal conditions in pregnancy has been encouraging. Studies have been carried out to investigate interventions in the pre- and periconceptual periods, as well as in the antenatal period, to prevent adverse pregnancy disorders related to oxidative stress, particularly preeclampsia because of its impact on both morbidity and mortality in both mother and fetus. Oxidative stress has also been implicated in fertility and miscarriage. This chapter reviews the most recent evidence available about the clinical potential of antioxidants in the prevention of some common and serious conditions in pregnancy.

FERTILITY

Human sperm is vulnerable to oxidative stress because of its high contents of polyunsaturated fatty acids, which leads to the destruction of its DNA strands [1]. Defective DNA strands in sperm can cause impaired fertility, abnormal embryonic development, high rates of miscarriage, and an increased risk of defects in offspring. Antioxidants have been found in the epididymis (extracellular superoxide dismutase, selenocysteine-independent glutathione peroxidase, GPx5), seminal fluid (vitamin C, uric acid, tryptophan, spermine, and taurine), and in the male reproductive tract that help reverse the effects of oxidative stress [2]. Smoking, alcohol intake, and obesity can all increase oxidative stress and therefore deplete the antioxidant stores, causing male subfertility. A recent Cochrane review of 34 randomized controlled trials, but only involving 2876 couples, suggests that antioxidant supplements such as vitamin C and E can increase live births in male factor subfertility [3]. A large, well-designed, robust placebo-controlled clinical trial needs to be carried out to confirm these findings.

The oocyte is also prone to oxidative stress induced by reactive oxygen species (ROS), and high levels in smokers and women with increased alcohol consumption have been reported. Low levels of ROS are necessary for the induction of oocytes (meiosis I), and high levels of ROS impair oocyte maturation, ovulation, and fertilization [1].

A study has shown that older women (aged 39–45 years) have increased ROS and reduced antioxidants compared with younger women (aged 27–32 years), and therefore reduced antioxidant capacity to neutralize the amount of ROS in the follicular fluid of ovarian follicles. This could cause mitochondrial DNA changes and chromosomal aneuploidy, possibly leading to a higher risk of miscarriage and fetal anomaly, explaining this age-related morbidity [4].

Although male subfertility has been found to improve with antioxidant supplements, less robust clinical evidence is available to recommend antioxidant supplements to treat female subfertility. Antioxidant supplementation, in certain cases, can cause adverse effects in women, but usually only in very high doses [5].

MISCARRIAGE

Studies have shown an increase in placental oxygenation from 8 to 12 weeks' gestation corresponding to placental perfusion before early miscarriage. It was also shown that markers of oxidative stress were increased in the placenta of women with early miscarriage compared with controls. Therefore, it has been hypothesized that they resulted from premature placental perfusion. Another study demonstrated an increased amount of ROS and reduced antioxidants in the peritoneal cavity of women with miscarriages. Sperm DNA damage could cause miscarriage [6]; however, studies showing potential treatment with antioxidants are very limited.

Increased natural killer cells are found in the endometrium of women with recurrent miscarriage. Natural killer cells release angiogenic factors in the endometrium, causing increased preimplantation angiogenesis. This causes abnormal placentation, early intraplacental maternal circulation, and increased oxidative stress possibly leading to miscarriages [7]. ROS (plasma lipid peroxidase, reduced glutathione [GSH], malondialdehyde [MDA]) have been found elevated while antioxidant enzymes (GPx, superoxide dismutase and catalase, vitamin E, β-carotene) are decreased in women with recurrent miscarriages [4]. However, meta-analyses of studies to date with periconceptual and early pregnancy supplementation of vitamins or antioxidants have shown no benefit in the prevention of early miscarriage [1,8].

PREECLAMPSIA

Preeclampsia is a syndrome that can occur after 20 weeks' gestation, with multiorgan involvement characterized by new onset of hypertension ($\geq$140/90 mm Hg), proteinuria ($\geq$300 mg/24 h), and symptoms such as visual disturbances, epigastric pain, or headache. The incidence of preeclampsia is around 2–7% of all pregnancies [1]. The spectrum of preeclampsia includes HELLP syndrome and eclampsia. HELLP is manifested as a deranged liver function test, breakdown of hemoglobin (hemolysis), and low platelet count. Eclampsia is described as seizure activity with hypertension that can be life-threatening to both mother and fetus. Other complications of preeclampsia include pulmonary edema, liver and renal failure, stroke, and thromboembolism. Moreover, of the women who die, many will not have a seizure; that is, eclampsia is not the inevitable endpoint of the untreated disease. Preeclampsia can also affect fetal growth *in utero*, causing growth restriction, low birth weight fetus, and often the need for premature birth and sometimes stillbirth. Preeclampsia, therefore, can have a devastating effect in terms of morbidity and mortality in both mother and fetus.

The mechanism of preeclampsia is unknown but is thought to occur because of defective placental implantation. After fertilization, trophoblast forms two layers called cytotrophoblast and syncytiotrophoblast. The cytotrophoblast invades the decidua and remodels the spiral arteries by breaking down the smooth muscle layer to enable low resistance blood flow to the placental bed. In preeclampsia, the spiral arteries do not break down completely, causing persistent high resistance blood flow. This causes reduced perfusion leading to hypoxia. Intermittent reperfusion of the placenta is thought to cause the release of ROS, which have been found in elevated levels in the placentas of women with preeclampsia [1]. Placental villi are also found to be less well developed in preeclamptic placenta, with fewer branches and less complex vascular loops, compared with a placenta with a normal pregnancy outcome [9].

Antioxidant supplementation during pregnancy, therefore, would theoretically be able to reduce oxidative stress in the placenta and may be able to prevent preeclampsia. Meta-analyses of 10 trials involving 6533 women found no reduction in preeclampsia, high blood pressure, or preterm birth with antioxidant supplementation [10]. Antioxidant supplementation has been reported to cause a small increase in the risk of low birth weight [1]. Therefore, routine antioxidant supplementation in pregnancy is not recommended.

INTRAUTERINE GROWTH RESTRICTION

As described in the pathogenesis of preeclampsia, abnormal placentation due to oxidative stress is thought to be the cause of intrauterine growth restriction (IUGR). Owing to reduced perfusion from defective spiral arteries, there is utero–placental insufficiency leading to restricted growth of the fetus. Raised ROS like lipid peroxides [11], MDA, and xanthine oxidase [12] with low antioxidants have been found in plasma, placenta, and umbilical cord of women with IUGR. There is little evidence that supplementation aids this process, but little research has been done.

PRETERM LABOR

Preterm labor is defined as cervical change with strong, regular uterine contractions leading to delivery before 37 weeks' gestation. Worldwide, the rate of preterm birth ranges between 5% and 18% of babies, but is increasing [13]. Preterm delivery, which causes significant mortality and morbidity in newborns, can be categorized into spontaneous or indicated [4]. Causes of spontaneous preterm labor include uterine overdistension, infection, cervical disease, and endocrine disorders. However, the exact mechanism and pathway leading to preterm labor is not clear. Various studies have been and still are being done to find answers, with the hope of finding treatment or prevention.

Raised oxidative stress markers like MDA and 8-hydroxydeoxyguanosine with lower antioxidant levels such as GPx, GSH, and selenium [14] are found in women with preterm labor. Activities of FKBP12 rapamycin-associated protein and glutathione S-transferase (providing defense against oxidative stress) are also reduced in women with preterm labor. Other study findings also indicate inflammation and oxidative stress with lower antioxidant levels, demonstrating a reduced capacity to counter oxidative stress as a cause of preterm labor [4]. However, a recent randomized controlled trial using vitamin C and E supplementation in low-risk pregnant women showed no significant difference in the incidence of preterm labor [11,15]. Vitamin C supplementation in pregnancy may even increase the risk of preterm labor [16].

PRETERM PREMATURE RUPTURE OF MEMBRANE

There are postulations that preterm premature rupture of membrane (PPROM) stems from ROS and pro-inflammatory cytokines that cause collagen remodeling [17] and the activation of collagenolytic enzymes [18,19], leading to reduced strength and integrity of the fetal membrane. In vivo and in vitro studies of vitamin C and E in the strengthening of fetal membrane showed that a combination of vitamin C and E did not prevent the weakening of the fetal membrane and, unexpectedly, vitamin C supplementation alone can cause weakening of the fetal membrane in vitro [17]. A controlled double-blind trial of 109 patients found that daily supplementation of 100 mg vitamin C reduced the incidence of premature rupture of membrane [20]. A larger placebo-controlled double-blinded randomized controlled trial of 697 women at risk of preeclampsia reported that supplementation of vitamin C and E at doses of 1000 mg and 400 IU, respectively, was associated with increased risk of both premature rupture of membrane (i.e., occurring at term) and PPROM [21].

A recent prospective randomized controlled study, looking at prolonging the latency period after PPROM with vitamin C and E supplementation and maternal and neonatal outcome, demonstrated that supplementation does prolong the latency period after PPROM with no significant difference in adverse maternal and neonatal outcome [22,23]. These studies are still preliminary, and routine vitamin C and E supplementation after PPROM in the general population is not currently recommended.

GESTATIONAL DIABETES MELLITUS

Elevated levels of ROS and low antioxidant levels are found in women with gestational diabetes mellitus, which could be related to the pathogenesis or complication of hyperglycemia [24–27]. The placenta of women with gestational diabetes mellitus are found to have increased antioxidant gene expression but is less responsive to exogenous oxidative stress compared with tissues of normal pregnant women, possibly owing to the protective or adaptive mechanism in response to the increased oxidative stress [28].

CONCLUSION

Oxidative stress has been implicated in many important disorders in pregnancy; however, studies to date have failed to show significant benefit in antioxidant supplementation in pregnancy. Antioxidant supplementation is, therefore, not recommended for the prevention or treatment of disorders in pregnancy currently. However, there is little doubt that oxidative stress is implicated in the pathophysiology of certain disorders in pregnancy. Vitamin C and E have been most commonly used as antioxidant supplements in trials to date. Further trials should look into different doses, regimens, and other types of antioxidant supplements. More research and robust large placebo-controlled clinical trials are needed to investigate the role of oxidative stress in pregnancy disorders, and the safety and benefit of antioxidant supplementation in pregnancy.

REFERENCES

1. Poston, L., Igosheva, N., Mistry, H.D., Seed, P.T., Shennan, A.H., Rana, S., Karumanchi, S.A., Chappell, L.C. Role of oxidative stress and antioxidant supplementation in pregnancy disorders. *Am J Clin Nutr.* 2011;94(6 Suppl):1980S–1985S. Epub May 25, 2011.
2. Aitken, R.J., Koppers, A.J. Apoptosis and DNA damage in human spermatozoa. *Asian J Androl.* 2011;13:36–42. Epub August 30, 2010.
3. Showell, M.G., Brown, J., Yazdani, A., Stankiewicz, M.T., Hart, R.J. Antioxidants for male subfertility. *Cochrane Database Syst Rev.* 2011;19(1):CD007411.
4. Agarwal, A., Aponte-Mellado, A., Premkumar, B.J., Shaman, A., Gupta, S. The effects of oxidative stress on female reproduction: A review. *Reprod Biol Endocrinol.* 2012;10:49.
5. Zadák, Z., Hyspler, R., Tichá, A., Hronek, M., Fikrová, P., Rathouská, J., Hrnciariková, D., Stetina, R. Antioxidants and vitamins in clinical conditions. *Physiol Res.* 2009;58 Suppl 1:S13–S17.
6. Robinson, L., Gallos, I.D., Conner, S.J., Rajkhowa, M., Miller, D., Lewis, S., Kirkman-Brown, J., Coomarasamy, A. The effect of sperm DNA fragmentation on miscarriage rates: A systematic review and meta-analysis. *Hum Reprod.* 2012;27(10):2908–2917. Epub July 12, 2012.
7. Quenby, S., Nik, H., Innes, B., Lash, G., Turner, M., Drury, J., Bulmer, J. Uterine natural killer cells and angiogenesis in recurrent reproductive failure. *Hum Reprod.* 2009;24(1):45–54.
8. Rumbold, A., Middleton, P., Pan, N., Crowther, C.A. Vitamin supplementation for preventing miscarriage. *Cochrane Database Syst Rev.* 2011;(1):CD004073.
9. Ruder, E.H., Hartman, T.J., Blumberg, J., Goldman, M.B. Oxidative stress and antioxidants: Exposure and impact on female fertility. *Hum Reprod Update.* 2008;14(4):345–357.
10. Rumbold, A., Duley, L., Crowther, C.A., Haslam, R.R. Antioxidants for preventing preeclampsia. *Cochrane Database Syst Rev.* 2008;(1):CD004227.
11. Karowicz-Bilińska, A. Lipid peroxides concentration in women with intrauterine growth restriction. *Ginekol Pol.* 2004;75(1):6–9.

12. Biri, A., Bozkurt, N., Turp, A., Kavutcu, M., Himmetoglu, O., Durak, I. Role of oxidative stress in intrauterine growth restriction. *Gynecol Obstet Invest.* 2007;64(4):187–192.
13. World Health Organization (WHO). Preterm birth. 2014. Available at http://www.who .int/mediacentre/factsheets/fs363/en/.
14. Rayman, M.P., Wijnen, H., Vader, H., Kooistra, L., Pop, V. Maternal selenium status during early gestation and risk for preterm birth. *CMAJ.* 2011;183(5):549–555.
15. Hauth, J.C., Clifton, R.G., Roberts, J.M., Spong, C.Y., Myatt, L., Leveno, K.J., Pearson, G.D., Varner, M.W., Thorp, J.M. Jr., Mercer, B.M., Peaceman, A.M., Ramin, S.M., Sciscione, A., Harper, M., Tolosa, J.E., Saade, G., Sorokin, Y., Anderson, G.B. Vitamin C and E supplementation to prevent spontaneous preterm birth: A randomized controlled trial. *Obstet Gynecol.* 2010;116(3):653–658.
16. Rumbold, A., Crowther, C.A. Vitamin C supplementation in pregnancy. *Cochrane Database Syst Rev.* 2005;(2):CD004072.
17. Mercer, B.M., Abdelrahim, A., Moore, M.R., Novak, J., Kumar, D., Mansour, J.M., Perez-Fournier, M., Milluzzi, C.J., Moore, J.J. The impact of vitamin C supplementation in pregnancy and *in vitro* upon fetal membrane strength and remodeling. *Reprod Sci.* 2010;17(7):685–695.
18. Woods, J.R. Jr., Plessinger, M.A., Miller, R.K. Vitamins C and E: Missing links in preventing preterm premature rupture of membranes? *Am J Obstet Gynecol.* 2001;185(1):5–10.
19. Wall, P.D., Pressman, E.K., Woods, J.R. Jr. Preterm premature rupture of the membranes and antioxidants: The free radical connection. *J Perinat Med.* 2002;30(6):447–457.
20. Casanueva, E., Ripoll, C., Tolentino, M., Morales, R.M., Pfeffer, F., Vilchis, P., Vadillo-Ortega, F. Vitamin C supplementation to prevent premature rupture of the chorioamniotic membranes: A randomized trial. *Am J Clin Nutr.* 2005;81(4):859–863.
21. Spinnato, J.A., Freire, S., Pinto e Silva, J.L., Rudge, M.V.C., Martins-Costa, S., Koch, M.A., Goco, N., Santos Cde B., Cecatti, J.G., Costa, R., Ramos, J.G., Moss, N., Sibai, B.M. Antioxidant supplementation and premature rupture of the membranes: A planned secondary analysis. *Am J Obstet Gynecol.* 2008;199(4):433.e1–433.e8.
22. Gungorduk, K., Asıcıoglu, O., Gungorduk, O.C., Yıldırım, G., Besimoğlu, B., Ark, C. Does vitamin C and vitamin E supplementation prolong the latency period before delivery following the preterm premature rupture of membranes? A randomized controlled study. *Am J Perinatol.* 2014;31(3):195–202. Epub April 16, 2013.
23. Borna, S., Borna, H., Daneshbodie, B. Vitamins C and E in the latency period in women with preterm premature rupture of membranes. *Int J Gynaecol Obstet.* 2005;90(1):16–20.
24. Dey, P., Gupta, P., Acharya, N.K., Rao, S.N., Ray, S. et al. Antioxidants and lipid peroxidation in gestational diabetes—A preliminary study. *Indian J Physiol Pharmacol.* 2008;52(2):149–156.
25. Chaudhari, L., Tandon, O.P., Vaney, N., Agarwal, N. Lipid peroxidation and antioxidant enzymes in gestational diabetics. *Indian J Physiol Pharmacol.* 2003;47(4):441–446.
26. López-Tinoco, C., Roca, M., García-Valero, A., Murri, M., Tinahones, F.J., Segundo, C., Bartha, J.L., Aguilar-Diosdado, M. Oxidative stress and antioxidant status in patients with late-onset gestational diabetes mellitus. *Acta Diabetol.* 2013;50(2):201–208. Epub February 17, 2011.
27. Suhail, M., Patil, S., Khan, S., Siddiqui, S. Antioxidant vitamins and lipoperoxidation in non-pregnant, pregnant, and gestational diabetic women: Erythrocytes osmotic fragility profiles. *J Clin Med Res.* 2010;2(6):266–273. Epub November 19, 2010.
28. Lappas, M., Mitton, A., Permezel, M. In response to oxidative stress, the expression of inflammatory cytokines and antioxidant enzymes are impaired in placenta, but not adipose tissue, of women with gestational diabetes. *J Endocrinol.* 2010;204(1):75–84. Epub October 15, 2009.

4 The Role of Antioxidants in Children's Growth and Development

Fátima Pérez de Heredia, Ligia Esperanza Díaz,
Aurora Hernández, Ana María Veses,
Sonia Gómez-Martínez, and Ascensión Marcos

CONTENTS

Introduction 53
    Micronutrients and Early Development 53
    Oxidative Stress and Children's Health 54
Antioxidants, Growth, and Physical Development 56
    Antioxidants and Growth 56
    Antioxidants in the Treatment of Deficiency Diseases 58
    Antioxidants, Asthma, and Allergies 59
    Antioxidants and Obesity 59
Antioxidants, Cognitive Function, Behavior, and Mental Development 60
    Antioxidants and Brain Development 60
    Antioxidants and Behavioral/Cognitive Alterations: ADHD 61
    Antioxidants in Autism Spectrum Disorders 62
    Antioxidants in Down Syndrome 63
Conclusions 64
Acknowledgments 65
References 65

INTRODUCTION

MICRONUTRIENTS AND EARLY DEVELOPMENT

The first years of life are crucial for the adequate physical, cognitive, and emotional development of children and future adults. Childhood is the life period with the highest developmental rate, and a continuous, adequate, and balanced provision of nutrients is essential to ensure optimal development and health. However, the presence of undernourishment during childhood is still a matter of great concern worldwide. Data from the United Nations Children's Fund (UNICEF, 2006) show that one in four children are underweight and at increased risk for disease and mortality. This is a major problem in developing countries, where access to food is limited and child malnutrition has been traditionally caused by energy and/or macronutrient (mainly protein) deficiency, leading to impaired growth and development (Figure 4.1). In recent years, however, the concern for underweight has been paralleled by another, not less important, issue: the steep rise in pediatric overweight and obesity in both industrialized and developing countries. The increase in overweight children should not mask another form of malnutrition—that which comes from an inadequate supply of nutrients in the diet. This fact can be the result of limited access to food, but also of the poorer nutritional values of current diets worldwide, promoted by the switch in dietary habits toward consumption of highly refined foods to the detriment of fresh products, the lower nutrient content of fresh foods due to modern growth and husbandry practices and long-distance transport, or the reluctance of children to eat certain foods such as fruits and vegetables (Maggini et al., 2010; Singh, 2004). The combined contributions of these factors may lead to suboptimal, if not overtly insufficient, provision of nutrients that are essential for maximum growth and development during childhood, such as vitamins and minerals. This, in turn, leads to clinical or subclinical deficiencies of not just isolated nutrients but rather a group of them (Thurlow et al., 2006), and that can be observed in children from developing countries as well as from the most industrialized ones (Maggini et al., 2010; Singh, 2004).

OXIDATIVE STRESS AND CHILDREN'S HEALTH

Oxidative stress results from an imbalance between the body's production of reactive oxygen species (ROS) and the antioxidant mechanisms in place. Generation of ROS can be the result of environmental injury (toxic chemicals, air pollutants, etc.); however, it is also a normal physiological process that can be part of the defense response against pathogens and abnormal cells, or a by-product of metabolism and respiration. However, when exceeding certain levels, ROS can oxidize cellular components, mainly membrane fatty acids, genetic material, and proteins, leading to (even irreversible) cell damage and loss of function. To keep ROS levels within a healthy physiological range, the organism depends on a series of enzymes, such as glutathione peroxidase (GSH-Px), with the capacity to protect the cell from oxidative damage (Granot and Kohen, 2004). Research conducted in the last decades suggests a role for oxidative stress in growth and development disturbances in children. For example, broncho-pulmonary diseases, enterocolitis, perinatal brain damage, and neonatal hemochromatosis in newborns, or asthma, cystic fibrosis, diarrhea, and kwashiorkor in older children, have all been associated with oxidative stress (revised by Granot and Kohen, 2004).

Vitamins such as A, E, or C; minerals like zinc or selenium; and certain phytochemical compounds such as polyphenols are known to be natural antioxidants, and as such they have been suggested to have a protective effect against some of the above-mentioned diseases. In fact, it has been reported that deficiencies in antioxidant vitamins and minerals during childhood may contribute to alterations in growth and physical and mental development, as we will discuss below. In addition, recent evidence suggests that other food components with antioxidant properties

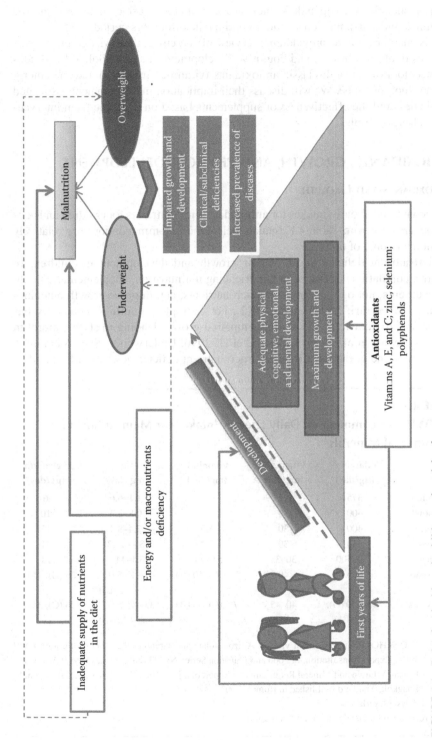

FIGURE 4.1 Role of antioxidants in child growth and development.

(i.e., polyphenols), for which deficiencies have not been described (and are therefore not named nutrients), may contribute to optimal health in this period of life.

This chapter aims to provide an overview of the current knowledge on the role of antioxidants in physical and cognitive development during childhood and adolescence, looking at both classic antioxidants (vitamins, minerals) and the emerging ones (polyphenols). We will discuss their implication in development-associated pathologies, and the effectiveness of supplements based on evidence from intervention studies and trials.

ANTIOXIDANTS, GROWTH, AND PHYSICAL DEVELOPMENT

ANTIOXIDANTS AND GROWTH

The recommended daily intakes for antioxidant micronutrients for children and adolescents are shown in Table 4.1. Intakes below the recommendations are relatively common for some of them.

Micronutrient deficiency can impair growth and development in children. In pediatric populations at risk of or experiencing malnutrition, supplementation with micronutrients, not only energy and macronutrients, can improve growth outcomes (Branca and Ferrari, 2002; Goyle, 2012). For example, vitamin A deficiency has been shown to contribute to stunting (impaired growth leading to short stature) in children (Beaton et al., 1993; Kirkwood et al., 1996; Underwood, 1994). Vitamin A deficiency is one of the most frequent micronutrient deficiencies. According to data

---

TABLE 4.1

FAO/WHO Recommended Daily Dietary Intakes for Main Antioxidant Vitamins and Minerals

Age	Vitamin A (µg/day)	Vitamin C (mg/day)	Vitamin E (mg/day)	Zinc (mg/day)[a]	Selenium (µg/day)
0–6 months	375	25	2.7	1.1–6.6	6
7–12 months	400	30	2.7	0.8–8.3	10
1–3 years	400	30	5.0	2.4–8.4	17
4–5 years	450	30	5.0	3.1–10.3	21
6–9 years	450–500	30–35	5.0–7.0	3.1–11.3	21
10–13 years	600	40	7.5 (G), 10 (B)	4.6–15.5 (G), 5.7–19.2 (B)	26 (G), 34 (B)
14–19 years	500–600 (G), 600 (B)	40–45	7.5 (G), 10 (B)	3.0–15.5 (G), 4.2–19.2 (B)	26 (G), 34 (B)

Source: FAO/WHO. Requirements of vitamin A, iron, folate and vitamin B12, Report of a joint FAO/WHO Expert Consultation. In Food and Nutrition Series No. 23 (ed.), Rome, 1988. FAO/WHO. Human Vitamin and Mineral Requirements. Report of a joint FAO/WHO expert consultation. In Bangkok, Thailand (published in Rome), 2002.

Note: B, boys; G, girls.

[a] Zinc recommendations depend on bioavailability.

from the World Health Organization (WHO) in 2005, its prevalence in regions at risk of hipovitaminosis A was estimated in 33.3% of preschool children, which translates to 190 million children worldwide (WHO, 2009). A prospective study on stunted Sudanese infants and children (6 months to 6 years of age) showed that the intake of vitamin A and carotenoids was associated with the extent of growth recovery with time, especially in the youngest children (Sedgh et al., 2000). Therefore, ensuring adequate levels of vitamin A in children is a goal to achieve.

Studies on vitamin A supplementation, however, suggest that this measure may be useful for stimulating growth only in those children with impaired growth at baseline or experiencing the specific deficiency. A study conducted in Indonesian preschool children showed that vitamin A supplementation (103,000 IU for children <2 years of age and 206,000 IU for older children, once every 4 months) could improve height and weight gain under certain conditions. For example, the effectiveness of the supplementation was influenced by age (more effective in older children) and breast-feeding (before 2 years of age, growth improvement was only observed in non-breast-fed children), but especially by nutritional status, as those children with serum retinol levels >0.35 $\mu mol/l$ showed no significant height or weight gain (Hadi et al., 2000). Another study in older (4–14 years) Brazilian children, on the contrary, found no significant effect of a similar single dose of vitamin A (200,000 IU) in growth during the 6 months after the intervention (Saccardo Sarni et al., 2003). The authors assessed the dietary intake of the participants and found that a considerable percentage of them (>60%) had intakes of retinol and carotenoids far below the recommendations; as they associated this low intake with an overall insufficient consumption of fruit and vegetables, they understandably concluded that such an unbalanced diet would result in multiple micronutrient deficiencies, making a single-nutrient supplement useless (Saccardo Sarni et al., 2003).

Another antioxidant deficiency that has been related to impaired growth is that of zinc, first described in the 1960s (Prasad et al., 1963). In addition, zinc deficiency is associated with delayed puberty, skin conditions, impaired wound healing, altered immune function, and increased susceptibility to infections (Maggini et al., 2010). Interestingly, the availability of zinc in human milk is higher than in cow's milk or infant formulae (Sandström et al., 1983), which indicates another way in which breast-feeding contributes to optimal growth in newborns during the first months of life.

Several studies have shown a benefit for zinc supplementation in improving children's weight and height (Brown et al., 2002; Lind et al., 2004; Umeta et al., 2000), with effects being more significant in those children who were underweight or stunted (Brown et al., 2002; Perrone et al., 1999; Sayeg et al., 2000; Umeta et al., 2000). Interestingly, the work by Lind and colleagues (2004) showed that while supplementation with zinc (10 mg/day) improved growth, and supplementation with iron (10 mg/day) improved cognitive development, the combination of both minerals did not have a significant effect on either outcome compared with placebo (Lind et al., 2004), due perhaps to the interactions between the minerals at the absorptive level (Sandström, 2001). However, in the study by Perrone and colleagues (1999), the combination of zinc and iron (12.5 mg/day + 12 mg/day, respectively) was more effective for improving growth than zinc alone; even more, zinc alone was effective only in those children with higher ferritin levels (i.e., better iron status). The different conclusions arising from Lind's and Perrone's studies might be perhaps explained by two important methodological differences: first, zinc and iron supplements in Perrone's study were provided 12 h apart, which could prevent interactions at the absorptive level, while in Lind's intervention both minerals were given together. Second, Perrone's study specified that all children were stunted, while this characteristic was not specifically stated in Lind's work (Lind et al., 2004; Perrone et al., 1999).

Recently, a new level has been revealed in the relationship between physical development and antioxidant levels according to the HELENA study results, where a significant association between vitamin status and cardiorespiratory and muscular fitness has been shown (Gracia-Marco et al., 2012). According to this study, after controlling for potential confounders, cardiorespiratory fitness in boys was positively associated with retinol and vitamin C serum concentrations, while muscular strength was associated with levels of retinol, carotenoids, and vitamin E. In girls, cardiorespiratory and muscular fitness were both positively correlated with carotenoid levels.

ANTIOXIDANTS IN THE TREATMENT OF DEFICIENCY DISEASES

Kwashiorkor, a typical protein-malnutrition disease, has been associated with low levels of antioxidant vitamins C, A, and E, and lower levels of GSH-Px and its cofactor selenium (Ashour et al., 1999; Fechner et al., 2001). However, despite the consistent findings linking kwashiorkor, oxidative stress, and low antioxidant (both endogenous and dietary) levels, intervention studies have not provided support for antioxidant supplementation in the treatment of the disease. Early work with vitamin E supplementation (10 mg/day) did not find any significant improvement in growth in children with kwashiorkor (Beau and Sy, 1996); later, another trial using multisupplementation (1.8/day mg riboflavin, 23 mg/day vitamin E, 55 µg/day selenium, and 300 mg/day N-acetylcysteine for 20 weeks) again found no significant increases in weight gain or height, or amelioration of disease-related symptoms (edema, diarrhea, or fever) when compared with placebo (Ciliberto et al., 2005). More recently, a systematic review of trials involving supplementation with riboflavin, vitamin E, selenium, and cysteine isolated or in combination demonstrated the lack of a significant difference in the prevalence of kwashiorkor or its associated mortality (Odigwe et al., 2010).

Anemia is another of the most common nutrition-related diseases in children, with prevalence ranging between 20% and 31% in school-aged children and between 46% and 49% in preschool children (WHO 2008, data from 2005). Although the main nutritional deficiency leading to anemia is that of iron, other micronutrients, and antioxidants in particular, like vitamins A, C, and zinc, have been associated with increased risk of anemia (Konomi and Yokoi, 2005 and Sommer et al., 2002 as cited in Chen et al., 2012; Maggini et al., 2010). Vitamin C, for example, contributes to optimal growth by reduction of non-heme iron from ferric to ferrous form, increasing its absorption by the intestinal epithelium (Sandström, 2001; Siegenberg et al., 1991). On the contrary, zinc and some polyphenols may sequester iron and reduce its bioavailability (Sandström, 2001; Siegenberg et al., 1991).

Supplementation with vitamin A has been found to improve markers of iron status and anemia. In China, preschool children (up to 6 years of age) were given supplements of vitamin A alone, vitamin A plus zinc, or vitamin A plus multivitamin/mineral cocktail, which included calcium, vitamin C, and B vitamins, for 6 months (Chen et al., 2012). The multinutrient supplementation proved to be the most effective for improving anemia, whereas the combination of vitamin A and zinc provided the best results in terms of stimulating growth (increased height). Similar results were obtained with another intervention with a multimicronutrient supplement including vitamin A, vitamin B-12, iron, and zinc, conducted in older children (6–11 years) in Haiti (Ianotti et al., 2014). Vitamin A alone can as well improve hemoglobin status; Mwanri and colleagues (2000), working with Tanzanite children, found that vitamin A (5000 IU, 3 days/week for 3 months) increased the beneficial effect of iron supplementation (200 mg ferrous sulfate) when given together. Similarly, both micronutrients alone improved height and weight gain when compared with placebo; however, the combination provided the best results (Mwanri et al., 2000).

ANTIOXIDANTS, ASTHMA, AND ALLERGIES

Particularly interesting is the role that antioxidants can play in the development and/ or treatment of asthma and allergies, two of the most prevalent diseases in childhood, with figures on the rise (Asher et al., 2006; Williams et al., 2008). Vitamins C and E, through their antioxidant and immunomodulatory actions, have been shown to improve lung function and hyperreactivity (Romieu and Trenga, 2001; Rubin et al., 2004). There is even evidence for a relationship between maternal antioxidant intake (vitamin E in particular) during pregnancy and the development of asthma later in childhood (Devereux et al., 2006). A study in Iraqi children showed reduced serum levels of vitamin C and E in those with asthma, when compared with healthy children, and also a negative association between serum antioxidants and the severity of asthma symptoms (Al-Abdulla et al., 2010). However, little information is available, to our knowledge, regarding the effectiveness of the use of dietary antioxidant supplements in the treatment of asthma and allergies in children.

Similarly, studies in the last two decades suggest beneficial actions of polyphenols (especially quercetin and catechins) in alleviating the symptoms of allergic diseases and immune hypersensitivity (revised by Singh et al., 2011). A role for polyphenols in reducing food allergies in children and associated asthma and rhinitis has been proposed; however, most data come from *in vitro* or animal studies, or from interventions in adults, and little is known about the potential or safety of these compounds in children.

ANTIOXIDANTS AND OBESITY

When considering the relationship between antioxidants and growth, the most immediate association arising is that between antioxidant deficits and impaired growth. However, antioxidants can contribute to the healthy growth of children by helping prevent overweight and obesity; in other words, deficiencies in antioxidant micronutrients have been linked to a higher risk of obesity in early ages.

Oxidative stress has been found to play a relevant role in the etiopathogenesis of obesity, which could be mediated by food intake (revised in Puchau et al., 2010).

Some authors have found overweight and obese children and adolescents to present lower serum levels of antioxidant vitamins and minerals, like zinc, selenium (Azab et al., 2014), vitamins C and E (García et al., 2013), carotenoids, and α-tocopherol (Gunanti et al., 2014). Interestingly, higher concentrations of vitamin A (García et al., 2013) and retinol (Gunanti et al., 2014) have been associated with higher adiposity.

Information from intervention studies in relation to the effect of supplementation on obesity in children is still scarce. Some trials that combined dietary treatments for obesity with antioxidant supplementation have reported improvements in markers of oxidative stress (Codoñer-Franch et al., 2010; D'Adamo et al., 2013; Murer et al., 2014) and obesity-related alterations, such as cardiometabolic risk parameters (D'Adamo et al., 2013; Hashemipour et al., 2009) or impaired liver function (Murer et al., 2014). However, none of these studies has reported a significant effect of supplementation on body weight or indices of adiposity, or else some have reported no significant effect on these measurements (Hashemipour et al., 2009). In fact, it is interesting to mention that voices have risen to warn about the potential detrimental effects of excessive or unnecessary vitamin supplementation on the risk of developing obesity in children (Zhou and Zhou, 2014). Some evidence suggest a relationship between vitamin intake (mainly B vitamins) and weight gain, and although this relationship has not been directly established with antioxidant vitamins, and it could well not be the case for them, it should be remembered that the most usual method of micronutrient supplementation is the administration of multivitamin–multimineral complexes. Therefore, further evidence is needed before a clear relationship between antioxidant status and pediatric obesity can be established, and especially before antioxidant supplementation can be considered as a therapeutic tool.

ANTIOXIDANTS, COGNITIVE FUNCTION, BEHAVIOR, AND MENTAL DEVELOPMENT

ANTIOXIDANTS AND BRAIN DEVELOPMENT

The high metabolic activity and demand for nutrients of the brain, combined with the lack of storage structures within it, make this organ highly dependent on dietary provision of energy and essential nutrients for its correct functioning. The first years of life are crucial with regard to brain plasticity and development; in consequence, diet plays a key role in cognitive development, behavior, and mental health in children and adolescents. In fact, quite often the nutritional deficiencies that impair physical growth are also associated with impaired cognitive function (it is the case, e.g., with iron-deficiency anemia; Falkingham et al., 2010).

Antioxidant micronutrients have multiple functions, and can act as coenzymes or prostatic parts of enzymes essential to brain growth and development (Benton, 2001). Zinc, for instance, is important for neurodevelopment, and research has shown that early (pre- or perinatal) deficiency may have permanent adverse effects on cognitive development (Benton, 2010). In addition, low zinc intakes have been associated with behavioral problems in children, such as attention-deficit hyperactivity disorder (ADHD) (DiGirolamo et al., 2010). However, results from intervention studies have not provided sound evidence in favor of zinc supplementation for improving cognitive abilities and/or mental health.

There have been attempts at using antioxidant supplements to improve cognitive and academic performance in children, but with uneven results (reviewed in Benton, 2001), and suggesting a significant effect mainly (or only) on those children who had learning difficulties or were malnourished. For example, in a study where children (9–14 years old) were given orange juice daily for 6 months, IQ was increased only in those with poor initial vitamin C status (Kubula and Katz, 1960, as cited in Benton, 2001). Interventions with multivitamin–multimineral supplements have provided positive results with regard to behavior and intellectual capacities (Benton, 2001, 2010); however, it is difficult to discern to which extent these benefits could be attributed to the antioxidants present in the supplements.

A special role can be attributed to vitamin E, not so much as a therapeutic agent in itself but as adjuvant of fatty acid supplementation for children with neurodevelopmental impairment. A growing body of evidence supports the use of polyunsaturated fatty acids (PUFA) of the ω-3 family in the treatment of disorders with either an inflammatory or a neurological component. Owing to their characteristic chemical structure, these fatty acids are essential for cell membrane formation, especially in the nervous and immune systems; in addition, they are precursors of anti-inflammatory eicosanoids. These properties make ω-3 PUFA important candidates for the treatment of neurodevelopmental disorders (Grassmann et al., 2013; Sinn, 2008). However, that same chemical nature makes them highly susceptible to lipid peroxidation, and that is where vitamin E exerts its protective action, preserving the integrity of the fatty acids. For that reason, combined supplementations of ω-3 PUFA and vitamin E have been proposed to treat neuronal alterations in children (Gumpricht and Rockway, 2013).

ANTIOXIDANTS AND BEHAVIORAL/COGNITIVE ALTERATIONS: ADHD

ADHD is characterized by impulsivity, excess of activity, and limited capacity to keep attention (American Psychiatric Association [APA], 1994). Its prevalence is estimated to be between 2% and 18% of children (Rowland et al., 2002), although these figures may rise with the new diagnostic criteria proposed by the APA in the DSM-V (Ghanizadeh, 2013). Both genetic and nongenetic factors are involved in the pathogenesis of ADHD. Among them, oxidative stress appears again as an important agent (Ross et al., 2003). Therefore, antioxidants are receiving growing interest for their potential to reduce oxidative stress in the brain, which may help in the treatment of ADHD and other neurodevelopmental disorders (Gumpricht and Rockway, 2013; Ng et al., 2008).

Observational studies have found an inverse relationship between zinc status in children and attention, including ADHD (Benton, 2010). Intervention studies also suggest a therapeutic potential for zinc supplementation. For example, 55 mg/day zinc sulfate in combination with the standard drug treatment with methylphenidate for 6 weeks seemed to improve parent- and teacher-reported behavior in children aged 5–11 years (Akhondzadeh et al., 2004), although these authors remained cautious about the need to replicate the study with different zinc doses. In the same year, a large controlled clinical trial was published showing how zinc supplementation

(150 mg/day zinc sulfate during 12 weeks) improved hyperactivity, impulsivity, and socialization, but not lack of attention (Bilici et al., 2004). On the contrary, although a significant negative association has been found between serum zinc levels and symptoms of depression or anxiety, no differences have been observed in those parameters between children receiving the supplement (10 mg ZnO/day for 5 days/week during 6 months) and their controls (DiGirolamo et al., 2010). Ghanizadeh and Berk (2013), in their systematic review of clinical trials, concluded that there is still not enough sound evidence of zinc supplements being useful for ameliorating ADHD in children and adolescents (Ghanizadeh and Berk, 2013).

Research with polyphenol supplements is still in a preliminary stage; however, the maritime pine bark extract known commercially as Pycnogenol®, rich in phenolic acids, catechin, taxifolin, and procyanidins, could be useful for treating the symptoms of ADHD. An intervention with this extract (1 mg/kg body weight/day for 4 weeks) caused a significant reduction of hyperactivity and improved attention, concentration, and visual–motor coordination in children with ADHD (Trebatická et al., 2006); however, further research is clearly needed.

ANTIOXIDANTS IN AUTISM SPECTRUM DISORDERS

Oxidative stress has been proposed to be also involved in the etiopathology of disorders of the autism spectrum, and, consequently, it could be a therapeutic target (Deth and Muratone, 2010; Ghanizadeh et al., 2012). There is evidence of lower levels of glutathione in children with these conditions, when compared with healthy ones (Geier et al., 2009). The antioxidant action of glutathione is important for protecting the brain tissue from oxidative stress and associated neuroinflammation in autism. Supplementation with glutathione in children with autism spectrum disorders has been shown to improve the levels of some of the transsulfuration metabolites (Kern et al., 2011); however, the effects on clinical symptoms still deserve further exploration.

The oxidative stress hypothesis has led to test the efficacy of dietary antioxidants, like zinc, to treat these disorders and/or their symptoms. In this line, recent studies have demonstrated that serum zinc concentrations are reduced in children with autism spectrum disorders (Faber et al., 2009; Yasuda et al., 2011), while other studies do not support such findings (Adams et al., 2011). We still lack results from clinical trials with zinc supplementation in children with autism spectrum disorders.

Similarly, supplementation with polyphenols can represent an option worth exploring in the future. Recently, results have been published from two interventions in which combinations of luteolin, quercetin, and rutin were given to children (ranging from 4 to 14 years) for at least 4 months (Theoharides et al., 2012) or for 6 months (Taliou et al., 2013). After the treatments, significant improvements were reported in communication skills, social interaction, and overall behavior in both studies (Taliou et al., 2013; Theoharides et al., 2012).

Also worth mentioning is the study by Gvozdjáková and co-workers (2014), in which children with autism were treated with the nondietary antioxidant ubiquinol (a reduced form of coenzyme Q10). Twenty-four children, aged 3–6 years, received

100 mg/day ubiquinol for 3 months; after that period, both coenzyme Q10 levels and various symptoms of autism were reported to be improved.

ANTIOXIDANTS IN DOWN SYNDROME

Down syndrome is one of the most frequent congenital conditions, with a prevalence of 1–2 in 1000 births (Weijerman and de Winter, 2010), and associated with learning disabilities and a higher risk of cognitive deterioration and of developing dementia at an earlier age (Thiel and Fowkes, 2005). As with the other diseases here mentioned, comorbidities of Down syndrome, especially cognitive impairment, have been proposed to be caused by oxidative stress. The gene that codifies one of the most relevant enzymes in ROS production, *superoxide dismutase* (SOD), is located in chromosome 21; because of the extra copy of this chromosome present in individuals with Down syndrome, this gene is overexpressed by up to 50%, and in consequence generation of ROS is increased in affected individuals. In addition, IQ has been positively associated with GSH-Px activity in individuals with Down syndrome (reviewed in Ani et al., 2000). This has led to the suggestion that nutritional supplementation could ameliorate oxidative stress in individuals with Down syndrome and improve some of the comorbidities of their condition, although evidence available provides inconclusive results. For example, serum zinc levels have been reported to be lower in Down syndrome, suggesting that supplementation with this mineral could be beneficial; however, clinical trials proving the efficacy of such supplements are lacking (Ani et al., 2000).

As a natural component of GSH-Px, selenium is one of the antioxidant micronutrients proposed for the treatment of Down syndrome. Back in 1990, Antila and co-workers gave selenium supplements (15–25 µg of selenium/kg/day) to individuals with Down syndrome and reported a 25% increase in the activity of GSH-Px and a 24% reduction in the SOD/GSH-Px ratio compared with corresponding controls (Antila et al., 1990). This intervention, however, was conducted on a very small sample (only seven subjects), varying greatly in age (1–54 years) and length of treatment (4–18 months); also, it did not report any measurements of cognitive function, making it difficult to draw conclusions regarding the effectiveness of selenium administration for treating the cognitive comorbidities of Down syndrome.

Almost two decades later, Ellis and coworkers (2008) provided an antioxidant cocktail (10 µg selenium + 5 mg zinc + 0.9 mg vitamin A + 100 mg vitamin E + 50 mg vitamin C daily) to 156 infants (up to 7 months of age) with Down syndrome. At 18 months follow-up, the authors failed to observe any significant effect on SOD activity or any of the cognitive outcomes measured, like locomotor activity or hearing and language development, when compared with placebo. Later on, Lott and colleagues (2011) conducted a similar intervention with adults (aged 40 years or older; 900 IU α-tocopherol, 200 mg ascorbic acid, and 600 mg α-lipoic acid per day), and again observed neither improvement in cognitive function nor a stabilization of cognitive decline compared with the controls (Lott et al., 2011).

Finally, as a summary, Figure 4.2 shows the potential effects of oxidative stress and antioxidants in child growth and development.

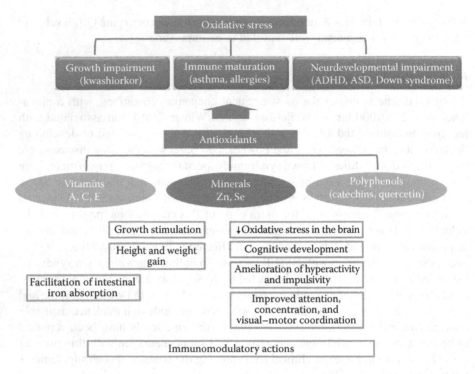

FIGURE 4.2 Potential impact of oxidative stress and antioxidants in child growth and development.

CONCLUSIONS

With the experimental evidence available thus far, there seems to be little doubt regarding the involvement of antioxidants, including dietary, in the physical and mental development of children, and of the role of antioxidant deficiencies in growth impairment and the occurrence of diseases that hinder children's physical and cognitive performance.

Less clear is the efficacy of antioxidant supplements for increasing growth and cognitive function in the early years of life, or for treating disease, except in those cases where specific nutritional deficiencies exist and must therefore be corrected.

It is also important to remark that vitamins, minerals, and polyphenols have pleiotropic roles in the body—in other words, one single compound will exert a wide range of functions other than sequestering ROS; for example, polyphenols have anti-inflammatory properties, and zinc is a cofactor for enzymes involved in gene transcription. It is therefore difficult to discern whether the effects of the antioxidants discussed in this chapter are due to their capacity to protect cells and molecules from oxidation, or to their other functions.

However, some areas of research, like those related to neurodevelopmental disorders in children, are still young but pointing at potentially interesting pathways to follow, like the use of zinc and polyphenol supplements, regardless of the actual mechanism of action involved in their effect.

ACKNOWLEDGMENTS

The authors would like to thank Bayer's contribution to the preparation of this chapter.

REFERENCES

Adams JB, Audhya T, McDonough-Means S, Rubin RA, Quig D, Geis E, Gehn E, Loresto M, Mitchell J, Atwood S, Barnhouse S, Lee W (2011) Nutritional and metabolic status of children with autism vs. neurotypical children, and the association with autism severity. *Nutr Metab (Lond)* 8(1): 34.

Akhondzadeh S, Mohammadi MR, Khademi M (2004) Zinc sulfate as an adjunct to methylphenidate for the treatment of attention deficit hyperactivity disorder in children: A double blind and randomized trial [ISRCTN64132371]. *BMC Psychiatry* 4: 9.

Al-Abdulla NO, Al Naama LM, Hassam MK (2010) Antioxidant status in acute asthmatic attack in children. *J Pak Med Assoc* 60: 1023–1027.

American Psychiatric Association (1994) *Diagnostic and Statistical Manual of Mental Disorders*, Fourth Edition. Washington, DC: American Psychiatric Association, pp. 112–119.

Ani C, Grantham-McGregor S, Muller D (2000) Nutritional supplementation in Down syndrome: Theoretical considerations and current status. *Dev Med Child Neurol* 42: 207–213.

Antila E, Nordberg U, Syväoja E, Westermarck T (1990) Selenium therapy in Down syndrome: A theory and a clinical trial. *Adv Exp Med Biol* 264: 183–186.

Asher MI, Montefort S, Björkstén B, Lai CKW, Strachan DP, Weiland SK, Williams H; the ISAAC Phase Three Study Group (2006) Worldwide time trends in the prevalence of symptoms of asthma, allergic rhinoconjunctivitis, and eczema in childhood: ISAAC phases one and three repeat multicountry cross-sectional surveys. *Lancet* 368(9537): 733–743.

Ashour MN, Salem SI, El-Gadban HM, Elwan NM, Basu TK (1999) Antioxidant status in children with protein–energy malnutrition (PEM) living in Cairo, Egypt. *Eur J Clin Nutr* 53(8): 669–673.

Azab SF, Saleh SH, Elsaeed WF, Elshafie MA, Sherief LM, Esh AM (2014) Serum trace elements in obese Egyptian children: A case–control study. *Ital J Pediatr* 40: 20.

Beaton GH, Martorell R, Aronson KJ, Edmonston B, McCabe G, Ross AC, Harvey B (1993) Effectiveness of vitamin A supplementation in the control of young child morbidity and mortality in developing countries. Nutrition policy discussion paper no. 13. Geneva, Switzerland: United Nations.

Beau JP, Sy A (1996) Vitamin E supplementation in Senegalese children with kwashiorkor. *Sante* 6: 209–212.

Benton D (2001) Micronutrient supplementation and the intelligence of children. *Neurosci Biobehav Rev* 25: 297–309.

Benton D (2010) The influence of dietary status on the cognitive performance of children. *Mol Nutr Food Res* 54: 457–470.

Bilici M, Yildirim F, Kandil S, Bekaroglu M, Yildirmis S, Yildirmiş S, Değer O, Ulgen M, Yildiran A, Aksu H (2004) Double-blind, placebo-controlled study of zinc sulfate in the treatment of attention deficit hyperactivity disorder. *Prog Neuropsychopharmacol Biol Psychiatry* 28: 181–190.

Branca F, Ferrari M (2002) Impact of micronutrient deficiencies on growth: The stunting syndrome. *Ann Nutr Metab* 46: 8–17.

Brown KH, Peerson JM, Rivera J, Allen LH (2002) Effect of supplemental zinc on the growth and serum zinc concentrations of prepubertal children: A meta-analysis of randomized controlled trials. *Am J Clin Nutr* 75: 1062–1071.

Chen L, Liu YF, Gong M, Jiang W, Fan Z, Qu P, Chen J, Liu YX, Li TY (2012) Effects of vitamin A, vitamin A plus zinc, and multiple micronutrients on anemia in preschool children in Chongqing, China. *Asia Pac J Clin Nutr* 21(1): 3–11.

Ciliberto H, Ciliberto M, Briend A, Ashorn P, Bier D, Manary M (2005) Antioxidant supplementation for the prevention of kwashiorkor in Malawian children: Randomised, double blind, placebo controlled Trial. *BMJ* 330(7500): 1109.

Codoñer-Franch P, López-Jaén AB, De La Mano-Hernández A, Sentandreu E, Simó-Jordá R, Valls-Bellés V (2010) Oxidative markers in children with severe obesity following low-calorie diets supplemented with mandarin juice. *Acta Paediatr* 99(12): 1841–1846.

D'Adamo E, Marcovecchio ML, Giannini C, de Giorgis T, Chiavaroli V, Chiarelli F, Mohn A (2013) Improved oxidative stress and cardio-metabolic status in obese prepubertal children with liver steatosis treated with lifestyle combined with vitamin E. *Free Radic Res* 47(3): 146–153.

Deth RC, Muratone CR (2010) The redox/methylation hypothesis of autism: A molecular mechanism for heavy metal-induced neurotoxicity. In: Chauhan A, Chauhan V, Brown WT, Eds. *Autism Oxidative Stress, Inflammation and Immune Abnormalities*. Boca Raton, FL: CRC Press.

Devereux G, Turner SW, Craig LCA, McNeill G, Martindale S, Harbour PJ, Helms PJ, Seaton A (2006) Low maternal vitamin E intake during pregnancy is associated with asthma in 5-year-old children. *Am J Respir Crit Care Med* 174: 499–507.

DiGirolamo AM, Ramirez-Zea M, Wang M, Flores-Ayala R, Martorell R, Neufeld LM, Ramakrishnan U, Sellen D, Black MM, Stein AD (2010) Randomized trial of the effect of zinc supplementation on the mental health of school-age children in Guatemala. *Am J Clin Nutr* 92(5): 1241–1250.

Ellis JM, Tan HK, Gilbert RE, Muller DP, Henley W, Moy R, Pumphrey R, Ani C, Davies S, Edwards V, Green H, Salt A, Logan S (2008) Supplementation with antioxidants and folinic acid for children with Down's syndrome: Randomised controlled trial. *BMJ* 336(7644): 594–597.

Faber S, Zinn GM, Kern JC II, Kingston HM (2009) The plasma zinc/serum copper ratio as a biomarker in children with autism spectrum disorders. *Biomarkers* 14: 171–180.

Falkingham M, Abdelhamid A, Curtis P, Fairweather-Tait S, Dye L, Hooper L (2010) The effects of oral iron supplementation on cognition in older children and adults: A systematic review and meta-analysis. *Nutr J* 9: 4.

Fechner A, Böhme C, Gromer S, Funk M, Schirmer R, Becker K (2001) Antioxidant status and nitric oxide in the malnutrition syndrome kwashiorkor. *Pediatr Res* 49(2): 237–243.

García OP, Ronquillo D, del Carmen Caamaño M, Martínez G, Camacho M, López V, Rosado JL (2013) Zinc, iron and vitamins A, C and E are associated with obesity, inflammation, lipid profile and insulin resistance in Mexican school-aged children. *Nutrients* 5(12): 5012–5030.

Geier DA, Kern JK, Garver CR, Adams JB, Audhya T, Geier MR (2009) A prospective study of transsulfuration biomarkers in autistic disorders. *Neurochem Res* 34: 386–393.

Ghanizadeh A (2013) Agreement between Diagnostic and Statistical Manual of Mental Disorders, Fourth Edition, and the proposed DSM-V attention deficit hyperactivity disorder diagnostic criteria: An exploratory study. *Compr Psychiatry* 54(1): 7–10.

Ghanizadeh A, Berk M (2013) Zinc for treating of children and adolescents with attention-deficit hyperactivity disorder: A systematic review of randomized controlled clinical trials. *Eur J Clin Nutr* 67: 122–124.

Ghanizadeh A, Akhondzadeh S, Hormozi M, Makarem A, Abotorabi-Zarchi M, Firoozabadi A (2012) Glutathione-related factors and oxidative stress in autism, a review. *Curr Med Chem* 19(23): 4000–4005.

Goyle A (2012) Effect of micronutrient fortified biscuit supplementation on the weight, height, and BMI of adolescent girls. *Coll Antropol* 36: 573–579.

Gracia-Marco L, Valtueña J, Ortega FB, Pérez-López FR, Vicente-Rodríguez G, Breidenassel C, Ferrari M, Molnar D, Widhalm K, de Henauw S, Kafatos A, Diaz LE, Gottrand F, Maiani G, Stehle P, Castillo MJ, Moreno LA, González-Gross M, HELENA Study Group (2012) Iron and vitamin status biomarkers and its association with physical fitness in adolescents: The HELENA study. *J Appl Physiol* 113: 566–573.

Granot E, Kohen R (2004) Oxidative stress in childhood—In health and disease states. *Clin Nutr* 23: 3–11.

Grassmann V, Santos-Galduróz RF, Galduróz JC (2013) Effects of low doses of polyunsaturated fatty acids on the attention deficit/hyperactivity disorder of children: A systematic review. *Curr Neuropharmacol* 11(2): 186–196.

Gumpricht E, Rockway S (2013) Can ω-3 fatty acids and tocotrienol-rich vitamin E reduce symptoms of neurodevelopmental disorders? *Nutrition* 30(7–8): 733–738.

Gunanti IR, Marks GC, Al-Mamun A, Long KZ (2014) Low serum concentrations of carotenoids and vitamin E are associated with high adiposity in Mexican-American children. *J Nutr* 144(4): 489–495.

Gvozdjáková A, Kucharská J, Ostatníková D, Babinská K, Nakládal D, Crane FL (2014) Ubiquinol improves symptoms in children with autism. *Oxid Med Cell Longev* 2014: 798957.

Hadi H, Stoltzfus RJ, Dibley MJ, Moulton LH, West KP Jr, Kjolhede CL, Sadjimin T (2000) Vitamin A supplementation selectively improves the linear growth of Indonesian preschool children: Results from a randomized controlled trial. *Am J Clin Nutr* 71(2): 507–513.

Hashemipour M, Kelishadi R, Shapouri J, Sarrafzadegan N, Amini M, Tavakoli N, Movahedian-Attar A, Mirmoghtadaee P, Poursafa P (2009) Effect of zinc supplementation on insulin resistance and components of the metabolic syndrome in prepubertal obese children. *Hormones (Athens)* 8(4): 279–285.

Ianotti LL, Dulience SJL, Green J, Joseph S, François J, Anténor ML, Lesorogol C, Mounce J, Nickerson NM (2014) Linear growth increased in young children in an urban slum of Haiti: A randomized controlled trial of a lipid-based nutrient supplement. *Am J Clin Nutr* 99: 198–208.

Kern JK, Geier DA, Adams JB, Garver CR, Audhya T, Geier MR (2011) A clinical trial of glutathione supplementation in autism spectrum disorders. *Med Sci Monit* 17(12): CR677–CR682.

Kirkwood BR, Ross DA, Arthur P, Morris SS, Dollimore N, Binka FN, Shier RP, Gyapong JO, Addy HA, Smith PG (1996) Effect of vitamin A supplementation on the growth of young children in northern Ghana. *Am J Clin Nutr* 63(5): 773–781.

Lind T, Lönnerdal B, Stenlund H, Gamayanti IL, Ismail D, Seswandhana R, Persson LA (2004) A community-based randomized controlled trial of iron and zinc supplementation in Indonesian infants: Effects on growth and development. *Am J Clin Nutr* 80: 729–736.

Lott IT, Doran E, Nguyen VQ, Tournay A, Head E, Gillen DL (2011) Down syndrome and dementia: A randomized, controlled trial of antioxidant supplementation. *Am J Med Genet* 155A: 1939–1948.

Maggini S, Wenzlaff S, Hornig D (2010) Essential role of vitamin C and zinc in child immunity and health. *J Intern Med Res* 38: 386–414.

Murer SB, Aeberli I, Braegger CP, Gittermann M, Hersberger M, Leonard SW, Taylor AW, Traber MG, Zimmermann MB (2014) Antioxidant supplements reduced oxidative stress and stabilized liver function tests but did not reduce inflammation in a randomized controlled trial in obese children and adolescents. *J Nutr* 144(2): 193–201.

Mwanri L, Worsley A, Ryan P, Masika J (2000) Supplemental vitamin A improves anemia and growth in anemic school children in Tanzania. *J Nutr* 130(11): 2691–2696.

Ng F, Berk M, Dean O, Bush A (2008) Oxidative stress in psychiatric disorders: Evidence base and therapeutic implications. *Int J Neuropsychopharmacol* 21: 1–26.

Odigwe CC, Smedslund G, Ejemot-Nwadiaro RI, Anyanechi CC, Krawinkel MB (2010) Supplementary vitamin E, selenium, cysteine and riboflavin for preventing kwashiorkor in preschool children in developing countries. *Cochrane Database Syst Rev* (4): CD008147.

Perrone L, Salerno M, Gialanella G, Feng SL, Moro R, Di Lascio R, Boccia E, Di Toro R (1999) Long-term zinc and iron supplementation in children of short stature: Effect of growth and on trace element content in tissues. *J Trace Elem Med Biol* 13(1–2): 51–56.

Prasad AS, Miale A, Farid Z, Sandstead HH, Schulert AR (1963) Zinc metabolism in patients with the syndrome of iron deficiency anemia, hepatosplenomegaly, dwarfism, and hypogonadism. *J Lab Clin Med* 61: 537–549.

Puchau B, Ochoa MC, Zulet MA, Marti A, Martínez JA, Members G (2010) Dietary total antioxidant capacity and obesity in children and adolescents. *Int J Food Sci Nutr* 61(7): 713–721.

Romieu I, Trenga C (2001) Diet and obstructive lung disease. *Epidemiol Rev* 23: 268–287.

Ross BM, McKenzie I, Glen I, Bennett CP (2003) Increased levels of ethane, a non-invasive marker of ω-3 fatty acid oxidation, in breath of children with attention deficit hyperactivity disorder. *Nutr Neurosci* 6: 277–281.

Rowland AS, Lesesne CA, Abramowitz AJ (2002) The epidemiology of attention-deficit/hyperactivity disorder: A public health view. *Ment Retard Dev Disabil Res Rev* 8: 162–170.

Rubin RN, Navon L, Cassano PA (2004) Relationship of serum antioxidants to asthma prevalence in youth. *Am J Respir Crit Care Med* 169: 393–398.

Saccardo Sarni R, Kochi C, Ramalho RA, Oliveira Schoeps D, Sato K, Mattoso L, Ximenes Pessotti CF, Suano Souza FI, Damiani FM, Catherino P (2003) Impact of vitamin A megadose supplementation on the anthropometry of children and adolescents with non-hormonal statural deficit: A double-blind and randomized clinical study. *Int J Vitam Nutr Res* 73(4): 303–311.

Sandström B (2001) Micronutrient interactions: Effects on absorption and bioavailability. *Br J Nutr* 85(Suppl 2): S181–S185.

Sandström B, Cederblad A, Lönnerdal B (1983) Zinc absorption from human milk, cow's milk, and infant formulas. *Am J Dis Child* 137: 726–729.

Sayeg Porto MA, Oliveira HP, Cunha AJ, Miranda G, Guimarães MM, Oliveira WA, dos Santos DM. (2000) Linear growth and zinc supplementation in children with short stature. *J Pediatr Endocrinol Metab* 13: 1121–1128.

Sedgh G, Herrera MG, Nestel P, el Amin A, Fawzy WW (2000) Dietary vitamin A intake and nondietary factors are associated with reversal of stunting in children. *J Nutr* 130: 2520–2526.

Siegenberg D, Baynes RD, Bothwell TH, Macfarlane BJ, Lamparelli RD, Car NG, MacPhail P, Schmidt U, Tal A, Mayet F (1991) Ascorbic acid prevents the dose-dependent inhibitory effects of polyphenols and phytates on non heme–iron absorption. *Am J Clin Nutr* 53: 537–541.

Singh A, Holvoet S, Mercenier A (2011) Dietary polyphenols in the prevention and treatment of allergic diseases. *Clin Exp Allergy* 41: 1346–1359.

Singh M (2004) Role of micronutrients for physical growth and mental development. *Indian J Pediatr* 71(1): 59–62.

Sinn N (2008) Nutritional and dietary influences on attention deficit hyperactivity disorder. *Nutr Rev* 66(10): 558–658.

Taliou A, Zintzaras E, Lykouras L, Francis K (2013) An open-label pilot study of a formulation containing the anti-inflammatory flavonoid luteolin and its effects on behavior in children with autism spectrum disorders. *Clin Ther* 35(5): 592–560.

Theoharides TC, Asadi S, Panagiotidou S (2012) A case series of a luteolin formulation (NeuroProtek®) in children with autism spectrum disorders. *Int J Immunopathol Pharmacol* 25(2): 317–323.

Thiel RJ, Fowkes SW (2005) Can cognitive deterioration associated with Down syndrome be reduced? *Med Hypotheses* 64(3): 524–532.

Thurlow RA, Winichagoon P, Pongcharoen T, Gowachirapant S, Boonpraderm A, Manger MS, Bailey KB, Wasantwisut E, Gibson RS (2006) Risk of zinc, iodine and other micronutrient deficiencies among school children in North East Thailand. *Eur J Clin Nutr* 60(5): 623–632.

Trebatická J, Kopasová S, Hradecná Z, Cinovský K, Skodácek I, Suba J, Muchová J, Zitnanová I, Waczulíková I, Rohdewald P, Duracková Z (2006) Treatment of ADHD with French maritime pine bark extract, Pycnogenol. *Eur Child Adolesc Psychiatry* 15(6): 329–335.

Umeta M, West CE, Haidar J, Deurenberg P, Hautvast JG (2000) Zinc supplementation and stunted infants in Ethiopia: A randomized controlled trial. *Lancet* 335: 2021–2026.

Underwood BA (1994) The role of vitamin A in child growth, development and survival. *Adv Exp Med Biol* 352: 201–208.

UNICEF (2006) Progress for children: A report card on nutrition, number 4. New York: UNICEF, May. Available at http://www.unicef.org/progressforchildren/2006n4/files /PFC4_EN_8X11.pdf.

Weijerman ME, de Winter JP (2010) Clinical practice. The care of children with Down syndrome. *Eur J Pediatr* 169(12): 1445–1452.

WHO (2008) Worldwide prevalence of anaemia 1993–2005: WHO global database on anaemia. In: De Benoist B, McLean E, Egli I, Cogswell M, Eds. Geneva: World Health Organization, pp. 1–40. Available at http://whqlibdoc.who.int/publications/2008/97892 41596657_eng.pdf?ua=1.

WHO (2009) Global prevalence of vitamin A deficiency in populations at risk 1995–2005. WHO global database on vitamin A deficiency. Geneva, Switzerland: World Health Organization. Available at http://whqlibdoc.who.int/publications/2009/9789241598019 _eng.pdf?ua=1.

Williams H, Stewart A, von Mutius E, Cookson W, Anderson HR; International Study of Asthma and Allergies in Childhood (ISAAC) Phase One and Three Study Groups (2008) Is eczema really on the increase worldwide? *J Allergy Clin Immunol* 121(4): 947–954.

Yasuda H, Yoshida K, Yasuda Y, Tsutsui T (2011) Infantile zinc deficiency: Association with autism spectrum disorders. *Sci Rep* 1: 129.

Zhou SS, Zhou Y (2014) Excess vitamin intake: An unrecognized risk factor for obesity. *World J Diabetes* 5(1): 1–13.

5 Adulthood and Old Age

Antonios E. Koutelidakis and Maria Kapsokefalou

CONTENTS

Dietary Antioxidants in Adulthood 71
    Adult Needs and Importance of Dietary Antioxidants 71
    Bioavailability of Natural Antioxidants and Its Effect on Antioxidant
    Biomarkers in Adults... 73
    Dietary Antioxidants and Disease Prevention in Adulthood 75
    Antioxidant Supplements and Adult Health.. 75
Dietary Antioxidants in the Elderly 76
    Special Needs of the Elderly and Importance of Dietary Antioxidants 76
    Dietary Antioxidant Consumption and Disease Prevention in the Elderly 77
References.. 79

DIETARY ANTIOXIDANTS IN ADULTHOOD

ADULT NEEDS AND IMPORTANCE OF DIETARY ANTIOXIDANTS

Adulthood is the longest period of human life. Scientific evidence supports that diet in this life period is correlated with possible progression of degenerative diseases in older age (Zampelas, 2003). Higher intake of antioxidant-rich foods is clearly associated with health improvement and longevity in adulthood. The specific mechanisms are under investigation; however, several studies have shown that a diet rich in plant-based, antioxidant-rich foods, herbs, and beverages may promote health and could decrease the risk of various age-related diseases (Benzie & Choi, 2014). Nevertheless, a major parameter that determines the final effect of natural antioxidants on the human body is their bioavailability. Antioxidant bioavailability, and consequently their bioactivity, is affected by multiple interactions in the lumen during digestion and may release a variety of metabolites with different pharmacokinetic actions (Kapsokefalou et al., 2006; Karabela et al., 2011; Koutelidakis et al., 2013).

Antioxidants are molecules that can interact with free radicals and terminate the chain reaction procedure before it destroys the vital molecules (Jacob, 1995). The ability of antioxidants to eliminate free radicals from the body and thus reduce the destruction of cellular organelles, such as lipids and DNA, may be the most important protective mechanism that prevents the pathophysiological processes of several diseases (Osawa et al., 1999; Saffari & Sadrzadeh, 2004; Sies et al., 2005). Although the human body has an enzymatic system (superoxide dismutase, catalase, glutathione peroxidase, etc.) with antioxidant scavenging/defense properties, the primary antioxidant defense of the body is dependent on dietary micronutrients such as vitamin E, vitamin C, β-carotene, and lycopene (Wootton-Beard & Ryan, 2011). In recent years, several studies have demonstrated the important role of the antioxidant selenium and the role of various phytochemicals such as polyphenols, and specifically flavonoids (Morton et al., 2000; Cabrera et al., 2006; Benfeito et al., 2013).

Ascorbic acid is a major plasma antioxidant factor that is needed for collagen synthesis. Humans must obtain an adequate intake of vitamin C to maintain its plasma and tissue levels. Current dietary recommendations suggest an ascorbic acid intake of at least 70 mg/day for women and 100 mg/day for men, with higher levels advised in pregnant women and in smokers, because of increased oxidative stress (Yoshihara et al., 2010; Doll & Ricou, 2013; Benzie & Choi, 2014). The typical concentration of ascorbic acid in fasting plasma is 10–60 μM, and its best food sources are fruits, particularly citrus, kiwi fruit, and strawberries (Benzie & Choi, 2014). The National Health and Nutrition Examination Surveys (NHANES) have shown that low serum levels of vitamin C is associated with an increased risk for all-cause mortality (Simon & Hudes, 1999). In contrast, the Nurses' Health Study did not find evidence for a protective effect of vitamin C against cardiovascular disease (Osganian et al., 2003).

Vitamin E is a fat-soluble antioxidant and has been proposed as the most important inhibitor of lipid peroxidation. Vitamin E prevents platelet activation and adhesion, and is the basic antioxidant factor of low-density lipoprotein (LDL). The recommended daily allowance (RDA) for men and for women is 15 mg/day α-tocopherol (Masella et al., 2004; Yoshihara et al., 2010). The typical concentration of α-tocopherol in fasting plasma is 16–40 μM (Benzie & Choi, 2014). Vitamin E consumption is difficult to assess as it depends on the processing and storage methods; however, the best food sources of tocopherols are plant oils, wheat germ, sunflower seeds, and nuts (Benfeito et al., 2012; Benzie & Choi, 2014). The Nurses' Health Study showed that supplemental vitamin E use for >2 years resulted in lower predicted cardiovascular disease risk; however, this beneficial effect was lost at lower doses and for shorter periods of use (Stampfer et al., 1993).

Carotenoids, such as lutein, zeaxanthin, and β-carotene, are lipophilic antioxidant compounds that are present in various plant and animal food sources. Their typical concentration in plasma ranges from 0.160 to 0.354 μM (Benzie & Choi, 2014), and they are linked to known mechanisms of action, such as protection from lipid peroxidation, immune function, DNA damage protection, and gene regulation. The recommended daily intakes for vitamin A are 900 μg retinoic acid (RA) and 700 μg retinol activity equivalents (RAE) for adult men and women, respectively (Pokorny et al., 2001). Another important dietary antioxidant is selenium, a nutrient associated with protein foods. The role of selenium is the defense against oxidation procedure and the regulation of thyroid hormone. The recommendation (RDA) for adults is 55 μg selenium per day, and the best food sources include seafood, meat, whole grains, and vegetables (depending on soil content) (Pokorny et al., 2001).

Recently, experimental data suggest the important role of polyphenols and especially of flavonoids on cell protection against oxidative stress (Benfeito et al., 2012). They can prevent or minimize oxidative damage processes by scavenging free radical species and enhancing the endogenous antioxidant system by stimulating the synthesis of endogenous antioxidants (Pokorny et al., 2001; Yoshihara et al., 2010; Benfeito et al., 2013). The typical concentration of anthocyanins in fasting plasma is 0.046 μM and that of quercetin is 0.001 μM (Benzie & Choi, 2014). It is also considered to confer further protective function owing to the synergistic action of different antioxidant components, such as flavonoids, into the food matrix (Koutelidakis et al., 2013). Nevertheless, there are no recommendations for daily flavonoid consumption because of the complex and multifactorial process of its absorption and because its metabolism differs among individuals. Furthermore, the European Food Safety Authority (EFSA) does not yet verify the nutritional or health claims for flavonoids and foods rich in antioxidants, such as herbal infusions (EFSA Panel on Dietetic Products, 2011).

BIOAVAILABILITY OF NATURAL ANTIOXIDANTS AND ITS EFFECT ON ANTIOXIDANT BIOMARKERS IN ADULTS

The antioxidant effect of several foods or beverages has been linked to the absorption and metabolism of its bioactive constituents; that is, a prerequisite for bioactivity is bioaccessibility and bioavailability. This means that food components must be absorbed into the enterocyte, and moved and distributed to the organ tissues. Absorption, metabolism, pharmacokinetics, tissue distribution, and rate of excretion in urine or feces reflect the bioavailability of the components and thus the biological role of food into the organism (Duthie et al., 2000; Scalbert et al., 2002; Manach et al., 2005; Koutelidakis & Kapsokefalou, 2012).

The holistic range of the possible health benefits of antioxidant-rich diets suggests their effect on various biomarkers in the human body (Koutelidakis et al., 2009; Koutelidakis & Kapsokefalou, 2012). The total antioxidant capacity of plasma, oxidized LDL, malondialdehyde, and oxidized DNA are some examples of biomarkers that indirectly indicate the synergistic effect of the antioxidant compounds on humans. Table 5.1 presents the effect of the consumption of several beverages, such as tea, cacao, or wine, on specific antioxidant biomarkers (Duffy et al., 2001; Erba et al., 2005; Hodgson et al., 2005; Widlansky et al., 2005).

Although many studies had indicated an increase of total antioxidant capacity or decrease of oxidized products after consumption of foods rich in antioxidants (Duffy et al., 2001; Erba et al., 2005), other studies suggest that natural antioxidants such as flavonoids are purely absorbed and have an extended metabolism in the body; thus, their contribution to serum total antioxidant activity and their final effect on organ tissues are controversial (Lotito & Frei, 2006). For example, the plasma concentration of all polyphenols, including catechins, quercetin, and anthocyanins, is only 1 mM, even with a diet that provides up to 1 g/day of polyphenols from fruits and vegetables (Manach et al., 2005). The plasma concentrations of ascorbic acid and α-tocopherol are 80 and 40 mM, respectively, while their daily consumption are 200 and 10 mg in healthy adults, respectively (Benzie & Choi, 2014).

According to the "EFSA Panel on Dietetic Products, Nutrition, and Allergies," it is not established that changes in the overall antioxidant capacity of plasma exert a beneficial physiological effect on humans, as required by Regulation (EC) No. 1924/2006. Furthermore, the induction of antioxidant enzymes, such as catalase or hyperoxide dismutase, cannot be used alone as evidence for claims related to the "antioxidant defense system" for nonessential food constituents. The EFSA panel

TABLE 5.1

Effect of Consumption of Various Foods on Plasma or Urine Antioxidant Biomarkers in Adults

Antioxidant Biomarkers in Plasma or Urine	Subjects	Study Design	Food Used	Study Duration	Results–Effect	References
MDA–LDL, vitamin C, total catechins, urinary 8-PGFa	Healthy	Water control–crossover	Green tea (*Camellia sinensis*)	2 weeks	No effect	Hirano-Ohmori et al., 2005
TAC, plasma flavonoids (HPLC), vitamin C	CAD	Water control–crossover	Green tea (*Camellia sinensis*)	4 weeks	Positive effect (flavonoids)	Duffy et al., 2001
α-Tocopherol, β-carotene, vitamin C	Healthy, smokers	Dosage effects	Black, green tea (*Camellia sinensis*)	4 weeks	Positive effect	de Maat et al., 2000
F2-isoprostanes (in plasma and urine)	Healthy, risk factors for CAD	Water control–crossover	Black, green tea (*Camellia sinensis*)	7 days	No effect	Hodgson et al., 2001
Plasma glutathione, DNA oxid., peroxides, TAC	Healthy	Controlled diet	Green tea (*Camellia sinensis*)	42 days	Positive	Erba et al., 2005
Cu oxid. LDL, TBARS, TAC, plasma phenolics	Healthy	Randomized–controlled	Red wine	2 weeks	Positive effect	Tsang et al., 2005
MDA, isoprostanes, DNA damage	Healthy	Randomized–controlled	Fruit juice	4 weeks	Positive effect	Weisel et al., 2006
Plasma total catechins, TAC	CAD	2 h after consumption	Black tea (*Camellia sinensis*)	Acute	No effect	Widlansky et al., 2004
Plasma F2-isoprostanes, MDA	Healthy	2, 4, and 6 h after consumption	Cocoa (*Theobroma cacao*)	Acute	Positive effect	Wiswedel et al., 2004

Note: CAD, cardiovascular disease; HPLC, high-performance liquid chromatography; LDL, low-density lipoprotein; MDA, malondialdehyde; TAC, total antioxidant capacity; TBARS, thiobarbituric acid reactive substances.

concludes that "for biomarkers relative to antioxidant capacity, changes in antioxidant status, oxidative damage to proteins, lipids and DNA, nonoxidative DNA damage and neoplastic degeneration of cells no definition has been provided of 'premature aging' or of 'healthy aging' in relation to the antioxidant properties of foods, and therefore the claimed effect is considered to be general and nonspecific, and thus does not comply with the criteria laid down in Regulation (EC) No. 1924/2006" (EFSA Panel on Dietetic Products, 2011).

DIETARY ANTIOXIDANTS AND DISEASE PREVENTION IN ADULTHOOD

Recent research data suggest that the beneficial biological role of natural antioxidants is focused not only on their antioxidant scavenging activity but also on their involvement in multiple metabolic signaling pathways at the cellular level. For example, flavonoids may influence the expression of genes encoding the overproduction or underproduction of substances associated with the pathophysiology of cancer and cardiovascular diseases. For example, tea catechins are possibly involved in the transcription of regulatory factors that determine the form of protein synthesized in cells of various tissues (Morton et al., 2000; Bauer et al., 2004; Ho et al., 2009).

Regarding atherosclerosis pathophysiology, several antioxidants have been shown to possibly alter metabolic pathways associated with endothelial function, inflammatory process, platelet aggregation, and hemostasis (Hodgson et al., 2005; Kaliora et al., 2005). In some cases, antioxidants such as catechins modify the expression of cyclooxygenase through suppressing factor AP-1; increasing the expression of an endogenous antioxidant of LDL, paraoxonase 1 (PON 1); deregulating the gene expression of inflammatory factors such as vascular endothelial growth factor, interferon-γ, and interleukin (IL)-4; and modulating the transcription factor nuclear factor (NF)-κB in endothelial cells and macrophages (Jochman et al., 2008).

Regarding cancer, antioxidants may affect genes associated with tumorigenesis. They may affect the cell cycle and act on the process of apoptosis. For example, flavonoids have been found to promote apoptosis in cancer cells via deregulation of the gene *p53*, which regulates the cell cycle phases. Flavonoids seem to inhibit the transcription of AP-1, preventing the transformation of DNA and affecting c-jun and c-foc expression. Thus, by promoting the expression of proteins associated with the c-jun-form heterodimers, they may decrease the activation of genes that cause cancer. Although for cardiovascular disease, research data show a direct effect of antioxidants and particular flavonoids in the pathophysiology of the disease, the data for the effect on cancer prevention are controversial, and further research is needed (Ahmad & Mukhtar, 1999).

ANTIOXIDANT SUPPLEMENTS AND ADULT HEALTH

Although the consumption of a diet rich in antioxidants is correlated with specific health benefits, there is no clear evidence supporting the claim that the intake of supplementary individual antioxidants exerts significant bioactivity (Benzie & Choi, 2014). This may be explained by the holistic antioxidant effect of a whole food or diet, which is the result of the synergistic action of specific antioxidants (Koutelidakis & Kapsokefalou, 2012).

TABLE 5.2

Recommended Dietary Allowance, Tolerable Upper Intake Level, Experimental Doses, and Regimen Used in Antioxidant Supplements

Antioxidant Supplements	RDA Men	RDA Women	TUIL	Experimental Doses	Median Doses	Regimen
β-Carotene	ND		ND	1.2–50 mg	15.5 mg	Daily or on alternate days
Vitamin A	900 µg	700 µg	3000 µg	400–7500 µg	1650 µg	Daily
Vitamin C	90 mg	70 mg	2000 mg	60–2000 mg	450 mg	Daily
Vitamin E	15 mg	15 mg	1000 mg	10–5000 mg	400 mg	Daily or on alternate days
Selenium	55 µg	55 µg	400 µg	20–200 µg	87.5 µg	Daily

Source: Bjelakovic, G., Nikolova, D., Gluud, L. L., Simonetti, R.G., and Gluud, C., *Cochrane Datab Syst Rev* 2, 2008.

Note: RDA, recommended dietary allowance; TUIL, tolerable upper intake level.

In a meta-analysis of the effect of antioxidant supplements for the prevention of mortality in healthy participants and patients with various diseases, Bjelakovic and coworkers showed that antioxidant supplements had no significant effect on mortality in a random-effects meta-analysis (RR, 1.02; 95% CI, 0.99–1.06), but significantly increased mortality in a fixed-effect model (RR, 1.04; 95% CI, 1.02–1.06). In trials with a low risk of bias, the antioxidant supplements significantly increased mortality (RR, 1.05; 95% CI, 1.02–1.08). When the different antioxidants were assessed separately, analyses found increased mortality with vitamin A, β-carotene, and vitamin E, but no significant detrimental effect of vitamin C (Bjelakovic et al., 2008). In another study, Kris-Etherton and coworkers (2004) suggested that the existing scientific databases do not justify the routine use of antioxidant supplements for the prevention and treatment of cardiovascular disease. Furthermore, *in vivo* studies have shown that the administration of vitamin E raised the plasma lipid peroxidation product levels in smokers on a high-fat diet and increased the fat content of livers in rats fed a high-fat diet plus ethanol (Yoshihara et al., 2010) (Table 5.2).

DIETARY ANTIOXIDANTS IN THE ELDERLY

SPECIAL NEEDS OF THE ELDERLY AND IMPORTANCE OF DIETARY ANTIOXIDANTS

Old people tend to be neglected by both their families and the health-care system, and they sometimes live in isolation in their final stage of life. They are usually unable to shop and cook properly, and only a small fraction of them consume the recommended levels of energy, essential trace elements, or vitamins A and D. Consumption of vegetables is usually low, and few of them manage to achieve the recommended five portions a day (Heinrich & Prieto, 2008). "Although health status has multiple contributing factors, nutrition is one of the major determinants of successful aging.

Many older adults have at least one or more chronic health condition. Disparities in health are believed to be the result of complex interaction among genetic variations, environmental factors, and cultural and health behaviors. Inequities in access to health care, income, and poverty, as well as food security also contribute to health disparities among older adults" (Bernstein & Munoz, 2012).

Nowadays there is a trend to increase the lifespan, and research is generally focused on dietary traditions or interventions that allow healthy aging. The antioxidant content of diet may play a pivotal role in the aging procedure and directly affect the appearance of neurodegenerative diseases (Heinrich & Prieto, 2008). The elderly life stage involves important physiological changes, including increased oxidative stress in tissues; thus, the antioxidant content of diets may decrease the impact of several pathophysiological processes (Zampelas, 2003; El Assar et al., 2013).

Vitamin A absorption is increased in the elderly; thus, the recommendations of 800 mg and 1000 mg for women and men, respectively, adequately cover the needs of old age. Furthermore, for the fat-soluble vitamin E, there is no risk of inefficiency in old age because it is stored in the liver. On the contrary, in old age, there is an extended metabolism of vitamin C, especially in men. Men need 150 mg ascorbic acid daily for a normal plasma concentration of 1 mg/dL, while women need the recommended amount of 75–80 mg (Zampelas, 2003). According to the Dietary Reference Intakes (DRIs), the RDA for men >70 years old is 900 µg/day vitamin A (as RAE), 90 mg/day vitamin C, and 20 µg/day vitamin E (as α-tocopherol). For females >70 years old, the RDA is 700 µg/day vitamin A, 75 mg/day vitamin C, and 20 µg/day vitamin E (Food and Nutrition Board, Institute of Medicine, National Academies, 2011).

Recent scientific reports suggest that adherence to a balanced diet rich in antioxidant components, such as the Mediterranean diet, could protect older adults from the progression of degenerative diseases. A balanced combination of antioxidant nutrients may be necessary to have a significant effect on the prevention of cognitive decline and dementia in the elderly. The Academy of Nutrition and Dietetics encourage older people to achieve intakes meeting the DRIs for antioxidant vitamins and minerals, and the recommendation of a multivitamin supplement only if food intake is low. High dietary intake of vitamins E and C was associated with a lower risk of Alzheimer's disease, while decreased vitamin E levels have been associated with memory deficit in old people (Benfeito et al., 2012).

Research on antioxidant intakes at supplemental levels is inconclusive, and the conflicting results may be the result of various genetic factors and prior nutrient deficiencies. Furthermore, there is no evidence demonstrating the effective action of antioxidant supplements in doses higher than the DRIs in the elderly. On the contrary, the high consumption of vitamins A and E may induce toxicity in older adults due to the increased absorption of these antioxidant compounds (Gillette et al., 2007; Bernstein & Munoz, 2012).

DIETARY ANTIOXIDANT CONSUMPTION AND DISEASE PREVENTION IN THE ELDERLY

The increasing oxidative stress during aging is correlated with the progression of various disease pathophysiologies such as cataract, arteriosclerosis, Alzheimer's disease, and Parkinson's disease (Lau et al., 2005; Lloret et al., 2011; El Assar et al.,

2013; Zampatti et al., 2014). Cataracts and age-related macular degeneration (AMD) are common diseases of older adults. Higher intakes of phytochemicals may help prevent or delay the development and progression of cataracts and AMD. Adequate intakes of flavonoids and carotenoids, especially lutein and zeaxanthin, through a diet rich in fruits and vegetables increase their serum concentrations and the macular pigment density, and may help in the prevention of AMD (Bernstein & Munoz, 2012; Zampatti et al., 2014). A balanced diet containing antioxidant compounds is considered a basic parameter for enhancing endogenous stress responses and could be effective during the aging process, favoring a successful vascular aging; thus, it may reduce the risk for cardiovascular disease (El Assar et al., 2013).

Human brain and nervous system cells are particularly sensitive to oxidative stress because (i) the brain constitutes 2% of the total weight and consumes 20% of recruited oxygen; (ii) it is rich in polyunsaturated fatty acids, which are easily oxidized; (iii) it contains large amounts of iron and ascorbate that catalyze lipid peroxidation; (iv) many neurotransmitters are auto-oxidized and produce reactive oxygen species; (v) in specific brain areas, neuronal mitosis promotes oxidative damage; and (vi) via activation of genes such as *Enos*, *IL-1β*, *TNF-α*, and *NF-κB*, inflammatory processes may occur in nerve cells, thereby producing free radicals and cytokines. Therefore, the brain and nerve cells being prone to oxidative process may lead to the aging process and the emergence of diseases such as Alzheimer's and Parkinson's (Sun et al., 2002; Lau et al., 2005).

In recent years, many scientific studies, mainly in animals and humans, have suggested a possible beneficial effect of several food antioxidants in the deceleration of aging process in the brain, which causes the neurodegenerative diseases of old age. Cognitive tests in mice with Alzheimer plaques showed that diet containing fruits and vegetables, which are rich in antioxidants, improved cognitive functions and increased the number of neuronal cells. Mice that ate fruits rich in polyphenols, such as berries, had increased memory, improved cognitive status, and showed proliferation of neuronal cells, which are attenuated during aging, due to the increased expression of *ERK* genes in synaptosomes (Lau et al., 2005). The main mechanisms of action of antioxidants in neurological diseases include the possible influence on specific genes, antioxidant scavenging, and the regulation of cellular pathway messaging (Sun et al., 2002; Lloret et al., 2011). For example, polyphenols have been found to inhibit free radicals in the brain, preventing the production of substances that promote neurological diseases, such as inflammatory cytokines and interleukins, in microglia and peripheral nerves. They may also activate the factor NF-kB and remove iron, which is found in large concentrations in synaptosomes and mitochondria in the brain of patients with Alzheimer's and Parkinson's and has been linked to the pathogenesis of those diseases. Dietary antioxidants may reduce lipid peroxidation induced in the presence of iron in the mitochondria of mouse brain cells. They also form complexes with iron that reduce the *in vitro* production of aldehydes, a contributing factor in the production of reactive oxygen species and toxicity in the dopaminergic system (Sun et al., 2002; Esposito et al., 2003; Weinreb et al., 2004).

Alzheimer's disease is a neurodegenerative process associated with oxidative stress. It is known that the intracellular amyloid β could play a pivotal role in the pathophysiology of the disease. Amyloid β binds to heme groups in mitochondrial membranes, causing electron transport chain impairment and loss of respiratory function. Although many clinical trials have investigated whether antioxidants are beneficial in the treatment of Alzheimer's, and there are some effective results from animal studies, there are no clear data confirming that antioxidants are an effective therapy; more research is necessary to clarify this point (Lloret et al., 2011). Findings from studies of antioxidant intake above RDA levels in subjects with diagnosed cognitive impairment or Alzheimer's disease demonstrated no difference in the delay of cognitive decline (Bernstein & Munoz, 2012).

REFERENCES

Ahmad, N. & Mukhtar, H. 1999. Green tea polyphenols and cancer: Biological mechanisms and practical implications. *Nutr Rev* 57(3):78–83.

Bauer, M., Hamm, A. & Pankratz, M. J. 2004. Linking nutrition to genomics. *Biol Chem* 385:593–6.

Benfeito, S., Oliveira, C., Soares, P. & Fernandes C. 2013. Antioxidant therapy: Still in search of the 'magic bullet'. *Mitochondrion* 13:427–35.

Benzie, F. F. & Choi, S.-W. 2014. Antioxidants in food: Content, measurement, significance, action, cautions, caveats, and research. *Adv Food Nutr Res* 71:1–53.

Bernstein, M. & Munoz, N. 2012. Position of the Academy of Nutrition and Dietetics: Food and nutrition for older adults: Promoting health and wellness. *J Acad Nutr Diet* 112:1255–77. doi: 10.1016/j.jand.2012.06.015.

Bjelakovic, G., Nikolova, D., Gluud, L. L., Simonetti, R. G. & Gluud, C. 2008. Antioxidant supplements for prevention of mortality in healthy participants and patients with various diseases. *Cochrane Database Syst Rev* 2.

Cabrera, A., Artacho, R. & Gimenez, R. 2006. Beneficial effects of green tea—A review. *J Am Coll Nutr* 25:79–99.

Doll, S. & Ricou, B. 2013. Severe vitamin C deficiency in a critically ill adult: A case report. *Eur J Clin Nutr* 67:881–2.

Duffy, S. J., Keaney, J. L., Holbrook, M. et al. 2001. Short- and long-term tea consumption reverses endothelial dysfunction in patients with coronary artery disease. *Circulation* 104:151–6.

Duthie, G. G., Duthie, S. J. & Kyle, A. M. 2000. Plant polyphenols in cancer and heart disease: Implications as nutritional antioxidants. *Nutr Res Rev* 13:340–57.

El Assar, M., Angulo, J. & Rodríguez-Mañas, L. 2013. Oxidative stress and vascular inflammation in aging. *Free Radic Biol Med* 65:380–401.

Erba, D., Riso, P., Bordoni, A., Foti, P., Biagi, P. L., & Testolin, G. 2005. Effectiveness of moderate green tea consumption on antioxidative status and plasma lipid profile in humans. *J Nutr Biochem* 16:144–9.

Esposito, K., Nappo, F., Giugliano, F., Marfella, R., & Giugliano, D. 2003. Effect of dietary antioxidants on postprandial endothelial dysfunction induced by a high-fat meal in healthy subjects. *Am J Clin Nutr* 77:139–43.

European Food Safety Authority Panel on Dietetic Products, Nutrition and Allergies (NDA). 2011. Scientific opinion. Guidance on the scientific requirements for health claims related to antioxidants, oxidative damage and cardiovascular health. *EFSA J* 9(12):247.

Food and Nutrition Board, Institute of Medicine, National Academies. 2011. Dietary Reference Intakes (DRIs). Available at http://iom.edu/Activities/Nutrition/SummaryDRIs/~/media /Files/Activity%20Files/Nutrition/DRIs/New%20Material/5DRI%20Values%20 SummaryTables%2014.pdf.

Food and Nutrition for Older Adults Promoting Health and Wellness Evidence Analysis Project. 2012. Academy of Nutrition and Dietetics Evidence Analysis Library website. Available at http://www.andevidencelibrary.com.

Gillette, G. S., Abellan, G., Van Kan, S. et al. 2007. IANA task force on nutrition and cognitive decline with aging. *J Nutr Health Aging* 11(2):132–52.

Heinrich, M. & Prieto, J. 2008. Diet and healthy ageing 2100: Will we globalise local knowledge systems? *Ageing Res Rev* 7:249–74.

Hirano-Ohmori, R., Takahashi, R., Momiyama, Y. et al. 2005. Green tea Consumption and serum malondialdehyde-modified LDL concentrations in healthy subjects. *Am Coll Nutr* 24(5):342–6.

Ho, C.-T., Lin, J.-K. & Shahidi, F. 2009. *Tea and Tea Products. Chemistry and Health-Promoting Properties*. CRC Press, Boca Raton, FL, pp. 1–20, 111–167.

Hodgson, J., Burke, V. & Puddey, I. 2005. Acute effects of tea on fasting and postprandial vascular function and blood pressure in humans. *J Hypertens* 23:47–54.

International Food Information Council Foundation. *Media Guide on Food Safety and Nutrition: 2004–2006*.

Jacob, R. 1995. The integrated antioxidant system. *Nutr Res* 15(5):755–66.

Jochman, N., Bauman, G. & Stangl, V. 2008. Green tea and cardiovascular disease: From molecular targets towards human health. *Curr Opin Clin Nutr Metab Care* 11:758–65.

Kaliora, A. C., Dedousis, G. V. Z. & Sehmid, H. 2005. Dietary antioxidants in preventing atherogenesis. *Atherosclerosis* 187(1):1–17.

Kapsokefalou, M., Zhu, L. & Miller, D. D. 2006. Adding iron to green tea modifies the antioxidant capacity in rats. *Nutr Res* 26:480–5.

Karabela, D., Koutelidakis, A., Proestos, H., Komaitis, M. & Kapsokefalou, M. 2011. Adding iron to white tea may decrease its antioxidant capacity in humans. *Trace Elem Electrolytes* 29(1):16–21.

Koutelidakis, A. & Kapsokefalou, M. 2012. Holistic approaches of tea bioactivity: Interactions of tea and meal components studied *in vitro* and *in vivo*. In *Tea in Health and Disease Prevention*, ed. Preedy, V. Elsevier, London.

Koutelidakis, A. E., Argyri, K., Serafini, M. et al. 2009. Green tea, white tea and *Pelargonium purpureum* increase the antioxidant capacity of plasma and some organs of mice. *Nutrition* 25:453–8.

Koutelidakis, A. E., Rallidis, L., Koniari, K. et al. 2013. Effect of green tea on postprandial antioxidant capacity, serum lipids, C reactive protein and glucose levels in patients with coronary artery disease. *Eur J Nutr* 53(2):479–86.

Kris-Etherton, P. M., Lichtenstein, A. H., Howard, B. V., Steinberg, D. & Witztum, J. L. 2004. Antioxidant vitamin supplements and cardiovascular disease. *Circulation* 110:637–41.

Lau, F. C., Shukitt-Hale, B. & Joseph, J. A. 2005. The beneficial effects of fruit polyphenols on brain aging. *Neurobiol Aging* 26:128–32.

Lloret, A., Giraldo, E. & Viña, J. 2011. Is antioxidant therapy effective to treat Alzheimer's disease? *Free Radic Antioxid* 1(4):8–14.

Lotito, S. & Frei, B. 2006. Consumption of flavonoid-rich foods and increased plasma antioxidant capacity in humans: Cause, consequence, or epiphenomena? *Free Radic Biol Med* 41:1727–46.

Manach, C., Williamson, G., Morand, C., Scalbert, A. & Remesy, C. 2005. Bioavailability and bioefficacy of polyphenols in humans. Review of 97 biovailability studies. *Am J Clin Nutr* 81:230–42.

Masella, R., Vari, R. & D'Archivio, M. 2004. Extra virgin olive oil biophenols inhibit cell-mediated oxidation of LDL by increasing the mRNA transcription of glutathione-related enzymes. *J Nutr* 134:785–91.

Morton, L. W., Caccetta, R. A.-A., Puddey, I. B. & Croft, K. D. 2000. Chemistry and biological effects of dietary phenolic compounds: Relevance to cardiovascular disease. *Clin Exp Pharmacol Physiol* 27(3):152–62.

Osawa, T. 1999. Protective role of dietary polyphenols in oxidative stress. *Mech Ageing Dev* 111:133–9.

Osganian, S. K., Stampfer, M. J., Rimm, E. et al. 2003. Vitamin C and risk of coronary heart disease in women. *J Am Coll Cardiol* 42:246–52.

Pokorny, J., Yanishlieva, N. & Gordon, M. 2001. *Antioxidants in Food: Practical Applications.* CRC Press, Boca Raton, FL.

Saffari, Y. & Sadrzadeh, S. M. H. 2004. Green tea metabolite EGCG protects menbranes against oxidative damage in vitro. *Life Sci* 74:1513–8.

Scalbert, A., Morand, C., Manach, C. & Remesy, C. 2002. Absorption and metabolism of polyphenols in the gut and impact on health. *Biomed Pharmacother* 56:276–82.

Sies, H., Stahl, W. & Sevanian, A. 2005. Nutritional, dietary and postprandial oxidative stress. *J Nutr* 135:969–72.

Simon, J. A. & Hudes, E. S. 1999. Serum ascorbic acid and cardiovascular disease prevalence in U.S. adults: The Third National Health and Nutrition Examination Survey (NHANES III). *Ann Epidemiol* 9:358–65.

Stampfer, M. J., Hennekens, C. H., Manson, J. E., Colditz, G. A., Rosner, B. & Willett, W. C. 1993. Vitamin E consumption and the risk of coronary heart disease in women. *N Engl J Med* 328:1444–9.

Sun, A. Y., Simonyl, A. & Sun, G. Y. 2002. The "French Paradox" and beyond: Neuroprotective effects of polyphenols. *Free Radic Biol Med* 32(4):314–8.

Tsang, C., Higgins, S., Duthie, G. G. et al. 2005. The influence of moderate red wine consumption on antioxidant status and indices of oxidative stress associated with CHD in healthy volunteers. *Br J Nutr* 93:233–40.

Weinreb, O., Mandel, S., Amit, T. & Youdim, M. B. II. 2004. Neurological mechanisms of green tea polyphenols in Alzheimer's and Parkinson's diseases. *J Nutr Biochem* 15:506–16.

Weisel, T., Baum, M., Eisenbrand, G. et al. 2006. An anthocyanin/polyphenolic-rich fruit juice reduces oxidative DNA damage and increases gluthathione levels in healthy probands. *Biotech J* 1:388–97.

Widlansky, M. E., Duffy, S. J., Hamburg, N. M. et al. 2005. Effects of black tea consumption on plasma catechins and markers of oxidative stress and inflammation in patients with coronary artery disease. *Free Radic Biol Med* 38:499–506.

Wootton-Beard, P. C. & Ryan, L. 2011. Improving public health?: The role of antioxidant-rich fruit and vegetable beverages. *Food Res Int* 44:3135–48.

Yoshihara, D., Fujiwara, N. & Suzuki, K. 2010. Antioxidants: Benefits and risks for long-term health. *Maturitas* 67:103–7.

Zampatti, S., Ricci, F., Cusumano, A. et al. 2014. Review of nutrient actions on age-related macular degeneration. *Nutr Res* 34:95–105.

Zampelas, A. 2003. *Nutrition During Lifetime.* Paschalidis Publications, Athens, Greece, p. 463.

6 Smoking, Oxidative Stress, and Antioxidant Intake

Aristea Baschali and Dimitrios Karayiannis

CONTENTS

Introduction 84
Interrelationship between Cigarette Smoke Chemistry and OS 85
    Radicals in Cigarette Tar 85
        Free Radicals (FRs) 85
        Quinones 86
        Trace Heavy Metals 86
    Radicals in Gas Phase 87
        Oxidative Radicals 87
        Peroxynitrite 87
        Glutathione Depletion 87
Effects of Cigarette Smoke on OS in Humans 88
Interrelationship between Smoking and Antioxidant Intake 89
    Dietary Antioxidants and Smoking 89
        Vitamins 91
        Minerals and Trace Elements 94
        Interaction of Smoking and Dietary Antioxidants 95
    Case of Natural Antioxidants 95
        Vitamin C 95
        Vitamin E 96
        Vitamin A and Non–Provitamin A Carotenoids 96
        Flavonoids 97
        Zinc 97
        Copper 97
        Selenium 98
        Iron 98
    Case of Antioxidants in Supplementation Studies 98
        Vitamin C Supplementation Studies 98
        Vitamin E Supplementation Studies 99
        Non–Provitamin A Carotenoid Supplementation Studies 99

Combined Antioxidant Supplementation Studies 99
Selenium Supplementation Studies...99
Conclusion 100
References..100

INTRODUCTION

Oxidative stress (OS) is a normal phenomenon in the body. The main contributors to OS, reactive oxygen species (ROS), are produced by living organisms as a result of normal cellular metabolism. Under normal conditions, physiologically important intracellular levels of ROS are maintained at low levels with various enzyme systems involved in redox homeostasis *in vivo* (Jakob and Reichmann 2013). At low to moderate concentrations, ROS function in normal cellular processes; however, at high concentrations, they produce undesirable changes in cellular components such as lipids, proteins, and DNA. The shift of the balance between oxidants/antioxidants is called "oxidative stress." For the past two decades, OS has been one of the hottest topics among biological researchers worldwide.

Several reasons may be given to justify the importance of knowledge on ROS and reactive nitrogen species (RNS) production and metabolism: identification of biomarkers for oxidative damage, evidence for the occurrence of serious of chronic health problems due to OS, identification of different dietary antioxidants present in vegetables such as bioactive molecules, and so forth. OS contributes to many disease states, including cancer, neurological disorders, atherosclerosis, hypertension, ischemia/perfusion diabetes, acute respiratory distress syndrome, idiopathic pulmonary fibrosis, chronic obstructive pulmonary disease, and asthma (Da Costa et al. 2012).

Cigarette smoke is a highly complex aerosol consisting of several thousands of chemical substances, approximately 4700 of which are distributed between the gas and particle phases. It is divided into mainstream smoke (inhaled smoke) and sidestream smoke. Mainstream smoke is divided into a solid particulate phase (tar) and a gas phase (toxic gases, volatile organic compounds, volatile organic compounds, free radicals [FRs], etc.) (Siasos et al. 2014, Wooten et al. 2006). Cigarette tar contains extremely high concentrations of stable FRs (about 10^{17} spins g^{-1}) with a very long lifetime. Sidestream smoke is divided into the solid and gas phases, and contains higher concentrations of toxic and carcinogenic compounds and other volatile and semivolatile compounds. FRs and antioxidants in the gaseous phase are present in a stable state that is continuously formed and destroyed, and the concentration increases as the smoke ages. The gaseous phase is about 0.4–0.5 g/cigarette and contains 500 volatile organic and inorganic compounds. The particulate phase (tar) consists of fine and very fine particles (0.1–1.0 micron, aerodynamic diameter) that penetrate deep into the alveoli. Some of the soluble components of aqueous cigarette tar (ACT) can generate superoxide anion (O_2^-) and then hydrogen peroxide (H_2O_2) and reactive hydroxyl radical (HO), which cause oxidative damage to cellular membrane lipids, proteins, enzymes, and DNA (Romero et al. 2013). Sidestream smoke is composed of similar chemical components in solid and gaseous phases, and is also rich in short-lived and highly reactive FRs. Passive smoking (or environmental tobacco [cigarette] smoke, ETS) has been shown to be a risk to the health of the nonsmoking population and contributes to major lung diseases (Widome et al. 2010, Wooten et al. 2006).

It is known that smoking is harmful to human health, from the results of many epidemiological studies linking smoking with high mortality from the onset of heart disease and cancer (Siasos et al. 2014). A large number of data on the composition of mainstream smoke have been published, and the matter has been examined in detail. The enormous complexity of cigarette smoke is the result of multiple thermolytic processes occurring during the combustion of the cigarette rod. These processes include distillation, pyrolysis, and combustion, and are influenced by factors including the design of the cigarette and the composition of tobacco. Numerous chemical classes of organic compounds present in cigarette smoke include saturated and unsaturated hydrocarbons, alcohols, aldehydes, ketones, carboxylic acids, esters, phenols, nitriles, terpenoids, and alkaloids. As the composition of cigarette smoke is complex, some components of tobacco have been scrutinized more than others have, either because of their greater relative abundance in tobacco (which makes them easy to analyze), their known pharmacological properties, and/or because they are believed to be carcinogenic or potentially harmful to smokers.

INTERRELATIONSHIP BETWEEN CIGARETTE SMOKE CHEMISTRY AND OS

There are a number of chemical classes of tobacco ingredients that have been reported to affect OS (Chalmers 1999). Owing to the complexity of cigarette smoke, it is impossible to be comprehensive, and much remains unknown. The components of smoke included in this chapter are compounds or metal ions that act as electrophiles, FRs, reactive anions or metal ions that act as reducing agents (donate an electron), or FRs or metal ions that act as oxidizing agents (accept an electron). ROS and RNS are generated when mainstream cigarette smoke interacts with aqueous media or physiological fluids. Some components of tobacco are involved in OS only when chemically modified by metabolic processes *in vivo*. Also, it is possible to distinguish between an oxidant from the direct action of the components of cigarette smoke and secondary antioxidants that occur as a reaction to inflammation resulting from smoking-related OS.

RADICALS IN CIGARETTE TAR

Free Radicals (FRs)
Studies have shown that the FRs in cigarette smoke originate not only from the combustion process but also from secondary reactions involving nitrogen oxide species (like nitric oxide [NO] and nitric dioxide [NO_2]) following smoke generation. These species are involved in the generation of oxygen-centered radicals via the addition of nitrogen dioxide to unsaturated compounds (i.e., reactive double bonds). This may lead to the generation of carbon-centered radicals that subsequently react with atmospheric oxygen to form oxygen-centered radicals (Wooten et al. 2006).

Mainstream tobacco smoke contains up to 700 ppm NO that is produced from nitrogen-containing compounds (like proteins and alkaloids) in tobacco. This high concentration of NO is partially responsible for the generation of FRs in cigarette smoke. There is also indirect evidence that NO_2 is involved in the generation of other radical species. By spin trapping the gas-phase FRs, the oxidation products derived from the corresponding spin trap can be clearly seen by electron paramagnetic resonance (EPR) spectroscopy (Chalmers 1999).

Oxygen-centered FRs such as alkoxyls and peroxyls have also been identified in cigarette smoke by spin trapping, or by using a nonreductive scavenging method. However, the EPR spectra for O-centered radicals in the literature are usually weak and complex because they are mixed with C-centered radicals, which are formed first and are more stable. By employing 5-diethoxyphosphoryl-5-methyl-1-pyrroline-N-oxide (DEPMPO), however, the lifetime of peroxyl radicals is increased by >15 times (Zuo et al. 2014). In the literature, N-t-butyl-α-phenylnitrone and 5,5-dimethyl-1-pyrroline-N-oxide have also been used as spin traps in cigarette smoke studies, although they are less suitable for O-centered radicals compared with DEPMPO. This work investigated some of the FRs in mainstream cigarette smoke in both the gas and particulate phases by combining spin-trapping techniques with EPR spectroscopy (Valavanidis et al. 2009).

Hydrogen peroxide is a naturally occurring by-product of OS, formed during normal breathing in living organisms by the catalytic disproportionation of superoxide by superoxide dismutase (SOD). Another enzyme, catalase, is very effective in converting H_2O_2 into "harmless products, water and molecular oxygen" (Wooten et al. 2006). If this cellular defense mechanism is overwhelmed, excess H_2O_2 can undergo disproportionation through the Fenton reaction to form hydroxyl radicals. The hydroxyl radicals from H_2O_2 are highly oxidizing species and are well known to cause oxidative damage to essential biomolecules, including DNA. H_2O_2 has been found in ACT and unbuffered aqueous solutions of catechin, a component of tobacco abundant in both ACT and total particulate matter (TPM). H_2O_2 concentration in smoke condensate has been shown to increase with age, temperature, and pH. H_2O_2 found in cigarette smoke and H_2O_2 formed as a physiological response to smoke constituents are considered to be a source of OS and/or damage to smokers.

Quinones

Quinones are easily formed by components of cigarette smoke that can undergo autoxidation. The toxicology of kinins has been studied extensively. Generally, the toxicity of quinones is believed to occur by two mechanisms: the mechanism of redox cycling, which produces excess ROS as by-products, and the formation of covalent bonds with the basic biological molecules (especially molecules containing thiol groups). Both mechanisms may contribute to the occurrence of OS (Valavanidis et al. 2009).

Trace Heavy Metals

Tobacco plants carry the metal ions from the soil through the roots into the sheets. Trace amounts of heavy metals are accumulated on the sheets, and they are known to transfer in trace amounts from the treated and processed sheets to the inhaled tobacco smoke. These metals include cadmium, lead, mercury, arsenic, iron, copper, chromium, nickel, and selenium. Both redox-active and redox-inactive metals could potentially cause an increase in ROS in smokers (Valavanidis et al. 2009).

RADICALS IN GAS PHASE

The gas phase of cigarette smoke contains high concentrations of inorganic gases (O_2, N_2, CO, NO, HCN, H_2S, and NH_3), as well as various alkanes, alkenes, alcohols, and saturated and unsaturated aldehydes as volatile products of organic combustion. More specifically, the main gas-phase constituents are oxidative radicals, peroxynitrite, and glutathione.

Oxidative Radicals

Cigarette smoke contains abundant oxidants in the gas vapor. Even if the NO is from the same root, it is neither reactive nor particularly toxic. NO combines slowly with molecular oxygen in the air (for a period of seconds) to form the toxic oxidant and nitrating agent NO_2. According to a proposed mechanism, NO_2 reacts rapidly with other smoke constituents, such as isoprene and butadiene, to form nitrosocarbon-centered radicals (Pryor et al. 1983). Atoms in the molecule are generally very reactive species. The gaseous-phase carbon in the molecule in tobacco reacts instantaneously with molecular oxygen to form peroxyl radicals that react with the NO gas phase of the smoke to form alkoxyl radicals and NO_2, thus creating a continuous cycle. There are two interesting effects of the above reaction scheme (Jakob and Reichmann 2013): (a) the oxidizing radicals in cigarette smoke are formed by reactions between the gas-phase constituents, and not primarily by pyrolysis or combustion reactions in the burning tobacco, and (b) the radicals collected inside an enclosed container of gas-phase smoke (Siasos et al. 2014) increase until the supply of NO· is depleted, persisting for several minutes.

Peroxynitrite

Peroxynitrite RNS is formed by the reaction of NO and superoxide. Peroxynitrite is itself an FR, which is derived from two FRs, but it is also a strong oxidant that has been shown to induce failure in key biomolecules in physiological media. Peroxynitrite has been recognized as an OS-inducing compound in aqueous fractions of cigarette smoke. After depletion of the intracellular reduced glutathione (GSH) content with electrophilic aldehydes, peroxynitrite interferes with specific target molecules, resulting in the activation of the stress associated with signal transduction and gene expression in cells treated with cigarette smoke *in vitro* (Wooten et al. 2006).

Glutathione Depletion

Glutathione is a tripeptide composed of glutamate, cysteine, and glycine, and is synthesized and utilized in every organ of the body. It is abundant in the cytoplasm, nuclei, and mitochondria, and is the main water-soluble antioxidant in these cell compartments in millimolar concentrations. Amendments of intracellular GSH with electrophiles in the vapor phase of cigarette smoke were first reported decades before it was reported that the concentration of protein sulfhydryl groups in plasma is about 500 µM. After exposure to cigarette smoke, the concentration of protein sulfhydryl groups decreased by about 60%. γ-Glutamylcysteine ligase is the rate-limiting enzyme involved in GSH synthesis, and its expression has been shown to be induced in response to cigarette smoke (Min et al. 2011). Cigarette smoke exposures evoke a powerful GSH adaptive response in the lung and systemically.

EFFECTS OF CIGARETTE SMOKE ON OS IN HUMANS

The acute effects of smoking (ACS) on OS markers have been mainly analyzed in exhaled air, bronchoalveolar lavage (BAL), and blood. Most studies have shown a direct increase in OS after ACS; however, in several studies, smoking had no effect (Wooten et al. 2006). Few studies have described the results of ACS in oxidative markers in exhaled breath condensate and air. In breath, the condensate 8-isoprostane, a product of lipid peroxidation, increased 15 min after ACS, and hydrogen peroxide increased 30 min after exposure. Smoke exhaled nitric oxide (eNO) was increased at 1 and 10 min but decreased 5 min after ACS in another study. This inconsistency probably reflects differences in eNO measurements and characteristics of individuals. No difference was observed in eNO at 15, 30, and 90 min after smoking. Breath condensate nitrate levels increased at 30 min after ACS; however, nitrite and nitrotyrosine levels did not change.

Another study has investigated the effects of smoking on markers of OS in BAL, indicating increased superoxide release from BAL fluid (BALF) leukocytes and increased Trolox equivalent antioxidant capacity (TEAC). The latter surprising result can be explained by the fact that the studied subjects were all chronic smokers already associated with high levels of BALF TEAC. No difference was found in intracellular GSH and oxidized glutathione (GSSG) in leukocytes, and thiobarbituric acid reactive substances (TBARS) in BALF and epithelial lining fluid.

Regarding peripheral blood, nitrate, nitrite, and cysteine levels were depressed for a short time just after smoking one cigarette (van der Vaart et al. 2004). No difference was observed in the production of reactive oxygen intermediates from neutrophils. Unlike in BALF, TBARS increased in plasma and plasma TEAC decreased 1 h after smoking. Levels of F2-isoprostane, another product of lipid peroxidation, showed no change in plasma, possibly because all subjects in this study were chronic smokers and already have high F2-isoprostane levels.

Generally, acute smoking increases markers of OS in all experimental models— human, animal, and *in vitro* (Rahal et al. 2014). NO and GSH are the only two parameters that have been investigated in all models. NO and its related substances increase within 24 h after smoke exposure. The GSH/GSSG ratio, reflecting the vital balance between oxidants and protecting antioxidants, decreased following acute smoke exposure in both animal and *in vitro* studies but not in the single study published in humans. This discrepancy can be explained by differences in species, smoke dose, or compartment (human BALF vs. animal lung homogenate).

Interestingly, ACS even results in damage of fatty acids in cell membranes, as measured by an increase in degradation products of lipid peroxidation in humans (exhaled air and plasma) and animals (BALF and lung tissue). No *in vitro* studies investigating the acute smoke effects on lipid peroxidation products have been found. Because different time points within 24 h have been studied, it is possible to observe a time response of OS (van der Vaart et al. 2004). In humans, all oxidative markers increase within the first hour after ACS and most markers returned to normal within 90 min. Exhaled air is the first compartment in which an increase in OS markers can be observed, followed by BALF and blood. In animals, most markers of OS change in the first 6 h after ACS and return to normal within 24 h. In all compartments (lung tissue, BALF, and blood), GSH or its derivatives are depressed in the same period, suggesting a generalized response to ACS.

As in humans, only a few time points have been studied in *in vitro* models. The initial depletion of GSH after ACS appeared to be followed by an increase in GSH 24 h later, suggesting a protective mechanism of cells against OS from smoke. The importance of the GSH/GSSG balance was shown in several studies. When GSH was added to the experiment, the OS and inflammatory response induced by cigarette smoke could be prevented. In summary, smoking immediately increases markers of OS in all models and even results in damage to the cell membrane.

INTERRELATIONSHIP BETWEEN SMOKING AND ANTIOXIDANT INTAKE

DIETARY ANTIOXIDANTS AND SMOKING

A great number of epidemiological studies state that the consumption of antioxidant-rich diets (fruits and vegetables) could reduce the risk of developing human degenerative diseases, by possibly protecting the organism more efficiently against OS (Da Costa et al. 2012). The most acceptable explanation was the presence of antioxidant nutrients, including vitamin C and E, carotenoids, flavonoids, selenium, etc., which protect against oxidative damage to the DNA, lipids, and proteins. Antioxidants are synthetic or natural substances, in low concentrations compared with the biomolecules that they should protect. Their protective role is provided by their reaction with ROS and inhibition of the oxidation chain reactions, reducing their accumulation and finally limiting the harmful effects of FRs (Romero et al. 2013). The human defense against OS includes endogenous and exogenous antioxidants. Endogenous antioxidants or endogenous radical scavengers, such as glutathione and coenzyme Q, are produced by the cell itself; however, the endogenous production is usually insufficient to inhibit OS (Kinnula 2005, Rahman et al. 2006). Exogenous antioxidants, including nutrients and phytochemicals entering the organism through the diet (found in specific foods) or through supplements with antioxidant formulations and cofactors such as copper, zinc, manganese, iron, and selenium, can strengthen the organism and help combat diseases.

Endogenous and exogenous antioxidants play an important role in the regulation of ROS in a physiological manner (Table 6.1). In special conditions such as excessive FR production, their synergistic effect may be insufficient to prevent oxidative damage (Figure 6.1). Furthermore, it is important to state that each person has a different capacity to defend against ROS and OS, which depends on the function of endogenous and exogenous antioxidant systems, their exposure to internal and external

TABLE 6.1
Examples of Endogenous and Exogenous (Dietary) Antioxidants

Endogenous Antioxidants	Exogenous (Dietary) Antioxidants
Enzymatic antioxidants	Vitamins
• Superoxide dismutase (SOD)	• C (ascorbic acid)
• Glutathione peroxidase (GPx)	• E (tocopherols, tocotrienols)
• Glutathione reductase (GRx)	Carotenoids
• Catalase (CAT)	• β-Carotene
Metabolic antioxidants (nonenzymatic)	• Lutein
• Glutathione	• Zeaxanthin
• Lipoic acid	• Lycopene
• Uric acid	• β-Cryptoxanthin
• Bilirubin	Trace elements
• Melatonin	• Selenium
• L-Arginine	• Zinc
• Coenzyme Q_{10}	Flavonols
• Metal-chelating proteins	• Quercetin
• Transferrin	• Kaempferol
	• Myricetin
	Phenolic acids
	• Chlorogenic acid
	• Gallic acid
	• Cafeic acid
	Flavanols
	• Proanthocyanidins
	• Catechins
	Antocyanidins
	• Cyanidin
	• Pelargonidin
	Isoflavones
	• Genistein
	• Daidzein
	• Glycitein
	Flavanones
	• Naringenin
	• Eriodictyol
	• Hesperetin
	Flavones
	• Luteolin
	• Apignen

Source: Da Costa, L.A. et al., *Prog Mol Biol Transl Sci*, 108, 179, 2012.

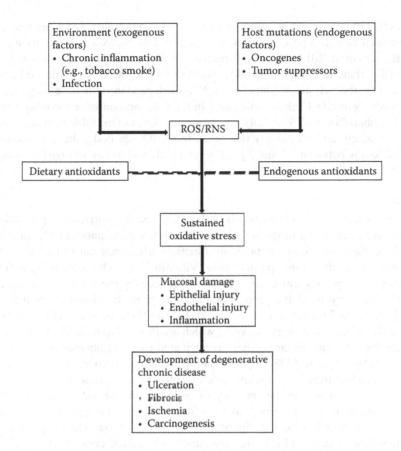

FIGURE 6.1 Interaction of reactive oxygen species (ROS), reactive nitrogen species (RNS), dietary and endogenous antioxidants, oxidative stress, and degenerative chronic disease. (From Da Costa, L.A. et al., *Prog Mol Biol Transl Sci*, 108, 179, 2012.)

stimuli (e.g., inflammation and smoking), and finally genetic variation (Comandini et al. 2010). The interaction of these factors may affect an individual's ability to manage OS and determine antioxidant status.

Vitamins

Vitamin C

Vitamin C, also known as ascorbic acid or ascorbate, is the primary and one of the most abundant water-soluble dietary antioxidants. Experimental and epidemiological evidence suggests that vitamin C is a powerful antioxidant, both *in vivo* and *in vitro*, in biological systems (Da Costa et al. 2012, Kelly 2003). Its health benefits refer to its anticarcinogenic, immunoregulatory, anti-inflammatory, and neuroprotector effects. It also plays an important physiological role as an electron donor, which explains its ability to neutralize FRs. Furthermore, it is an effective scavenger of the superoxide anion (O_2^-), singlet oxygen ($^1O_2$), and hydroxyl radicals (OH^-), and it protects lipids, proteins, and DNA from oxidative damage. However, vitamin C is not an effective scavenger or neutralizer of hydrogen peroxide (H_2O_2) and may play an important role as a prooxidant in combination with redox-active metals such as iron (Romero et al. 2013). Vitamin C reacts with ROS and RNS to synthesize semi-dehydroascorbate (ascorbate FR) and dehydroascorbate, which are reduced back to ascorbate by the actions of glutathione, NADH-dependent reductase enzymes, or thioredoxin. Vitamin C also participates in the regeneration of α-tocopherol from the α-tocopherol radical. The daily recommended doses of ascorbic acid are 75 mg/day (for women) and 90 mg/day (for men). In the human body, the availability of ascorbic acid is between 1.2 and 2 g (20 mg/kg body weight) and its half-life ranges from 10 to 20 days.

Vitamin E

Vitamin E (α, β, γ, and δ tocopherols and α, β, γ, and δ tocotrienols), particularly α-tocopherol, acts as an intra- and extracellular liposoluble antioxidant; since it is a lipid-soluble molecule, its antioxidant functions are important in the protection of membrane lipids against peroxidation. Vitamin E is a chain-breaking antioxidant that interrupts radical chain reactions produced by the lipid peroxy radicals (LOO⁻), thus preventing the propagation of damage to the biological membranes that give rise to FRs (Da Costa et al. 2012). Additionally, it directly scavenges superoxide radicals and singlet oxygen, which are thought to be initiators of oxidation reactions. Its antioxidant activity is attributed to its chromanol rings, capable of donating hydrogen to ROS. In particular, the tocopherols concentrate on protecting the polyunsaturated fatty acids of cell membrane phospholipids from cellular peroxidation, maintaining the integrity of biological membranes and other reactive compounds (e.g., vitamins A and C) from oxidative damage. It also inhibits the peroxidation of low-density lipoproteins (LDLs), oxidizes the oxygen singlet, neutralizes peroxides, and captures the superoxide anion, converting it into less reactive forms (Kelly 2002a). In addition, tocopherols play an important role in cell respiration and in DNA and coenzyme Q biosynthesis. Regarding the dietary requirements of vitamin E, it is important to state that 1 international unit (IU) vitamin E is equal to 1 mg α-tocopherol, and 1 IU vitamin E is equal to 0.67 mg vitamin E. In adults specifically, the minimum daily requirement for vitamin E is 15 mg/day, and the range between 200 and 600 mg/day is safe as it would not cause any disorder (Romero et al. 2013).

Vitamin A and Non–Provitamin A Carotenoids

Vitamin A is a family of essential liposoluble compounds, named retinoids, including retinol, retinal, retinoic acid, and retinyl esters, which have a structural relationship and share their biological activity (Da Costa et al. 2012). In the human diet, the two different forms of vitamin A that are available are the preformed vitamin A (retinol and its esterified form, retinyl ester) and provitamin A carotenoids (β-carotene [the most important form], α-carotene, and β-cryptoxanthin) (National Institutes of Health 2013). The most well-studied function of carotenoids is their role as precursors for vitamin A. This characterization applies only to the carotenes and cryptoxanthins, as lutein, zeaxanthin, and lycopene cannot be converted to retinol and are known as non–provitamin A carotenoids. Both retinyl esters and provitamin

A carotenoids are metabolized intracellularly to retinol, which is oxidized to retinal and then to retinoic acid, the active forms of vitamin A, to exert the vitamin's important biological functions.

Many roles have been proposed for carotenoids, including inhibition of tumor growth, protection against genotoxicity, and modulation of the immune system (Kelly 2002b). Vitamin A and carotenoids are characterized as antioxidant vitamins and are effective FR scavengers, inhibiting the activity of FR, protecting the DNA from their mutagenic action, and thus preventing cellular aging. Their oxygen sensitivity is due to the large amount of double loops present in their structure.

As carotenoids are lipid soluble, their antioxidant properties may be particularly important for protection of lipids and may work synergistically with vitamin E to prevent lipid peroxidation. Their bioavailability increases with the presence of vitamin E and other antioxidants. Carotenoids may also play an important role in the protection of DNA damage from ROS attack while additionally modulating DNA repair mechanisms. Particularly for lycopene, which is a non–provitamin A carotenoid (not converted into vitamin A in the human body), evidence supports their very high antioxidant properties. High consumption of lycopene has been related with the prevention of some cancer types, specifically that of the prostate (Romero et al. 2013).

Flavonoids

Flavonoids belong to an aromatic group, with heterocyclic pigments that contain oxygen, which can be found among plants and especially the majority of yellow, red, and blue fruits (Da Costa et al. 2012). Several properties have been attributed to flavonoids, such as anti-inflammatory, antimicrobial, antithrombotic, antiallergic, antitumor, anticarcinogenic, and antioxidant properties. The following are examples of flavonoids:

1. Elegiac acid
2. Anthocyanidines
3. Catechins
4. Citroflavonoids
5. Isoflavonoids, such as genestein and daidzein
6. Kaempferol
7. Proanthocyanidines

Flavonoids are easily oxidized substances; for this reason, a fundamental characteristic of these substances responsible for many of their beneficial effects is their antioxidant capacity (Braun et al. 2011). Quercetin protects primary human osteoblasts exposed to cigarette smoke. Quercetins are characterized by their low toxicity, and they exert a protector effect of the vascular wall. They can also inhibit lipid peroxidation, have antimutagenic effects, and possess the capacity to inhibit diverse enzymes. The antioxidant function of flavonoids relies mainly on their capacity to sequester FRs; chelate transition metals such as Fe^{2+}, Cu^{2+}, or Zn^{2+}; impede the catalytic actions of FR; and they also act by inhibiting the enzyme systems related with vascular functionality (Braun et al. 2011, Romero et al. 2013). Furthermore, it has been suggested that they also indirectly inhibit oxidative pathways, such as phospho-lipase A2, while stimulating others with recognized antioxidant properties, such as catalase and SOD.

Among the >4000 varieties of flavonoids, quercetin is the natural flavonoid widely distributed in a healthy human diet that exerts an effective antioxidant function. It is present in five times higher amounts than vitamins A and C, and additionally is also hydrophilic like vitamin C. Flavonoids have been shown to exert antioxidant capacity by reducing OS-dependent damage and ROS formation, not only *in vitro* (e.g., ethanol-treated primary human hepatocytes) but also *in vivo* in rats exposed to methyl-mercury. Furthermore, recent studies have shown that various flavonoids may positively influence the negative effects of cigarette-associated tissue damage in humans (Braun et al. 2011). Specifically, rutin (quercetin-3-β-D-rutinoside) has a synergic effect with all of the vita-mins to which we have alluded. Ascorbic acid also reduces the oxidation of quercetin, allowing the flavonoids to maintain their functions for a longer time. Quercetin also pro-tects vitamin E from oxidation. The flavonoids remove reactive oxygen, especially in the form of SOD, hydroxyl radicals, hydroperoxides, and lipid peroxides, inhibiting the harmful effects of these compounds on cells.

Some flavonoids, such as the anthocyanidines, cause low oxidation potentials (EP/2), which allow them to reduce Fe^{3+} and Cu^{2+}, and thus they undergo autooxidation or become involved in the redox recycling pathway; acting in this manner, they work as pro-oxidant agents (Da Costa et al. 2012). Another potential mechanism is the autooxida-tion of the aroxyl radical and generation of the superoxide anion (O_2^-) that becomes the harmful hydroxyl radical (HO). The determinant of the antioxidant or prooxidant charac-ter is the redox stability/lability of the radical compound that forms a part of the original flavonoid. The prooxidant actions are exerted when the flavonoid doses are very high.

Minerals and Trace Elements

Minerals and trace elements such as copper, manganese, selenium, zinc, and iron may exert antioxidant properties. These substances act as potent antioxidant in a variety of metabolic processes and pathways in the human body (Da Costa et al. 2012).

Zinc

Zinc is a trace element that takes part in >200 enzymatic reactions. In case of defi-ciency, there is an increase in the production of oxidant species and OS (Romero et al. 2013).

Copper

Copper is a mineral that acts as an antioxidant through its participation in functions of the enzyme SOD, which eliminates the superoxide anion. Its antioxidant effect is exerted through the protection of cells from the toxic effects of FR and the facilita-tion of calcium and phosphorous fixation (Da Costa et al. 2012).

Selenium

Selenium is a trace element that is involved in the process of the synthesis of enzymes related with oxidative function, including glutathione peroxidase. This enzyme eliminates peroxide groups such as oxygen peroxide. Selenium is attached to proteins, forming the denominated selenoproteins. With this action, it contributes to the prevention of cell damage (Da Costa et al. 2012).

Iron

Iron takes part in the organism's antioxidant defense processes, as it intervenes in the elimination of the peroxide groups. Furthermore, its ability to change valence with ease (2+/3+) means that it can also be involved in the formation of FRs (Da Costa et al. 2012).

Interaction of Smoking and Dietary Antioxidants

The reviewed literature proposes that smokers have lower circulating concentrations of many micronutrients, including ascorbic acid, β-carotene, α-carotene, and cryptoxanthin (Vardavas et al. 2008). There is a complex relationship between smoking and the circulating concentrations of micronutrients, and scientific evidence is conflicting concerning the antioxidant capacity of certain micronutrients, e.g., β-carotene. Taking into consideration that antioxidants may act as potential prooxidants, possible lower concentrations of antioxidants in smokers compared with nonsmokers may be a defensive adaptation to the pro-inflammatory environment in smokers' tissues. Furthermore, another explanation for these disparities may be the differences in dietary intakes.

CASE OF NATURAL ANTIOXIDANTS

Vitamin C

A great number of studies have shown that smoking reduces the plasma vitamin C level (Alberg 2002, Kelly 2003, Northrop-Clewes and Thurnham 2007). Specifically, one study that investigated the relationship between smoking status and serum and dietary micronutrient concentrations revealed that current smoking status affected the dietary nutrient intake (lower dietary intake) of vitamin C, but not of vitamin A and E (Vardavas et al. 2008). Epidemiological evidence also supports the idea that low-plasma vitamin C is a risk factor for coronary heart disease (May 2000, Northrop-Clewes and Thurnham 2007). The early and more recent research has suggested that adverse changes in the intake, absorption, transport, utilization, turnover, and excretion of vitamin C are associated with exposure to cigarette smoke. Vitamin C status may also play a role in modulating the action and metabolism of components of smoke and will be discussed in the following sections (Northrop-Clewes and Thurnham 2007).

Regarding the dietary intake of vitamin C and its interrelation with blood concentrations, some studies propose that the low concentrations of circulating vitamin C in smokers could be explained from alterations in the metabolism of this vitamin. Other studies suggest that this is due to low dietary intake of the nutrient. Most of the studies have shown that plasma and leukocyte concentrations of vitamin C are lower in smokers than in nonsmokers. Furthermore, it is stated that smokers have a nicotine-induced decrease in the efficiency of intestinal absorption, a decreased urinary excretion rate, and a higher metabolic turnover of vitamin C. Although evidence suggests that administration of vitamin C can result in decreases in markers of OS, a recommended dietary allowance derived from a direct antioxidant function of vitamin C could not be calculated and proposed. This is due to the lack of a quantitative relationship between any antioxidant function and a health-related endpoint (Northrop-Clewes and Thurnham 2007). Concerning the turnover of vitamin C, a great number of studies support the idea that there is increased turnover in response to the high and sustained oxidant load from smoking.

Vitamin E

In regard to vitamin E status, α-tocopherol concentrations usually do not differ in the serum of smokers and nonsmokers, in contrast to β-carotene and vitamin C, which are lower in cigarette smokers (Northrop-Clewes and Thurnham 2007). Older smokers may also have lower blood vitamin E concentrations than younger smokers (Alberg 2002). In a cohort analysis study, it was found that higher α-tocopherol concentrations may be protective against pancreatic carcinogenesis in male smokers (Stolzenberg et al. 2009). Furthermore, in one study, α-tocopherol concentration was negatively correlated with a smoking index (cigarettes/day × years of smoking). Pharmacokinetic data from different studies suggest that α-tocopherol metabolism might differ between smokers and nonsmokers (Bruno and Maret 2005).

With respect to the dietary intake of vitamin E, it is not clear whether the increase in vitamin E turnover is due to smoking-induced inflammatory changes or OS. It is also proposed that if the turnover of vitamin E is faster in smokers than in nonsmokers and, and if plasma concentrations are not adversely affected in smokers, the intake of vitamin E for smokers in industrialized countries should be adequate enough to enable them to deal with the added oxidative smoking-induced stress. Nicotine in cigarettes could cause the difference in vitamin E intake, which has an influence on taste and appetite (Northrop-Clewes and Thurnham 2007). However, the effects of smoking on appetite do not affect the intake of vitamin E–containing foods in the way and extent that smoking influences the intake of carotene and vitamin C.

Vitamin A and Non–Provitamin A Carotenoids

The serum retinol concentrations in smokers are usually similar to those of nonsmokers. This suggests that the inflammation associated with smoking is not sufficient to disturb the normal homeostatic control of retinol in plasma. Also, the evidence on total dietary intake of vitamin A of smokers appears to be inconsistent, suggesting the need for further study (Alberg 2002, Northrop-Clewes and Thurnham 2007).

With respect to the β-carotene status of cigarette smokers and comparison of plasma/serum concentrations of β-carotene between heavy smokers (≥20 cigarettes/day or ≥10 years of smoking) and nonsmokers, the data revealed lower plasma β-carotene concentrations in smokers than in nonsmokers. The data also revealed that in heavy smokers, the increase in plasma β-carotene concentrations associated with higher intakes was smaller than in nonsmokers or light smokers (Northrop-Clewes and Thurnham 2007).

Regarding the dietary intake of β-carotene and its relationship with blood concentrations and disease, scientific evidence has shown that the concentration of plasma β-carotene is mainly determined by dietary intake. Epidemiological evidence also proposes that cigarette smokers consume less fruit and vegetables than nonsmokers. Low plasma β-carotene concentrations commonly found in smokers suggest that higher intakes of dietary carotenoids are probably needed to achieve optimal concentrations of plasma carotenoids in this population (Northrop-Clewes and Thurnham 2007). In the case of carotenoids other than β-carotene, there are only small amounts in the diet and blood, and differences in intakes of vegetables and fruits may obscure the effects of smoking on both diet and blood concentrations.

Concerning lycopene, the major carotenoid present in tomato, its consumption may prevent smoke-induced cell damage; however, the mechanisms are still unclear. Beneficial effects of tomato lycopene on the risk of smoke-related diseases, including cancer and cardiovascular injury, have been stated in epidemiological studies. However, the experimental basis for such health benefits is not fully understood (Alberg 2002).

Flavonoids

Results of meta-analyses of various studies revealed that total dietary flavonoids and several flavonoid subclasses were associated with reduced risks of smoking-related cancers (Hae and Jeongseon 2013). In only the case–control studies, flavones, flavanones, isoflavones, and flavonol quercetin (a natural flavonoid widely distributed in a healthy human diet) were inversely associated with the risk of smoking-related cancers. The beneficial effects of flavonoids on cancer risk were more prominent among smokers than nonsmokers. Although the protective effects of dietary flavonoids may differ by cancer site among the smoking-related cancers, the results of each flavonoid subclasses were similar. Total flavonols and flavonol quercetin may be the most powerful agents for smoking-induced carcinogenesis. Generally, it is proposed that smokers might benefit from a flavonoid-rich diet. Another study also found that quercetin might be used not only in supporting bone regeneration in smokers but also in strengthening the bone metabolism in different pathogenesis (Braun et al. 2011).

Zinc

The reported differences in serum zinc concentrations between smokers and nonsmokers can reflect the duration and amount of smoking exposure. In one study, it was found that plasma zinc concentrations were unaffected by smoking; however, CuZn–SOD activity was higher in smokers. In another study, it was found that mean serum zinc was significantly lower in the smoking group than in the nonsmokers. In this study, it was suggested that lower serum zinc concentrations could reduce the zinc available for incorporation into CuZn–SOD and increase the risk of oxidative damage (Northrop-Clewes and Thurnham 2007).

Copper

Serum ceruloplasmin concentrations and erythrocyte CuZn–SOD activity are the two main indices of copper status that can be influenced by smoking. Scientific evidence has revealed that CuZn–SOD activity is consistently higher in smokers than nonsmokers, and the increases may have been part of the body's anti-inflammatory response to smoking. One explanation is that it has been shown to act as an acute-phase protein with antioxidant and anti-inflammatory properties; however, it is not clear yet (Northrop-Clewes and Thurnham 2007).

Selenium

The relationship between smoking and selenium status has not been studied extensively, and generally, it was found that lower plasma concentrations are associated with increased cigarette use. Specifically, it has been suggested that the lower activity of erythrocyte GSHPx in smokers may occur due to the lower concentrations of plasma selenium. These low concentrations may be influenced by several other factors, such as the negative impact of cadmium, a toxic heavy metal found in tobacco, on the bioavailability of dietary selenium and the increased expression of inflammatory mediators such as interleukin-1 (IL-1), IL-2, IL-6, and IL-8 in response to smoking, which can have an effect on the concentrations of plasma selenium (Northrop-Clewes and Thurnham 2007). There is some evidence to suggest that the lower serum selenium concentrations are associated with inflammation.

Iron

There is scientific interest in the direction that high iron status may have an etiological role in cardiovascular disease (CVD) and various cancers, since iron can promote the formation of FRs. Smoking appears to affect iron homeostasis mainly by causing changes in blood hemoglobin concentration. Serum iron, transferrin receptor (TfR), and ferritin concentrations are unaffected by smoking except in pregnancy, where there is evidence of increased erythropoiesis. Increased erythopoiesis causes lower iron saturation of plasma transferrin and probably results in lowering of iron stores (Northrop-Clewes and Thurnham 2007).

CASE OF ANTIOXIDANTS IN SUPPLEMENTATION STUDIES

Although observational studies have provided support for the potential health benefits of antioxidants to smokers, we still have relatively little direct experimental evidence from randomized trials. In this section, we present data from supplementation studies with antioxidants, alone or in combination.

Vitamin C Supplementation Studies

Several studies have demonstrated that a moderately large dose of vitamin C prevents cigarette smoke–induced oxidative damage, inflammation, and apoptosis by reducing and thereby inactivating p-benzoquinone (p-BQ) (Archita et al. 2012). Other studies in humans have looked at the effect of vitamin C supplementation on the ability of oxidation of LDLs, which is a risk factor for CVD. However, the supplementation is often in combination with supplements of vitamin E or β-carotene. The study group in these studies includes smokers and nonsmokers, and a significant reduction in the ability of oxidation of LDLs has been revealed. However, because of the use of multiple nutrients in the supplements, it is difficult to clarify and quantify the contribution of vitamin C. Where vitamin C was the only given nutrient in supplement dose, some studies found no effect while others found a significant reduction in the ability of oxidation of LDLs. The conclusion is that supplementing smokers with vitamin C might provide some protection against atherosclerosis; however, no biomarker can be related to any health endpoint.

Vitamin E Supplementation Studies

According to the results from the ATBC (Alpha-Tocopherol Beta-Carotene Cancer Prevention) study, no reduction in lung cancer or major coronary events was found in male smokers receiving α-tocopherol. In another study, the HOPE (Heart Outcomes Prevention Evaluation) study, the subgroup analysis of data showed that vitamin E alone had no apparent effect on cardiovascular or myocardial infarction outcomes or deaths from coronary heart disease or stroke among smokers. In a meta-analysis studying the effects of vitamin E on myocardial infarction, stroke, or death from cardiovascular causes in smokers from four large trials: ATBC, CHAOS (Cambridge Heart Antioxidant Study), GISSI (Gruppo Italiano per lo Studio della Sopravvivenza nell'Infarto Miocardico), and HOPE, it was found that the overall relative risk (RR) was 0.97 (95% CI, 0.9–1.02) during a 4–6-year period of supplementation, and thus, there was little effect on the outcomes measured (Mondul et al. 2011). However, in another study, γ-tocopherol-rich supplementation in combination with smoking cessation improved vascular endothelial function (Mah et al. 2013).

Non–Provitamin A Carotenoid Supplementation Studies

Scientific evidence suggests that lycopene may be protective against smoke-induced cell damage and has an important role in inflammatory processes. The results of one study with 2 μM lycopene indicated that this non–provitamin A carotenoid prevented cigarette smoke extract–induced IL-8 production through the inactivation of nuclear factor-κB (Rossella et al. 2014).

Combined Antioxidant Supplementation Studies

It has been stated that pharmacological interventions with nonselective antioxidants usually fail to be an effective strategy for the prevention and treatment of CVD caused by smoking; thus, a combined application of antioxidants may be needed (Bernhard and Wang 2007). Data from a study with combined α-tocopherol and ascorbic acid supplementation showed protective effects against smoking-induced lung lesions in ferrets (Kim et al. 2012). Another study showed that oral supplementation (with commonly available antioxidants, vitamins, and omega-3 fatty acids) induced metabolomic changes in cigarette smokers, and these effects were different between smokers and nonsmokers (Spitale et al. 2012).

Selenium Supplementation Studies

Data from the Nutritional Prevention of Cancer Trial, a randomized clinical trial designed to evaluate the efficacy of selenium in preventing nonmelanoma skin cancer in the United States, stated that supplementation with 200 μg selenium daily was associated with a significantly lower risk of both total and prostate cancer incidence in former smokers; nonsignificantly lower risks were found in current and nonsmokers who were supplemented (Northrop-Clewes and Thurnham 2007).

CONCLUSION

It is increasingly evident that a good diet influences the development and treatment of diseases. Furthermore, epidemiological studies have shown the association between moderate consumption of certain foods and reduced incidence of various diseases. These observations have attracted considerable interest in studying the properties of substances inherent in the chemical composition of food. Among the characteristics of these substances is their antioxidant activity, associated with the elimination of FRs and therefore with the prevention of the early stages that can trigger degenerative diseases. In this regard, it is important to continue the study of dietary antioxidants concerning the activity they may have in human diseases, paying attention to the substances, primarily natural antioxidants of food, and the synthetic way to assess their protective effect on the body. Finally, a novel strategy for the prevention and treatment of diseases caused by smoking, relying on a combined application of antioxidants, substitution of important factors for human oxidant defense, and metal-detoxifying agents, may be proposed.

REFERENCES

Alberg, A. 2002. The influence of cigarette smoking on circulating concentrations of antioxidant micronutrients. *Toxicology.* 180(2):121–37.

Archita, D. et al. 2012. Molecular and cellular mechanisms of cigarette smoke-induced myocardial injury: Prevention by vitamin C. *Public Lib Sci.* 7(9):e44151.

Bernhard, D., Wang, X.L. 2007. Smoking, oxidative stress and cardiovascular diseases—Do anti-oxidative therapies fail? *Curr Med Chem.* 14(16):1703–12.

Braun, K.F. et al. 2011. Quercetin protects primary human osteoblasts exposed to cigarette smoke through activation of the antioxidative enzymes HO-1 and SOD-1. *Sci World J.* 11:2348–57. doi: 10.1100/2011/471426.

Bruno, R.S., Maret, G.T. 2005. Cigarette smoke alters human vitamin E requirements. *J Nutr.* 135(4):671–4.

Chalmers, A. 1999. Smoking and oxidative stress. *Am J Clin Nutr.* 69(3):572.

Comandini, A. et al. 2010. Markers of anti-oxidant response in tobacco smoke exposed subjects: A data-mining review. *Pulm Pharmacol Ther.* 23(6):482–92. doi: 10.1016/j.pupt.2010.05.006.

Da Costa, L.A. et al. 2012. Genetic determinants of dietary antioxidant status. *Prog Mol Biol Transl Sci.* 108:179–200. doi: 10.1016/B978-0-12-398397-8.00008-3.pdf.

Hae, D.W., Jeongseon, K. 2013. Dietary flavonoid intake and smoking-related cancer risk: A meta-analysis. *PLoS One.* 8:e75604. doi: 10.1371/journal.pone.0075604.

Jakob, U., Reichmann, D. 2013. *Oxidative Stress and Redox Regulation.* Springer, New York.

Kelly, G. 2002a. The interaction of cigarette smoking and antioxidants. Part 2: Alpha-tocopherol. *Altern Med Rev.* 7(6):500–11.

Kelly, G. 2002b. The interaction of cigarette smoking and antioxidants. Part I: Diet and carotenoids. *Altern Med Rev.* 7(5):370–88.

Kelly, G. 2003. The interaction of cigarette smoking and antioxidants. Part III: Ascorbic acid. *Altern Med Rev.* 8(1):43–54.

Kim, Y. et al. 2012. Combined α-tocopherol and ascorbic acid protects against smoke-induced lung squamous metaplasia in ferrets. *Lung Cancer.* 75(1):15–23. doi: 10.1016/j.lungcan.2011.05.017.

Kinnula, V.L. 2005. Focus on antioxidant enzymes and antioxidant strategies in smoking related airway diseases. *Thorax.* 60(8):693–700.

Mah, E. et al. 2013. γ-Tocopherol-rich supplementation additively improves vascular endothelial function during smoking cessation. *Free Radic Biol Med.* 65:1291–9. doi: 10.1016/j.freeradbiomed.2013.09.016.

May, J.M. 2000. How does ascorbic acid prevent endothelial dysfunction? *Free Radic Biol Med.* 28(9):1421–9.

Min, E. et al. 2011. Lung glutathione adaptive responses to cigarette smoke exposure. *Respir Res.* 7(12):133. doi: 10.1186/1465-9921-12-133.

Mondul, A.M. et al. 2011. Supplementation with alpha-tocopherol or beta-carotene reduces serum concentrations of vascular endothelial growth factor-D, but Not -A or -C, in male smokers. *J Nutr.* 141(11):2030–4. doi: 10.3945/jn.111.143669.

National Institutes of Health. 2013. *Vitamin A. Fact Sheet for Health Professionals.* Available at: http://ods.od.nih.gov/factsheets/VitaminA-HealthProfessional/.

Northrop-Clewes, C.A., Thurnham, D.I. 2007. Monitoring micronutrients in cigarette smokers. *Clin Chim Acta.* 377:14–38. doi: 10.1016/j.cca.2006.08.028.

Pryor, W.A. et al. 1983. Electron-spin resonance study of mainstream and sidestream cigarette smoke: Nature of the free radicals in gas-phase smoke and in cigarette tar. *Environ Health Perspect.* 47:345–55.

Rahal, A. et al. 2014. Oxidative stress, prooxidants, and antioxidants: The interplay. *BioMed Res Int* 2014:761264, 19 pp.

Rahman, I. et al. 2006. Oxidant and antioxidant balance in the airways and airway diseases. *Eur J Pharmacol.* 533(1–3):222–39.

Romero, C.A. et al. 2013. The exogenous antioxidants. In *Oxidative Stress and Chronic Degenerative Diseases—A Role For Antioxidants*, ed. J.A. Morales-González. doi: 10.5772/52490. InTech, Rijeka, Croatia. Available at http://www.intechopen.com/books/oxidative-stress-and-chronic-degenerative-diseases-a-role-for-antioxidants/the-exogenous-antioxidants.

Rossella, E.S. et al. 2014. Retraction: Lycopene inhibits NF-kB-mediated IL-8 expression and changes redox and PPARγ signalling in cigarette smoke–stimulated macrophages. *PLoS One.* 9(7):e102411. doi: 10.1371/journal.pone.0102411.

Siasos, G. et al. 2014. Smoking and atherosclerosis: Mechanisms of disease and new therapeutic approaches. *Curr Med Chem.* 21(34):3936–48.

Spitale, R.C. et al. 2012. Differential effects of dietary supplements on metabolomic profile of smokers versus non-smokers. *Genome Med.* 4(2):14. doi: 10.1186/gm313.

Stolzenberg, R.Z. et al. 2009. Vitamin E intake, a-tocopherol status, and pancreatic cancer in a cohort of male smokers. *Am J Clin Nutr.* 89:584–91.

Valavanidis, A. et al. 2009. Tobacco smoke: Involvement of reactive oxygen species and stable free radicals in mechanisms of oxidative damage, carcinogenesis and synergistic effects with other respirable particles. *Int J Environ Res Public Health.* 6(2):445–62.

van der Vaart, H. et al. 2004. Acute effects of cigarette smoke on inflammation and oxidative stress: A review. *Thorax.* 59:713–21.

Vardavas, C.I. et al. 2008. Smoking status in relation to serum folate and dietary vitamin intake. *Tob Induc Dis.* 4:8. doi: 10.1186/1617-9625-4-8.

Widome, R. et al. 2010. Passive smoke exposure and circulating carotenoids in the CARDIA study. *Ann Nutr Metab.* 56(2):113–8. doi: 10.1159/000277662.

Wooten, J.B., Chouchane, S., and McGrath, T.E. 2006. Tobacco smoke constituents affecting oxidative stress. In *Cigarette Smoke and Oxidative Stress*, eds. B. Halliwell, H. Poulson. Springer, New York. pp. 6–46.

Zuo, L. et al. 2014. Interrelated role of cigarette smoking, oxidative stress, and immune response in COPD and corresponding treatments. *Am J Physiol Lung Cell Mol Physiol.* 307(3):L205–18.

7 Physical Exercise

Mustafa Atalay, Jani Lappalainen,
Ayhan Korkmaz, and Chandan K. Sen

CONTENTS

Introduction 103
Antioxidants and General Health 104
Need for Antioxidant Supplementation for Physically Active Individuals 104
Endogenous Antioxidants 106
    Glutathione 106
    Lipoic Acid 107
Exogenous Antioxidants 109
    Vitamins C and E 109
    Flavonoids 110
Conclusions 111
References 111

INTRODUCTION

Physical exercise is a cornerstone of good health, and it also plays a key role in the primary prevention of lifestyle-related diseases. Generation of reactive oxygen species (ROS) is a constant process of normal cellular function. Oxidative stress, an imbalance of the generation of ROS and antioxidant defense capacity, and perturbation of redox control of cellular events, is closely related to physiological aging and the pathophysiology of a wide range of diseases (Radak et al. 2013; Sen and Packer 2000). During heavy physical exercise, the oxygen flux to active skeletal muscles is remarkably increased. Such acceleration in the oxidative metabolism is associated with increased production of ROS that are hazardous to living organisms. Oxidative insult is not only mediated by macromolecular oxidative damage but also through the disruption of the cellular redox homeostasis. At moderate concentrations, however, ROS and other related reactive molecules play an important role in the regulation of cellular signaling. ROS act as secondary messengers to control a variety of vital processes. Therefore, many of the ROS-mediated responses protect against oxidative and metabolic stress and constitute a "redox homeostasis" (Sen 2001).

In biological systems, a variety of endogenous antioxidants have evolved to cope with oxidative stress, acting in concert to quench ROS and to maintain redox homeostasis and tissue protection. This synergism between several endogenous and dietary antioxidants is essential for an effective protection. Although no solid scientific evidence exists on the benefits of antioxidant supplementations to exercise performance, multivitamins are widely used among athletes in hope that these agents may be effective (Atalay et al. 2006). The aim of this chapter is to briefly discuss the role of endogenous and exogenous antioxidants on physical exercise and human performance. Specifically, we will focus on the need, advantages, and disadvantages of antioxidant supplements for the physically active population and give a special emphasis on thiol antioxidants, which play a key role in cellular redox regulation.

ANTIOXIDANTS AND GENERAL HEALTH

There is a general consensus in the mechanistic and epidemiologic studies that an adequate and balanced intake of dietary antioxidants prevents the formation of ROS and contributes to lowering the risk of several common diseases. The frequent use of natural sources of antioxidant nutrients in the Mediterranean diet, together with unsaturated fats, low proportion of simple sugars, and high content of dietary fibers, appear to account for a lower risk of certain types of cancer as well as chronic heart disease (Castro-Quezada et al. 2014). Epidemiological evidence suggests protection of cardiovascular disease by dietary intake of flavonoids (Basu et al. 2010). Although several epidemiological studies have pointed out an inverse association between dietary intake of vitamin C, vitamin E, and β-carotene and cardiovascular disease (Whayne and Maulik 2012), the overall results of published trials of vitamin E and β-carotene supplementations have failed to confirm any protective effect on mortality. In agreement with previous reports, a meta-analysis of 68 randomized antioxidant supplement trials (a total of 232,606 human participants) concluded that dietary supplementation with β-carotene, vitamin A, and vitamin E above the recommended daily allowance (RDA) does not improve health outcomes and may increase mortality (Bjelakovic et al. 2007). In contrast, a recent meta-analysis of 15 trials reporting data on 188,209 participants indicated that antioxidant vitamin supplementation as compared with placebo did not provide any overall protection against major cardiovascular events (Ye et al. 2013). Therefore, in contrast to the benefits of adequate antioxidant intake through a balanced and healthy diet, the use of antioxidant supplements may even exert a negative impact on general health.

NEED FOR ANTIOXIDANT SUPPLEMENTATION FOR PHYSICALLY ACTIVE INDIVIDUALS

It is a common practice for athletes to use antioxidant supplements with the notion that they prevent the deleterious effects of exercise-induced oxidative stress, hasten the recovery of muscle function, and improve performance (Atalay et al. 2006; Peternelj and Coombes 2011). Athletes may have ambiguous perceptions and receive misinformation about antioxidant supplementation in the public press: most of the physically active persons believe that they may have higher requirements of antioxidants than those who are sedentary. Therefore, physically active persons are more likely to use diverse antioxidant supplements compared with the overall prevalence in the general population (Rock 2007). In a recent study, 30% of athletes were reported to use more than two supplements (Tscholl et al. 2010). Most surprisingly, among elite athletes aged 12 to 21 years, the average supplement use was even higher than what was observed in adult athletes with, on an average, 2.96 products used (Dascombe et al. 2010). Although a supplement may contain a dosage close to the RDA, the use of multiple supplements may result in cumulative, and sometimes an excess, intake of one or more nutrients. Despite the frequent use of antioxidant supplements among the physically active population, until now there has been no convincing scientific evidence to prove the presumption that antioxidant supplementations enhance sport performance, increase the health benefits of exercise, or decrease sports injuries. Furthermore, the obtained results are conflicting, and because of the diverse structure and biological effects of the antioxidant compounds, generalizing any individual supplementation result to all antioxidant supplements may be problematic. The reasons behind the null findings or inconsistent results among the studies employing simultaneous exercise and supplementation interventions could be explained by several factors: differences in exercise protocols; characteristics of the subject population, including sex, age, prior training, and physical activity status; dosage, form, duration, and timing of the supplementation; and the method used to assess the outcomes of the intervention.

Up until now, there has been no solid evidence in the literature demonstrating a higher need for antioxidants in athletes. Most of the nutrition surveys in the United States indicate that athletes have adequate intake of vitamin C. The vitamin C consumption for male athletes ranges from 95 to 520 mg/day, whereas the consumption range for females is from 55 to 230 mg/day (Lukaski 2004), while the current dietary reference intakes (DRIs) of vitamin C are 90 mg/day for males and 75 mg/dL for females of different adult age groups (U.S. Department of Health and Human Services and the U.S. Department of Agriculture 2010). However, inadequate intake of vitamin C in certain athlete groups involved with heavy training load and exposed to physiologic stressors, including infection, cigarette smoke, high altitude, and extreme environmental temperatures, increase requirements for vitamin C (Lukaski 2004). Nonetheless, there has not been any solid evidence to support the idea that regular exercise increases the requirement for vitamin C in athletes (Peake 2003), and plasma vitamin C levels of athletes are usually within the normal ranges. Only a small fraction of athletes have plasma vitamin C values less than the lower limits or at the lower end of the range of normal values (Lukaski 2004). Regarding the vitamin E levels according to the National Health and Nutrition Examination Survey III (NHANES III) (Ford and Sowell 1999), mean intakes of α-tocopherol of the U.S. population meet and probably exceed the RDA of 15 mg/day when corrections are applied for underreporting of food intake. Although physically active people generally consume vitamin E within the limits of DRI or higher (Economos et al. 1993), an early study showed that vitamin E intake was greater among athletes than sedentary people (Guilland et al. 1989). Nevertheless, a certain group of athletes having limitation of their food intake for esthetical purposes or competitive limitations may have inadequate intake of vitamin E (Guilland et al. 1989; Lukaski 2004). Although physical activity and increased intake of polyunsaturated fatty acids may induce oxidative stress and increase the need for vitamin E, its deficiency is rare among the physically active population and athletes consuming balanced diets.

ENDOGENOUS ANTIOXIDANTS

GLUTATHIONE

The endogenous thiols, specifically glutathione (GSH), play a central role in the antioxidant defenses that control cellular events and regulate protection against oxidative stress (Radak et al. 2013), a condition that alters normal redox control of cellular signaling, more specifically by disruption of thiol redox circuits (Jones 2006). In addition to its central role in supporting a large network of antioxidant defense, GSH has various biological functions, including regulation of receptors, enzyme activity, short-term storage of cysteine, protein structure, cell growth, proliferation, apoptosis, transcription factors, and ultimately redox-sensitive signal transduction (Sen 2000).

Glutathione (L-γ-glutamyl-L-cysteinylglycine) is the predominant intracellular thiol. GSH plays an essential role in antioxidant protection and provides an appropriate reducing milieu inside the cell directly, and also by regenerating crucial exogenous antioxidants such as vitamins E and C from their respective oxidized forms (Radak et al. 2013). During strenuous physical exercise where the oxygen consumption is increased many fold, when ROS is detoxified, GSH is oxidized, and, as a consequence, the disulfide glutathione (GSSG) accumulates. The balance of oxidized to reduced glutathione (GSSG/GSH) acts as a "redox control node" to regulate "sulfur switches" for responses to acute exercise-induced oxidative stress, and also to develop adaptations of various defense mechanisms during regular physical training.

GSH can either directly scavenge ROS, or enzymatically via GSH peroxidases (GSHPx) and GSH transhydrogenases, while GSH itself is oxidized to GSSG. Intracellular GSSG, thus formed, may be reduced back to GSH by GSSG reductase, or released to the extracellular compartment (Sen 2000). Most of the GSHPx, but not all, are selenium dependent. Because selenium is a cofactor of most of the subtypes of GSHPx, it has gained considerable attention as a key antioxidant. Nevertheless, one has to keep in mind that selenium itself is not a potent antioxidant but only a component of GSH-dependent antioxidant defense. Supplementation of selenium and other trace minerals is not generally necessary in well-nourished populations; however, possible deficiencies of selenium should be avoided.

GSH is synthesized in the liver and also in skeletal muscle; however, intact GSH is usually not transportable to intracellular compartments, and therefore, strategies to increase tissue GSH levels through various administration protocols have ended in failures. Furthermore, data on the role of endogenous glutathione on exercise performance, especially for the endurance capacity, are limited. In an early work of our group, we investigated the relative role of exogenous GSH and N-acetylcysteine (NAC), as well as endogenous GSH, on exercise-induced oxidative stress and exercise performance in rats. Intraperitoneal administration of GSH neither affected tissue GSH levels nor reduced oxidative stress. Furthermore, GSH and NAC administration did not influence exercise performance measured as time to exhaustion during treadmill running. In contrast, GSH depletion in rats decreased endurance time to exhaustion by half with concomitant increase of oxidative stress in all the tissues examined (Sen et al. 1994). Although there is a controversial report in the literature regarding the impact of GSH deficiency on prolonged swimming performance in mice (Leeuwenburgh and Ji 1995), one may still postulate that endogenous GSH not only plays a critical role in the tissue protection against exercise-induced oxidative stress but also determines exercise performance.

ROS act as important mediators of the signal transduction pathways for several physiological functions, including immune response and inflammation. In several studies, cytokine response was represented with the commonly studied cytokine interleukin-6 (IL-6). In addition to inflammatory and immune modulatory functions, IL-6 is also a skeletal muscle secreted myokine and tightly related with the skeletal muscle energy availability during strenuous exercise (Pedersen 2012). In an early study, antioxidant supplementation with vitamins E, A, and C, allopurinol, and NAC attenuated plasma IL-6 and other cytokine responses to exercise in humans (Vassilakopoulos et al. 2003). In agreement with these findings, we have observed that α-lipoic acid decreased hydrogen peroxide-induced IL-6 secretion from L6 myoblasts (Atalay et al. unpublished observations). Hence, the blunting effect of antioxidants on IL-6 levels may not only be interpreted as an anti-inflammatory effect; instead, antioxidants can decrease energy availability to working muscle and may potentially decrease exercise performance. Similarly, excess availability of antioxidants may suppress other adaptive responses of physical training, such as stress protein expression. Heat shock proteins (HSPs), a group of stress-regulated proteins that contribute to cellular protection and promote cell survival, are induced by various stresses, including exhaustive physical exercise (Fehrenbach and Northoff 2001). A large number of studies showed that both acute exercise and endurance training induce HSP expression and enhance tissue protection (Atalay et al. 2004). Previous studies of our group and others showed that antioxidant supplementations blunt exercise induced increases of HSPs (Khassaf et al. 2003; Oksala et al. 2006). Vitamin C supplementation increased baseline expression but attenuated acute exercise-induced HSP expression in humans (Khassaf et al. 2003). Co-supplementation of vitamins C and E attenuated moderately exercise-induced HSP72 expression in the elderly population (Simar et al. 2012).

Lipoic Acid

α-Lipoic acid is a natural thiol antioxidant and redox modulator that has been widely used as a therapeutic agent in many oxidative stress-associated diseases, including diabetes and diabetic complications. α-Lipoic acid plays an important role in antioxidant defense; in addition to its potent antioxidant properties as a direct scavenger of various ROS, it also increases GSH synthesis and act together with vitamin C to contribute to the regeneration of vitamin E. As an essential coenzyme for pyruvate dehydrogenase and α-ketoglutarate dehydrogenase, α-lipoic acid plays a critical role in mitochondrial energy metabolism, ultimately resulting in the production of adenosine triphosphate, ATP (Petersen Shay et al. 2008). The effects of α-lipoic acid on stress protein response were diverse in our studies using different animal models and different dosages of α-lipoic acid. In rats, high dosages of α-lipoic acid (150 mg/kg intragastrically) decreased the levels of skeletal muscle, liver, and kidney HSP72 and of the antioxidant stress protein heme oxygenase-1 (HSP32, HO-1) in healthy as well in diabetic rats (our unpublished observations); however, α-lipoic acid supplementation increased hepatic HSP60 levels (Oksala et al. 2006). On the other hand, in regularly trained horses, 5-week supplementation of low-dose α-lipoic acid (25 mg/kg body weight/day) enhanced the skeletal muscle HSP response (Kinnunen et al. 2009a). One can postulate that high doses of antioxidant supplementations may result in a decline in HSP response to exercise, which may impair tissue protection and increase tissue damage that ultimately reduces the health benefits of exercise.

Despite the reported unfavorable effects of antioxidant supplementations to decrease health benefits and adaptations of exercise training, we observed beneficial effects of low-dose α-lipoic acid supplementation (25 mg/kg body weight/day) on performance and exercise-induced muscle damage in horse (Kinnunen et al. 2009b). As a result of 5-week α-lipoic acid supplementation, we found a decreased rate of lactate formation during exercise and simultaneously increased skeletal muscle citrate synthase activity, a key indicator of muscle oxidative metabolism. These observations may be explained by the impact of α-lipoic acid on the enzymes of oxidative metabolism in mitochondria: by improving their cofactor availability, which, in turn, may increase oxidative capacity of the skeletal muscle and lead to improved performance in endurance events (Sen and Packer 2000). However, our group has previously reported that intragastrically supplemented high doses of α-lipoic acid (150 mg/kg) did not increase the levels of lipoyllysine in rat skeletal muscle (Khanna et al. 1998). Lipoyllysine is the bound form of α-lipoic acid and a cofactor of pyruvate dehydrogenase and α-ketoglutarate dehydrogenase in skeletal muscle (Khanna et al. 1998). On the other hand, α-lipoic acid enhances glucose uptake by the muscle cells by increasing glucose transporters in the plasma membrane (Sen and Packer 2000). Enhanced glucose metabolism, in turn, may increase pyruvate availability for the tricarboxylic acid cycle and result in increased oxidative capacity of the muscles (Savitha et al. 2005). In addition, low-dose α-lipoic acid supplementation attenuated plasma creatine kinase levels after exercise and during recovery, which indicates a less exercise-induced muscle damage (Kinnunen et al. 2009b). In addition, α-lipoic acid supplementation attenuated exercise-induced oxidative stress as evident by directly measured lower free radical signals and also by lower lipid peroxidation by-products in horses (Kinnunen et al. 2009b) and in humans (Zembron-Lacny et al. 2007).

On the other hand, in another study (Matsumoto et al. 2012), the effects of 14 weeks of cosupplementation of α-lipoic acid with α-tocopherol and treadmill exercise on myocardial and vascular endothelium gene expression were investigated in rats. Antioxidant supplementation upregulated and exercise downregulated the expression of the *RAS homolog gene family member A* (*RhoA*), a gene involved in cardiovascular disease progression. The combination of supplementation and exercise abolished the exercise-mediated downregulation of *RhoA* expression. These findings pointed out an unfavorable effect of antioxidant supplementation on exercise-induced cardiovascular protection. Consistent with these findings, antioxidant supplementation of vitamins C and E and α-lipoic acid reversed the beneficial effect of 6 weeks of knee-extensor exercise training that had reduced systolic blood pressure and also blunted training-induced improvements in vascular function, measured as flow-mediated vasodilation (Wray et al. 2009).

Furthermore, in a recent study, the therapeutic role of α-lipoic acid supplementation in combination with moderate-intensity aerobic exercise on metabolic disturbances was examined in obese subjects with impaired glucose tolerance (McNeilly et al. 2011). Surprisingly, a 12-week supplementation period with a relatively high dose of α-lipoic acid (1 g/day) increased low-density lipoprotein (LDL) oxidation, which indicates increased atherogenesis. Nevertheless, exercise training and α-lipoic acid in combination attenuated LDL oxidation. Therefore, apart from the general trend of results that antioxidants diminish the health benefits of exercise, in this study, exercise training offset the adverse effect of antioxidant supplementation on LDL atherogenicity. However, because there was no exercise training group independent of antioxidant supplementation, one cannot make any conclusion whether α-lipoic acid supplementation blunted or potentiated the health benefits of exercise training (McNeilly et al. 2011). In addition, the same study found no impact of α-lipoic acid alone or in combination with exercise training on glycemic control, which is in total disagreement with previous studies that have pointed out the beneficial role of α-lipoic acid on glucose transport and consequently on glycemic regulation (Estrada et al. 1996).

In early animal studies, allopurinol has been found to attenuate the exercise-induced increase of XO activity and ROS formation, which was associated with a decreased activation of mitogen-activated protein kinases (MAPKs) and blunted DNA-binding of nuclear factor kappa B (NF-κB) (Gomez-Cabrera et al. 2006). MAPKs regulate cell development and survival in response to extracellular stimuli, including oxidative stress. The transcription factor NF-κB is not only implicated in the regulation of inflammatory responses and innate immune response, but also control the enzymes such as Mn-superoxide dismutase (Mn SOD) and nitric oxide synthases (eNOS and iNOS). Therefore, impairing the effects of exercise training by antioxidant supplementation on MAPKs and NF-κB would affect these positive benefits. Consistent with these assumptions, administration of allopurinol before a marathon race suppressed the exercise-induced increase of antioxidant enzyme expression in humans (Gomez-Cabrera et al. 2006).

EXOGENOUS ANTIOXIDANTS

VITAMINS C AND E

The antioxidants vitamins C and E are among the most commonly consumed supplements (Kennedy et al. 2013), and often taken in large doses by athletes in belief of their potential protective effect against muscle damage. In the body, vitamins C and E act synergistically, with vitamin E acting as the primary antioxidant; the resulting vitamin E radical is regenerated back to vitamin E at the expense of vitamin C. Although vitamin C can decrease indices of oxidative stress taken at doses of 200 to 1000 mg/day (Braakhuis 2012), there is no convincing supporting evidence for a role of vitamin C and/or vitamin E in protecting against muscle damage (McGinley et al. 2009).

It could be speculated that higher intakes of vitamin C for short periods, such as onset of illness or during training camps, may provide health benefit for improved immunity. Indeed, a recent meta-analysis supports the notion that to reduce the incidence of colds, at least 200 mg of vitamin C per day may be useful for people exposed to brief periods of severe physical exercise (Hemila and Chalker 2013).

Antioxidant supplementation with vitamins C and E has shown to prevent the induction of molecular regulators of insulin sensitivity and endogenous antioxidant defense by physical exercise (Ristow et al. 2009). At large doses, e.g., ≥1000 mg/day, vitamin C appears to reduce training-induced adaptations by reducing mitochondrial biogenesis (Ristow et al. 2009), indicating that the exercise-induced increase in ROS is necessary for physiological adaptations. In a recent study by Paulsen et al. (2014), a combination of vitamin C and E supplementation ingested shortly before and after exercise training hampered cellular adaptions in the exercised muscles. Although this did not translate to changes in the physical performance outcomes, the authors advocate caution when considering antioxidant supplementation combined with endurance exercise. Although high doses of vitamin C have not been shown to result in impaired exercise performance outcomes (Roberts et al. 2011), there is growing evidence of the negative effects of antioxidant supplementation on exercise performance (Nikolaidis et al. 2012). It is likely that a smaller dose of about 200 to 500 mg/day vitamin C may be sufficient to reduce oxidative stress without hampering mitochondrial training adaptations (Braakhuis 2012; Yfanti et al. 2010).

As discussed by Nikolaidis et al. (2012), the inherent complexity of redox biochemistry signifies the difficulty in providing unidirectional predictions after antioxidant supplementation; thus, a permanent intake of supraphysiological dosages of vitamin C and/or E cannot be recommended to healthy, exercising individuals.

FLAVONOIDS

Flavonoids (plant polyphenols) are well-established antioxidants, with direct ROS-scavenging and chain-breaking properties. Current evidence indicates that the protective actions of polyphenols are mainly through the modulation of cellular signaling cascades by binding to specific target proteins and less via their potent antioxidant properties (Quideau et al. 2011). Among a large number of flavonoids, quercetin has been recognized with its several purported physiological benefits to health. Quercetin is not only a cardioprotective, anticarcinogenic, antioxidant, and antiapoptotic agent, but has also been proposed to exhibit ergogenic properties. On the other hand, human studies examining the effects of quercetin on exercise performance do not indicate a high level of efficacy. A recent meta-analysis indicated that quercetin supplementation in human subjects actually exerts a favorable effect on endurance capacity (calculated as combining VO_{2max} and endurance exercise performance). However, the ergogenic effect was small and corresponded to an approximately 3% improvement over placebo. In subgroup meta-analysis, no significant difference was found for the effects of quercetin on endurance exercise performance and VO_{2max}. Furthermore, meta-regression analyses showed that variation in the study effect size was not significantly associated with subjects' fitness level or plasma quercetin concentration (Kressler et al. 2011).

Sirtuins comprise a family of NAD^+-dependent deacylases that promote longevity and mediate many of the beneficial effects of calorie restriction. Recently, sirtuins have been postulated as redox-dependent metabolic sensors (Radak et al. 2013).

Among the polyphenolic compounds, resveratrol has been identified as the most potent inducer of sirtuin-1 (SIRT1) and AMP-activated protein kinase (AMPK), and reported to increase the lifespan of organisms via a wide range of processes, including suppression of apoptosis and inflammation or enhancing DNA repair (Hubbard and Sinclair 2014). Animal studies provided evidence that resveratrol has effects similar to those observed with exercise training: increases mitochondrial mass, increases endurance capacity, and induces muscle fiber shift to red type with greater aerobic capacity (Price et al. 2012). In human studies, the effect of resveratrol is controversial; in a recent study with healthy aged subjects, resveratrol did not elicit metabolic improvements but, in contrast, impaired the observed exercise training–induced improvements in the markers of inflammation and oxidative stress in skeletal muscle (Olesen et al. 2014).

CONCLUSIONS

Compelling evidence indicates that exercise-induced ROS production is crucial to develop training response and adaptations by promoting the expression of numerous skeletal muscle proteins, including antioxidant and HSP defenses, and regulating glucose homeostasis and mitochondrial function. Although epidemiological evidence suggests that adequate intakes of antioxidant micronutrients may help protect against life-threatening diseases, the general trend of published studies does not support the notion that antioxidant supplementation over a balanced diet rich in fruits and vegetables is beneficial to human health.

Despite a perceived need of antioxidant supplements to attenuate exercise-induced oxidative damage, a number of studies pointed out that excess antioxidant intake through antioxidant supplementation generally does not improve physical performance or potentiate health outcomes of physical exercise. In contrast, supraphysiological dosages of antioxidant supplementations may interfere with ROS-mediated cell signaling and blunt the positive effects of exercise. According to current knowledge, a nutritional approach of adequate intake of antioxidant nutrients through a healthy diet remains to be the safest strategy to minimize exercise-induced oxidative insult and sustain high performance.

REFERENCES

Atalay, M., Oksala, N. K. J., Laaksonen, D. E. et al. 2004. Exercise training modulates heat shock protein response in diabetic rats. *Journal of Applied Physiology* 97:605–11.

Atalay, M., Lappalainen, J. and Sen, C. K. 2006. Dietary antioxidants for the athlete. *Current Sports Medicine Reports* 5:182–6.

Basu, A., Rhone, M. and Lyons, T. J. 2010. Berries: Emerging impact on cardiovascular health. *Nutrition Reviews* 68:168–77.

Bjelakovic, G., Nikolova, D., Gluud, L. L., Simonetti, R. G. and Gluud, C. 2007. Mortality in randomized trials of antioxidant supplements for primary and secondary prevention: Systematic review and meta-analysis. *JAMA: The Journal of the American Medical Association* 297:842–57.

Braakhuis, A. J. 2012. Effect of vitamin C supplements on physical performance. *Current Sports Medicine Reports* 11:180–4.

Castro-Quezada, I., Roman-Vinas, B. and Serra-Majem, L. 2014. The Mediterranean diet and nutritional adequacy: A review. *Nutrients* 6:231–48.

Dascombe, B. J., Karunaratna, M., Cartoon, J., Fergie, B. and Goodman, C. 2010. Nutritional supplementation habits and perceptions of elite athletes within a state-based sporting institute. *Journal of Science and Medicine in Sport* 13:274–80.

Economos, C. D., Bortz, S. S. and Nelson, M. E. 1993. Nutritional practices of elite athletes. Practical recommendations. *Sports Medicine* 16:381–99.

Estrada, D. E., Ewart, H. S., Tsakiridis, T. et al. 1996. Stimulation of glucose uptake by the natural coenzyme alpha-lipoic acid/thioctic acid: Participation of elements of the insulin signaling pathway. *Diabetes* 45:1798–804.

Fehrenbach, E. and Northoff, H. 2001. Free radicals, exercise, apoptosis, and heat shock proteins. *Exercise Immunology Review* 7:66–89.

Ford, E. S. and Sowell, A. 1999. Serum alpha-tocopherol status in the United States population: Findings from the Third National Health and Nutrition Examination Survey. *American Journal of Epidemiology* 150:290–300.

Gomez-Cabrera, M. C., Martinez, A., Santangelo, G., Pallardo, F. V., Sastre, J. and Vina, J. 2006. Oxidative stress in marathon runners: Interest of antioxidant supplementation. *British Journal of Nutrition* 96 Suppl. 1:S31–3.

Guilland, J. C., Penaranda, T., Gallet, C., Boggio, V., Fuchs, F. and Klepping, J. 1989. Vitamin status of young athletes including the effects of supplementation. *Medicine and Science in Sports and Exercise* 21:441–9.

Hemila, H. and Chalker, E. 2013. Vitamin C for preventing and treating the common cold. *Cochrane Database Systematic Reviews* 1:CD000980.

Hubbard, B. P. and Sinclair, D. A. 2014. Small molecule SIRT1 activators for the treatment of aging and age-related diseases. *Trends in Pharmacological Sciences* 35:146–54.

Jones, D. P. 2006. Redefining oxidative stress. *Antioxidants and Redox Signaling* 8:1865–79.

Kennedy, E. T., Luo, H. and Houser, R. F. 2013. Dietary supplement use pattern of U.S. adult population in the 2007–2008 National Health and Nutrition Examination Survey (NHANES). *Ecological Food Nutrition* 52:76–84.

Khanna, S., Atalay, M., Lodge, J. K. et al. 1998. Skeletal muscle and liver lipoyllysine content in response to exercise, training and dietary alpha-lipoic acid supplementation. *Biochemistry and Molecular Biology International* 46:297–306.

Khassaf, M., McArdle, A., Esanu, C. et al. 2003. Effect of vitamin C supplements on antioxidant defence and stress proteins in human lymphocytes and skeletal muscle. *Journal of Physiology* 549:645–52.

Kinnunen, S., Hyyppa, S., Oksala, N. et al. 2009a. alpha-Lipoic acid supplementation enhances heat shock protein production and decreases post exercise lactic acid concentrations in exercised standardbred trotters. *Research in Veterinary Science* 87:462–7.

Kinnunen, S., Oksala, N., Hyyppa, S. et al. 2009b. alpha-Lipoic acid modulates thiol antioxidant defenses and attenuates exercise-induced oxidative stress in standardbred trotters. *Free Radical Research* 43:697–705.

Kressler, J., Millard-Stafford, M. and Warren, G. L. 2011. Quercetin and endurance exercise capacity: A systematic review and meta-analysis. *Medicine and Science in Sports and Exercise* 43:2396–404.

Leeuwenburgh, C. and Ji, L. L. 1995. Glutathione depletion in rested and exercised mice: Biochemical consequence and adaptation. *Archives of Biochemistry and Biophysics* 316:941–9.

Lukaski, H. C. 2004. Vitamin and mineral status: Effects on physical performance. *Nutrition* 20:632–44.

Matsumoto, A., Mason, S. R., Flatscher-Bader, T. et al. 2012. Effects of exercise and antioxidant supplementation on endothelial gene expression. *International Journal of Cardiology* 158:59–65.

McGinley, C., Shafat, A. and Donnelly, A. E. 2009. Does antioxidant vitamin supplementation protect against muscle damage? *Sports Medicine* 39:1011–32.

McNeilly, A. M., Davison, G. W., Murphy, M. H. et al. 2011. Effect of alpha-lipoic acid and exercise training on cardiovascular disease risk in obesity with impaired glucose tolerance. *Lipids in Health and Disease* 10:217.

Nikolaidis, M. G., Kerksick, C. M., Lamprecht, M. and McAnulty, S. R. 2012. Does vitamin C and E supplementation impair the favorable adaptations of regular exercise? *Oxidants in Medicine and Cell Longevity* 2012:707941.

Oksala, N. K., Laaksonen, D. E., Lappalainen, J. et al. 2006. Heat shock protein 60 response to exercise in diabetes: Effects of alpha-lipoic acid supplementation. *Journal of Diabetes and Its Complications* 20:257–61.

Olesen, J., Gliemann, L., Biensoe, R. S., Schmidt, J. F., Hellsten, Y. and Pilegaard, H. 2014. Exercise training, but not resveratrol, improves metabolic and inflammatory status in skeletal muscle of aged men. *Journal of Physiology* 592(Pt 8):1873–86.

Paulsen, G., Cumming, K. T., Holden, G. et al. 2014. Vitamin C and E supplementation hampers cellular adaptation to endurance training in humans: A double-blind randomized controlled trial. *Journal of Physiology* 592(Pt 8):1887–901.

Peake, J. M. 2003. Vitamin C: Effects of exercise and requirements with training. *International Journal of Sport Nutrition and Exercise Metabolism* 13:125–51.

Pedersen, B. K. 2012. Muscular interleukin-6 and its role as an energy sensor. *Medicine and Science in Sports and Exercise* 44:392–6.

Peternelj, T. T. and Coombes, J. S. 2011. Antioxidant supplementation during exercise training: Beneficial or detrimental? *Sports Medicine* 41:1043–69.

Petersen Shay, K., Moreau, R. F., Smith, E. J. and Hagen, T. M. 2008. Is alpha-lipoic acid a scavenger of reactive oxygen species in vivo? Evidence for its initiation of stress signaling pathways that promote endogenous antioxidant capacity. *IUBMB Life* 60:362–7.

Price, N. L., Gomes, A. P., Ling, A. J. et al. 2012. SIRT1 is required for AMPK activation and the beneficial effects of resveratrol on mitochondrial function. *Cell Metabolism* 15:675–90.

Quideau, S., Deffieux, D., Douat-Casassus, C. and Pouysegu, L. 2011. Plant polyphenols: Chemical properties, biological activities, and synthesis. *Angewandte Chemie International Edition in English* 50:586–621.

Radak, Z., Zhao, Z., Koltai, E., Ohno, H. and Atalay, M. 2013. Oxygen consumption and usage during physical exercise: The balance between oxidative stress and ROS-dependent adaptive signaling. *Antioxidants and Redox Signaling* 18:1208–46.

Ristow, M., Zarse, K., Oberbach, A. et al. 2009. Antioxidants prevent health-promoting effects of physical exercise in humans. *Proceedings of the National Academy of Sciences of the United States of America* 106:8665–70.

Roberts, L. A., Beattie, K., Close, G. L. and Morton, J. P. 2011. Vitamin C consumption does not impair training-induced improvements in exercise performance. *International Journal of Sports Physiology and Performance* 6:58–69.

Rock, C. L. 2007. Multivitamin–multimineral supplements: Who uses them? *American Journal of Clinical Nutrition* 85:277S–9S.

Savitha, S., Sivarajan, K., Haripriya, D., Kokilavani, V. and Panneerselvam, C. 2005. Efficacy of levo carnitine and alpha lipoic acid in ameliorating the decline in mitochondrial enzymes during aging. *Clinical Nutrition* 24:794–800.

Sen, C. K. 2000. Cellular thiols and redox-regulated signal transduction. *Current Topics in Cellular Regulation* 36:1–30.

Sen, C. K. 2001. Antioxidant and redox regulation of cellular signaling: Introduction. *Medicine and Science in Sports and Exercise* 33:368–70.

Sen, C. K. and Packer, L. 2000. Thiol homeostasis and supplements in physical exercise. *American Journal of Clinical Nutrition* 72:653S–69S.

Sen, C. K., Atalay, M. and Hanninen, O. 1994. Exercise-induced oxidative stress: Glutathione supplementation and deficiency. *Journal of Applied Physiology* 77:2177–87.

Simar, D., Malatesta, D., Mas, E., Delage, M. and Caillaud, C. 2012. Effect of an 8-week aerobic training program in elderly on oxidative stress and HSP72 expression in leukocytes during antioxidant supplementation. *Journal of Nutrition in Health and Aging* 16:155–61.

Tscholl, P., Alonso, J. M., Dolle, G., Junge, A. and Dvorak, J. 2010. The use of drugs and nutritional supplements in top-level track and field athletes. *American Journal of Sports Medicine* 38:133–40.

U.S. Department of Health and Human Services and the U.S. Department of Agriculture. 2010. *Dietary Guidelines for Americans 2010*. Washington, DC: U.S. Government Printing Office.

Vassilakopoulos, T., Karatza, M. H., Katsaounou, P., Kollintza, A., Zakynthinos, S. and Roussos, C. 2003. Antioxidants attenuate the plasma cytokine response to exercise in humans. *Journal of Applied Physiology* 94:1025–32.

Whayne, T. F., Jr. and Maulik, N. 2012. Nutrition and the healthy heart with an exercise boost. *Canadian Journal of Physiology and Pharmacology* 90:967–76.

Wray, D. W., Uberoi, A., Lawrenson, L., Bailey, D. M. and Richardson, R. S. 2009. Oral antioxidants and cardiovascular health in the exercise-trained and untrained elderly: A radically different outcome. *Clinical Science (London)* 116:433–41.

Ye, Y., Li, J. and Yuan, Z. 2013. Effect of antioxidant vitamin supplementation on cardiovascular outcomes: A meta-analysis of randomized controlled trials. *PLoS One* 8:e56803.

Yfanti, C., Akerstrom, T., Nielsen, S. et al. 2010. Antioxidant supplementation does not alter endurance training adaptation. *Medicine and Science in Sports and Exercise* 42:1388–95.

Zembron-Lacny, A., Szyszka, K. and Szygula, Z. 2007. Effect of cysteine derivatives administration in healthy men exposed to intense resistance exercise by evaluation of pro-antioxidant ratio. *Journal of Physiological Science* 57:343–8.

Section III

Antioxidants in Various
Disease States

8 Coronary Heart Disease and Stroke

Antonis Zampelas and Ioannis Dimakopoulos

CONTENTS

Introduction 117
    Risk Factors Associated with CHD and Stroke 118
    Antioxidant Hypothesis 119
Antioxidants 120
    Vitamin E 120
    Vitamin C 129
    Carotenoids 130
    Selenium 139
    Polyphenols 140
    Resveratrol 141
    Lycopene 142
Conclusion 143
References 143

INTRODUCTION

Noncommunicable diseases (NCDs) or chronic diseases generally progress slowly and have a long duration (World Health Organization [WHO] 2013a). NCDs account for 64% of all annual deaths (WHO 2013a). The four major types of NCDs are cardiovascular diseases (CVDs), cancer, chronic respiratory diseases, and diabetes. CVD is the number one cause of death globally (WHO 2011a). CVDs are a group of disorders that include coronary heart disease (CHD), cerebrovascular disease, peripheral arterial disease (PAD), rheumatic heart disease, congenital heart disease, deep vein thrombosis, and pulmonary embolism (WHO 2013b).

The majority of CVDs result from complications of atherosclerosis (Singh et al. 2005). Atherosclerosis is a disease in which plaque (fatty deposits) builds up inside the arteries and blood vessels and thus narrowing them, making it more difficult for blood to pass through and therefore limiting oxygen supply to the organs as well as other parts of the body (American Heart Association [AHA] 2013b). Heart attacks and strokes are acute events mainly caused by a blood clot that blocks the blood supply to the heart or brain, respectively (WHO 2013b). Of the 17.3 million people that have died globally due to CVD, 7.3 million died due to CHD and 6.2 million due to stroke (WHO 2011a), and it is estimated that by 2030 this number will increase to 23.3 million deaths annually (WHO 2011b).

CHD occurs when plaque builds up in the coronary arteries that supply oxygenated blood to the heart muscle, therefore limiting blood supply (National Institutes of Health 2013). This is called ischemia and can be chronic, caused by narrowing of the coronary artery, or it can be acute as a result of a plaque that suddenly ruptures (AHA 2013a).

The most common type of stroke is ischemic stroke, which occurs when a blood vessel that supplies the brain is blocked and when blood supply to a part of the brain is shut off, leading to the death of brain cells (AHA 2013b). On the other hand, a hemorrhagic stroke occurs when a blood vessel within the brain bursts (AHA 2013b). Stroke remains the second leading cause of death globally and the most common cause of disability in adults in most regions (Chen et al. 2013a). Every year, 795,000 people experience a new or recurrent stroke and, on average, every 40 s, someone in the United States has a stroke and dies of one approximately every 4 min (Go et al. 2013). In Europe, CVD is responsible for nearly half of all deaths each year, and due to its high mortality and morbidity CVD is estimated to cost the European Union €190 billion a year (Allender et al. 2008).

RISK FACTORS ASSOCIATED WITH CHD AND STROKE

There is a multitude of risk factors associated with CHD and stroke that can be differentiated to modifiable and nonmodifiable risk factors. The most important modifiable risk factors are the following: unhealthy diet, physical inactivity, smoking, and harmful use of alcohol (WHO 2013b). The effects that risk factors can exert on CVD may be shown via the so-called intermediate risk factors such as hypertension, increased levels of blood glucose and/or lipids, and increased body weight (WHO 2013b). Changes in health behavior associated with those risk factors (e.g., maintaining a healthy body weight, increasing physical activity levels, consumption of fruits and vegetables, and smoking cessation) have been shown to reduce the risk of CVD (WHO 2013b). In addition to modifiable risk factors, there are nonmodifiable risk factors, including family history, ethnicity, and being postmenopausal for women and age older than 45 years for men, that also exert an effect on CVD (AHA 2013b; World Heart Federation [WHF] 2013).

As a risk factor, diet plays an important role in the maintenance of optimal cardiovascular health, and there is consistent evidence from observational cohort studies showing that increased consumption of fruits and vegetables, as well as other plant foods, is associated with lower overall mortality rates and lower death rates from CVD (He et al. 2006, Dauchet et al. 2009, WHO 2013b). Furthermore, according to estimates, if an individual increases fruit and vegetable intake to 600 g/day, the global burden of disease could be reduced by 31% for ischemic heart disease and 19% for ischemic stroke (Lock et al. 2005). In addition, it is estimated that 74% of coronary events among nonsmokers might have been prevented by eating a healthy diet, maintaining a healthy body weight, exercising regularly for ≥30 min/day, and consuming a moderate amount of alcohol (Hu and Willett 2002). However, the difficulty of individuals to reduce and maintain a normal body weight, as well as make healthier food choices in the long term, made the hypothesis of counteracting this with antioxidants, among other nutrients, attractive (Traber 2007).

ANTIOXIDANT HYPOTHESIS

Evidence for the association between CVD and fruit and vegetable consumption has led to the hypothesis that specific components of fruits and vegetables are responsible for the health benefits observed, although it is not yet known which molecules found in fruits and vegetables contribute more to their cardioprotective effect (Chong-Han 2010). One very popular hypothesis is that antioxidant nutrients prevent atherosclerosis via their beneficial effect against reactive oxygen species (ROS) (Stanner et al. 2004). ROS include free radicals, oxygen ions, and peroxides, both organic and inorganic (Taverne et al. 2013). They are produced as a by-product of oxidative phosphorylation but can also be produced through physiological biochemical reactions (Taverne et al. 2013).

Physiologically, ROS are found in low levels and this enables them to function as messengers in signal transduction for vascular homeostasis and cell signaling (Taverne et al. 2013). When ROS are excessively produced, when they are not controlled, or when antioxidants are depleted, they can damage lipids, proteins, and DNA (Taverne et al. 2013). This imbalance between oxidation and reduction is called oxidative stress and can contribute to the development as well as progression of CVD (Taverne et al. 2013). In addition, common characteristics of CVD risk factors, such as obesity, dyslipidemia, insulin resistance, and hypertension are the elevated levels of oxidative stress (Griendling and FitzGerald 2003a,b). Therefore, as the majority of CVDs are a result of atherosclerosis (Taverne et al. 2013), and oxidative damage contributes to atherosclerosis (Ozkanlar and Akcay 2012), antioxidant supplementation could be an important step toward the prevention and treatment of CVD. It has been shown that antioxidants can protect against atherosclerosis by blocking low-density lipoprotein (LDL) oxidation, positively influencing plaque stability, vasomotor function, and tendency for thrombosis, among other possible protective mechanisms (Bin et al. 2011). The oxidative modification hypothesis (Figure 8.1) supports the idea that the oxidation of LDL is a crucial step in atherogenesis (Maiolino et al. 2013). In fact, a series of biological properties of oxidized LDLs that are thought to promote atherosclerosis are the following: recruitment/activation and proliferation of monocytes/macrophages in the arterial wall, increased production of growth factors, stimulation of collagen production, cytotoxic activity in vascular cells, promotion of apoptosis, and stimulation of platelet adhesion and aggregation (Maiolino et al. 2013). However, although the oxidized LDL hypothesis of atherogenesis seems plausible, human observational studies have shown conflicting results (Maiolino et al. 2013). Furthermore, researchers believe that LDL oxidation alone does not explain the complex mechanism of atherosclerosis and other mechanisms have also been proposed, like, for example, a mechanism involving oxidized LDL and nitric oxide (Ozkanlar and Akcay 2012). It has also been shown that plasma vitamin E is inversely correlated with mortality from ischemic heart disease (Gey et al. 1991), and therefore supplemental intake of antioxidants might be a treatment option for CVD (Taverne et al. 2013).

In contrast to the available evidence from animal studies and data from prospective human studies for fruits and vegetables, data from randomized controlled trials (RCTs) have not reported consistent benefit from the use of antioxidant supplements on CVD risk (Bhupathiraju and Tucker 2011), and some trials have reported harm

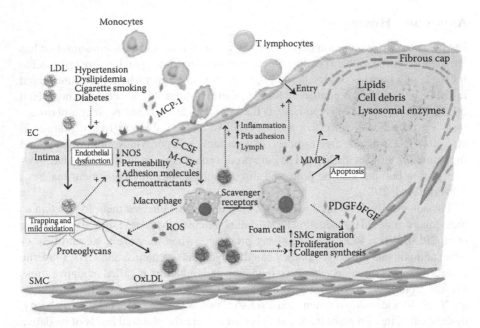

FIGURE 8.1 Putative pathway of oxidized low-density lipoprotein (OxLDL) in the athero-genetic process according to the oxidative hypothesis of atherosclerosis. SMC, smooth muscle cell; MMPs, matrix metalloproteinases; NOS, nitric oxide synthase; G-CSF, granulocyte colony stimulating factor; M-CSF, macrophage colony stimulating factor; MCP-1, monocyte chemoattractant protein-1; PDGF, platelet derived growth factor; bFGF, basic fibroblast growth factor. (From Maiolino, G. et al., *Mediators Inflamm* 2013, 1, 2013.)

with high doses of antioxidant supplements. In addition, the effects of different anti-oxidants to CVD are further perplexed, as there is lack of knowledge with regard to the optimal dose. For example, oral supplementation of some antioxidants like vitamin C can decrease its bioavailability, and lack of clinical improvement in RCTs might be a result of the characteristics of the population being studied (Taverne et al. 2013). In addition, in many RCTs, participants have been diagnosed with CVD, and this might be the reason why a beneficial effect is not observed with supplementation.

ANTIOXIDANTS

Antioxidants are molecules that interact with and protect the body from free radi-cals, the molecules that induce oxidative stress, thus preventing them from causing damage (National Cancer Institute 2013). The major dietary antioxidants include the following: vitamin E, vitamin C, carotenoids, flavonoids, selenium, polyphenols, resveratrol, and lycopene.

Vitamin E

Vitamin E is a lipid-soluble vitamin with the ability to inhibit lipid peroxidation by acting as a scavenger for ROS and preserving cell membranes (Schurks et al. 2010).

In vitro studies have proposed that antioxidants, including vitamin E, reduce lipid peroxidation and the damage by free radicals, therefore postponing the development of atherosclerosis (Bleys et al. 2006).

In addition, some observational epidemiological evidence suggests that increased consumption of dietary or supplementary vitamin E has a protective effect against CHD (Rimm et al. 1993, Stampfer and Rimm 1995). This might partly explain the fact that before the availability of evidence from RCTs, about 25% of adults were taking vitamin E supplements in the United States (Eidelman et al. 2004). However, findings from observational studies are inconsistent (Knekt et al. 2004, Ye and Song 2008). This might have occurred owing to the few CHD cases reported in some of the studies detecting associations, not controlling for confounding factors, inability to investigate subpopulations, and misclassification of antioxidants taken (Knekt et al. 2004). Given these limitations, meta-analyses of prospective cohort studies were conducted to examine the effects of vitamin E on CVD.

A meta-analysis of nine prospective cohort studies suggests that dietary intake of antioxidant vitamins was only weakly related to reduced CHD risk and that supplemental vitamin E intake is not significantly related to CHD (Knekt et al. 2004). Another meta-analysis of 15 prospective cohort studies, of >7000 incident CHD cases and 370,000 participants, reported that increased vitamin E is significantly associated with reduced CHD risk irrespective of study size, sex, duration of follow-up, and type of vitamins taken (dietary or supplemental) (Ye and Song 2008). It also suggests that each 30 IU/day increase in vitamin E could decrease CHD risk by 4% (Ye and Song 2008). However, due to limitations in the included prospective cohort studies (e.g., inability to adjust for some confounding factors) as well as the limitations associated with observational studies in general, it is suggested that the observed relationship still needs careful consideration (Ye and Song 2008). To illustrate this last point, further participants taking supplements might also have other healthy habits that have an effect on CVD risk factors, therefore confounding the relationship (Ye and Song 2008).

Apart from laboratory and observational studies, several RCTs (Table 8.1) and meta-analyses of RCTs (Eidelman et al. 2004, Shekelle et al. 2004, Bleys et al. 2006, Schurks et al. 2010, Bin et al. 2011, Myung et al. 2013, Ye et al. 2013) have been conducted to examine the effect of vitamin E intake on CVD outcomes.

A recent meta-analysis, of 13 RCTs that included 166,282 participants, was conducted by Bin et al. (2011) to evaluate the role of vitamin E supplementation in the prevention of stroke. The pooled results showed no significant benefit in the vitamin E group with respect to any type of stroke—hemorrhagic stroke, ischemic stroke, fatal stroke, and nonfatal stroke (Bin et al. 2011).

This discrepancy between studies evaluating the association of increased fruit and vegetable consumption vs. studies evaluating supplemental intake with regard to risk of stroke might be explained by the fact that supplemental intake and diet are different types of intake of antioxidants, and their effects on CVD might be different (Bin et al. 2011). In addition, although observational studies usually involve healthy participants whereas RCTs mostly study participants at high risk of macrovascular disease or who are diseased, in a subanalysis of healthy participants in three RCTs, performed by Bin et al. (2011), the pooled result showed similar effects.

TABLE 8.1
Randomized Controlled Trials of Supplemental Antioxidant Intake and Risk of Major CVD Outcomes

Trial/Author, Country	Study Design	N	Age (years)	Health Status	Follow-Up	Vitamin	Daily Dosage	CVD Outcomes	CVD Outcome, RR (95% CI), p-Value
Vitamin E									
CHAOS, UK 1996 (Stephens et al. 1996)	Double blind	2002	61.8 (Mean)	Angiography-proven coronary atherosclerosis	1.5 (Median)	α-Tocopherol	400 or 800 IU	CVD death and nonfatal MI, nonfatal MI alone	CVD death and nonfatal MI, 0.53 (0.34–0.83), 0.005
ATBC, Finland 1997 (Rapola et al. 1997)	Double blind	1862	50–69	Smokers with previous MI	5.3 (Median)	α-Tocopherol	50 mg	Nonfatal MI, fatal CHD	Nonfatal MI, 0.62 (0.41–0.96), S
ATBC, Finland 1998 (Virtamo et al. 1998)	Double blind	27,271	50–69	Smokers, no history of MI	6.1 (Median)	α-Tocopherol	50 mg	Nonfatal MI, fatal CHD	NS
GISSI, Italy 1999 (GISSI 1999)	Open label	11,324	59.4	Patients with recent MI	3.5	α-Tocopherol	300 mg	Death, nonfatal MI, stroke	NS
SPACE, Israel 2000 (Boaz et al. 2000)	Double blind	196	40–75	Hemodialysis patients	2	α-Tocopherol	800 IU	MI, ischemic stroke, PVD, unstable angina	Total CVD, 0.46 (0.27–0.78), 0.014
ATBC, Finland 2000 (Leppala et al. 2000)	Double blind	28,519	50–69	Smokers	6 (Median)	α-Tocopherol	50 mg	Stroke (SH, IH, CI), incidence and mortality	CI incidence, 0.86 (0.75–0.99), 0.03; SH mortality, 2.81 (1.37–5.79), 0.005

(Continued)

TABLE 8.1 (CONTINUED)
Randomized Controlled Trials of Supplemental Antioxidant Intake and Risk of Major CVD Outcomes

Trial/Author, Country	Study Design	N	Age (years)	Health Status	Follow-Up	Vitamin	Daily Dosage	CVD Outcomes	CVD Outcome, RR (95% CI), p-Value
					Vitamin E				
PPP, 2001 (de Gaetano 2001)	Open label	4495	64.6 (Mean)	With at least one major CVD risk factor	3.6 (Mean)	α-Tocopherol	300 mg	CVD death, nonfatal MI, nonfatal stroke, angina pectoris, TIA, PAD, revascularization procedures	PAD, 0.54 (0.30–0.99), 0.043
HATS, USA, and Canada 2001 (Brown et al. 2001)	Double blind	160	<63 (M), <70 (F)	With coronary disease	3.2	D-α-Tocopherol Vitamin C β-Carotene Selenium	800 IU 1000 mg 25 mg 100 mg	CVD mortality, MI, stroke, revascularization	NS
SUVIMAX, France 2004 (Hercberg et al. 2004)	Double blind	13,017	46.6 (F), 51.3 (M)	Adults	7.5 (Median)	Ascorbic acid Vitamin E β-Carotene Selenium Zinc	120 mg 30 mg 6 mg 100 μg 20 mg	Fatal and nonfatal ischemic CVD events	NS
WHS, USA 2005 (Lee et al. 2005)	Double blind	39,876	54.6 (Mean)	Healthy women	10.1 (Mean)	α-Tocopherol	600 IU (every other day)	Nonfatal MI, nonfatal stroke, CVD death	CVD mortality, 0.76 (0.59–0.98), 0.03

(Continued)

TABLE 8.1 (CONTINUED)
Randomized Controlled Trials of Supplemental Antioxidant Intake and Risk of Major CVD Outcomes

Trial/Author, Country	Study Design	N	Age (years)	Health Status	Follow-Up	Vitamin	Daily Dosage	CVD Outcomes	CVD Outcome, RR (95% CI), p-Value
Vitamin E									
HOPE and HOPE-TOO, Canada 2005 (Lonn et al. 2005)	Double blind	9541	66 (Mean)	With vascular disease or diabetes	7 (Median)	RRR-α-tocopheryl-acetate	400 IU	MI, stroke, death from CVD	NS
WACS, USA 2007 (Cook et al. 2007)	Double blind	8171	60.6 (Mean)	CVD history or at high risk	9.4 (Mean)	D-α-Tocopherol-acetate	600 IU (every other day)	MI, stroke, CABG, PTCA, CVD mortality	NS
PHS II, USA 2008 (Sesso et al. 2008)	Double blind	14,641	64.3 (Mean)	Physicians with prevalent CVD	8 (Mean)	α-Tocopherol	400 IU (every other day)	Nonfatal MI, nonfatal stroke, CVD death	Hemorrhagic stroke, 1.74 (1.04–2.91), 0.036
Milman et al. 2008, Israel (Milman et al. 2008)	Double blind	1434	≥55	Diabetes mellitus, Hp 2-2 genotype	1.5	D-α-Tocopherol	400 IU	Composite endpoint (CVD mortality, MI, stroke)	Composite endpoint, 0.30 (0.16–0.70), 0.003
Vitamin C									
HATS, USA and Canada 2001 (Brown et al. 2001)	Double blind	160	<63 (M), <70 (F)	With coronary disease	3.2	D-α-Tocopherol, Vitamin C, β-Carotene, Selenium	800 IU, 1000 mg, 25 mg, 100 mg	CVD mortality, MI, stroke, revascularization	NS

(Continued)

TABLE 8.1 (CONTINUED)
Randomized Controlled Trials of Supplemental Antioxidant Intake and Risk of Major CVD Outcomes

Trial/Author, Country	Study Design	N	Age (years)	Health Status	Follow-Up	Vitamin	Daily Dosage	CVD Outcomes	CVD Outcome, RR (95% CI), p-Value
Vitamin C									
SUVIMAX, France 2004 (Hercberg et al. 2004)	Double blind	13,017	46.6 (F), 51.3 (M)	Adults	7.5 (Median)	Ascorbic acid Vitamin E β-Carotene Selenium Zinc	120 mg 30 mg 6 mg 100 μg 20 mg	Fatal and nonfatal ischemic CVD events	NS
WACS, USA 2007 (Cook et al. 2007)	Double blind	8171	60.6	CVD history or at high risk	9.4 (Mean)	Synthetic ascorbic acid	500 mg	MI, stroke, CABG, PTCA, CVD mortality	NS
PHS II, USA 2008 (Sesso et al. 2008)	Double blind	14,641	64.3	Physicians with prevalent CVD	8 (Mean)	Synthetic ascorbic acid	500 mg	Nonfatal MI, nonfatal stroke, CVD death	NS
β-Carotene									
PHS, USA 1996 (Hennekens et al. 1996)	Double blind	22,071	40–84	Physicians with no history of cancer, MI, stroke, or transient ischemia	12 (Mean)	β-Carotene	50 mg (every other day)	MI, stroke, CVD mortality	NS
CARET, USA 1996 (Omenn et al. 1996)	Double blind	18,314	45–74	Smokers, former workers, and workers exposed to asbestos	4	β-Carotene Retinol	30 mg 25,000 IU	CVD mortality	NS

(Continued)

TABLE 8.1 (CONTINUED)
Randomized Controlled Trials of Supplemental Antioxidant Intake and Risk of Major CVD Outcomes

Trial/Author, Country	Study Design	N	Age (years)	Health Status	Follow-Up	Vitamin	Daily Dosage	CVD Outcomes	CVD Outcome, RR (95% CI), p-Value
					β-Carotene				
ATBC, Finland 1997 (Rapola et al. 1997)	Double blind	1862	50–69	Smokers with previous MI	5.3 (Median)	β-Carotene	20 mg	Nonfatal MI, fatal CHD	Fatal CHD, 1.75 (1.16–2.64), 0.012
ATBC, Finland 1998 (Virtamo et al. 1998)	Double blind	27,271	50–69	Smokers with no history of MI	6.1 (Median)	β-Carotene	20 mg	Nonfatal MI, fatal CHD	Major coronary events, 0.69 (0.50–0.94), 0.03; fatal CHD, 0.64 (0.41–1.00), 0.02
WHS, USA 1999 (Lee et al. 1999)	Double blind	39,876	≥45	Healthy women	4.1 (Median)	β-Carotene	50 mg (every other day)	MI, stroke, or CVD mortality	NS
ATBC, Finland 2000 (Leppala et al. 2000)	Double blind	28,519	50–69	Smokers without a history of stroke	6	β-Carotene	20 mg	Stroke (SH, IH, CI)	IH, 1.62 (1.10–2.36), 0.01
HATS, USA and Canada 2001 (Brown et al. 2001)	Double blind	160	<63 (M), <70 (F)	With coronary disease	3.2	D-α-Tocopherol Vitamin C β-Carotene Selenium	800 IU 1000 mg 25 mg 100 mg	CVD mortality, MI, stroke, revascularization	NS

(Continued)

TABLE 8.1 (CONTINUED)
Randomized Controlled Trials of Supplemental Antioxidant Intake and Risk of Major CVD Outcomes

Trial/Author, Country	Study Design	N	Age (years)	Health Status	Follow-Up	Vitamin	Daily Dosage	CVD Outcomes	CVD Outcome, RR (95% CI), p-Value
β-Carotene									
SUVIMAX, France 2004 (Hercberg et al. 2004)	Double blind	13,017	46.6 (F), 51.3 (M)	Adults	7.5 (Median)	Ascorbic acid, Vitamin E, β-Carotene, Selenium, Zinc	120 mg, 30 mg, 6 mg, 100 µg, 20 mg	Fatal and nonfatal ischemic CVD events	NS
WACS, USA 2007 (Cook et al. 2007)	Double blind	8171	60.6	CVD history or at high risk	9.4 (Mean)	β-Carotene	50 mg (every other day)	MI, stroke, CABG, CVD mortality	NS
Selenium									
HATS, USA, and Canada 2001 (Brown et al. 2001)	Double blind	160	<63 (M), <70 (F)	With coronary disease	3.2	D-α-Tocopherol, Vitamin C, β-Carotene, Selenium	800 IU, 1000 mg, 25 mg, 100 µg	CVD mortality, MI, stroke, revascularization	NS
SUVIMAX, France 2004 (Hercberg et al. 2004)	Double blind	13,017	46.6 (F), 51.3 (M)	Adults	7.5 (Median)	Ascorbic acid, Vitamin E, β-Carotene, Selenium, Zinc	120 mg, 30 mg, 6 mg, 100 µg, 20 mg	Fatal and nonfatal ischemic CVD events	NS

(Continued)

TABLE 8.1 (CONTINUED)
Randomized Controlled Trials of Supplemental Antioxidant Intake and Risk of Major CVD Outcomes

Trial/Author, Country	Study Design	N	Age (years)	Health Status	Follow-Up	Vitamin	Daily Dosage	CVD Outcomes	CVD Outcome, RR (95% CI), p-Value
					Selenium				
NPC, USA 2006 (Stranges et al. 2006)	Double blind	1312	62 (Mean)	Confirmed history of nonmelanoma skin cancer	7.6	Selenium	200 µg	Fatal and nonfatal MI, CABG, PTCA, stroke, CVD mortality	NS

Note: ATBC, Alpha-Tocopherol Beta-Carotene Cancer Prevention Study; BHF, British Heart Foundation; CABG, coronary artery bypass grafting; CARET, Beta-Carotene and Retinol Efficacy Trial; CD, coronary disease; CHAOS, Cambridge Heart Antioxidant Study; CHD, coronary heart disease; CI, cerebral infarction; CVD, cardiovascular disease; F, female; GISSI, Gruppo Italiano per lo Studio della Sopravvivenza nell'Infarto Miocardico; HATS, HDL Atherosclerosis Treatment Study; HOPE, Heart Outcomes Prevention Evaluation; HOPE-TOO, HOPE The Ongoing Outcomes; IH, intracerebral hemorrhage; M, male; MI, myocardial infarction; MRC, Medical Research Council; NPC, Nutrition Prevention Cancer; NS, nonsignificant; PAD, peripheral arterial disease; PHS, Physician's Health Study; PPP, primary prevention project; PTCA, percutaneous transluminal coronary angioplasty; S, significant; SH, subarachnoid hemorrhage; SPACE, Secondary Prevention with Antioxidants of Cardiovascular Disease in Endstage Renal Disease; SUVIMAX, Supplementation en Vitamines et Mineraux Antioxydants; WACS, Women's Antioxidant Cardiovascular Study; WHS, Women's Health Study.

An earlier meta-analysis on the effects of vitamin E on stroke subtypes concluded that vitamin E increases the risk of hemorrhagic stroke by 22% and reduces the risk of ischemic stroke by 10%, results that are obscured when examining total stroke (Schurks et al. 2010). Owing to the small risk reduction of ischemic stroke and the increased risk of hemorrhagic stroke, as noted in the meta-analysis by Schurks et al. (2010), widespread use of vitamin E is not suggested. Furthermore, apart from vitamin E supplementation, there are other strategies that can effectively and substantially reduce the risk of stroke, such as antihypertensive or lipid-lowering medication, as well as cessation of smoking, maintaining a healthy weight, having a healthy diet, and regularly exercising (Schurks et al. 2010).

A very recent meta-analysis that included 50 RCTs concluded that there was no evidence to support the use of vitamin and antioxidant supplements for the prevention of CVD irrespective of the type of prevention, type of vitamins and antioxidants, type of CVD outcomes, study design, methodological quality, duration of treatment, funding source, provider of supplements, type of control, number of participants in each trial, and supplements given singly or in combination with other supplements (Myung et al. 2013). In addition, another meta-analysis of RCTs has shown that there is no effect of vitamin–mineral supplementation on the progression of atherosclerosis (Bleys et al. 2006). This is in agreement with previous meta-analyses that also report that there is good evidence that vitamin E supplementation does not have an effect on CVD (Vivekananthan et al. 2003, Shekelle et al. 2004).

Overall, the evidence does not support the long-term use of vitamin E for CVD prevention or progression of atherosclerosis.

VITAMIN C

Vitamin C, also known as ascorbic acid, is a hydrophilic vitamin and acts as an antioxidant in hydrophilic media (Wang et al. 2012). Vitamin C regenerates tocopheryl from its oxidized form (Wang et al. 2012). As described previously, vitamin C may have a beneficial effect on atherogenesis as it is a strong antioxidant and has been shown to decrease the oxidation of LDL, inhibit proliferation of smooth muscle cells, and protect membranes from peroxidation (Chen et al. 2000, 2013a).

Similar to vitamin E, vitamin C has also been extensively investigated with regard to its effect on CVD outcomes (Ye and Song 2008); however, results are inconsistent. Meta-analysis of nine prospective cohort studies suggested a reduced incidence of major CHD events at high supplementation of vitamin C in men and women, whereas dietary vitamin C intake was not related to CHD incidence (Knekt et al. 2004). In more detail, participants in the highest quintile of vitamin C intake had 24% lower risk compared with those in the lowest quintile, and a dose–response association was observed. Adjustment for confounding factors did not affect the association. Although the results of this meta-analysis suggest the use of vitamin C supplementation to reduce CHD incidence, as the effects of high antioxidant vitamin intake are not fully understood, there is no adequate support for recommending high doses of vitamin C supplementation.

In contrast, a later meta-analysis of 15 prospective cohort studies suggests that dietary vitamin C has an inverse association with CHD risk, whereas supplement use of vitamin C is not significantly associated with the risk of CHD (Ye and Song 2008). Given the inconsistencies observed in prospective cohort studies and the limitations associated with their study design, RCTs have been conducted to evaluate the effect of vitamin C on CVD outcomes.

A meta-analysis of RCTs concluded that antioxidant vitamin supplementation (including vitamin C) does not affect major CVD events such as myocardial infarction, stroke, CVD mortality, CHD, angina, congestive heart failure, and revascularization (Ye et al. 2013). Furthermore, the authors found that subgroup analysis also supported the same conclusions. These results have also been replicated in other meta-analyses of RCTs (Chen et al. 2013a, Myung et al. 2013). Another meta-analysis has also shown that there is no evidence of a protective effect of antioxidant vitamin supplementation, including vitamin C, on the progression of atherosclerosis (Bleys et al. 2006). In contrast, dietary vitamin C is significantly and inversely associated with the risk of stroke in a dose–response manner (Chen et al. 2013a).

Apart from the examined effect of vitamin C on CVD outcomes, RCTs have also been conducted to examine the effect of vitamin C on intermediate risk factors such as blood pressure. A recent meta-analysis of RCTs about the effects of vitamin C supplementation on blood pressure showed that in short-term trials, vitamin C significantly reduced systolic and diastolic blood pressure (Juraschek et al. 2012) by −3.84 mm Hg and −1.48 mm Hg, respectively; however, there is lack of long-term clinical trial evidence. The authors of this meta-analysis also note that the included trials were small, and there was significant heterogeneity of effects across studies, which leads to the conclusion that additional trials are needed, with larger sample sizes and with attention to the quality of blood pressure assessment.

In summary, vitamin C supplementation is not recommended for the prevention or treatment of CVD.

CAROTENOIDS

There are 600 naturally occurring carotenoids; however, six carotenoids (lutein, lycopene, zeaxanthin, β-cryptoxanthin, β-carotene, and α-carotene) represent >95% of carotenoids in plasma and are associated with health benefits (Wang et al. 2013). Table 8.2 provides an overview of observational studies of dietary and supplemental intake of carotenoids and their association with major CVD outcomes.

Most of the observational studies of dietary carotenoid intake have examined the effect of β-carotene on CVD outcomes. In the Nurses' Health Study, dietary α- and β-carotene were inversely associated with coronary artery disease; the same was not observed for intake of other carotenoids (Osganian et al. 2003). In addition, in the Health Professionals' Follow-up Study, current and former smokers had significantly lower CHD risk; however, the same was not observed for nonsmokers (Rimm et al. 1993). In the same cohort study, only lutein was shown to be inversely associated with the risk of stroke (Ascherio et al. 1999).

A meta-analysis of nine prospective cohort studies suggested that the risk reduction of carotenoids was only weakly associated with major CHD events (Knekt et al. 2004). In more detail, significant inverse associations were observed between dietary α-carotene, β-carotene, lutein, and β-cryptoxanthin with the incidence of all major

TABLE 8.2
Observational Studies on Intake of Antioxidants and Risk of Major CVD Outcomes

Trial/Author, Country	Population/Sex	N	Age (years)	Follow-Up (years)	Exposure (Plasma/Dietary/Supplements)	Outcomes, RR (Highest vs. Lowest) and (95% CI), p-Value
Vitamin E						
Rotterdam study, Netherlands 1999 (Klipstein-Grobusch et al. 1999)	Free of MI at baseline	4802	55–95	4 (Mean)	Dietary vitamin E	Risk of MI, 1.21 (0.75–1.98), 0.528
Kushi et al. 1996, USA (Kushi et al. 1996)	Postmenopausal women with no CVD	34,486	55–69	7	Total vitamin E intake Dietary vitamin E Supplemental vitamin E	CHD mortality, 0.96 (0.62–1.51), 0.27 CHD mortality, 0.38 (0.18–0.8), 0.004 CHD mortality, 1.09 (0.67–1.77), 0.39
HPFS, USA 1993 (Rimm et al. 1993)	Male health professionals	39,910	40–75	4	Dietary vitamin E Supplemental vitamin E Total vitamin E intake	CHD, 0.79 (0.54–1.15), 0.11 CHD, 0.70 (0.55–0.89), 0.22 CHD, 0.60 (0.44–0.81), 0.001
NHS, USA 1993 (Stampfer et al. 1993)	Female nurses	87,245	34–59	8	Total vitamin E intake Dietary vitamin E intake	CHD, 0.66 (0.50–0.87), <0.001 CHD, 0.95 (0.72–1.23), 0.99
Knekt et al. 1994, Finland (Knekt et al. 1994)	Men and women	5133	30–69	14 (Mean)	Dietary vitamin E	M: CHD mortality, 0.68 (0.42–1.11), 0.01 F: CHD mortality, 0.35 (0.14–0.88), <0.01
EPESE, USA 1996 (Losonczy et al. 1996)	Men and women	11,178	67–105	6	Supplemental vitamin E	CHD mortality, 0.37 (0.15–0.90), NS
Sahyoun et al. 1996, USA (Sahyoun et al. 1996)	Noninstitutionalized Massachusetts residents, men and women	725	≥60	9–12	Vitamin E intake	Mortality from HD, 0.75 (0.41–1.39), 0.40

(Continued)

TABLE 8.2 (CONTINUED)
Observational Studies on Intake of Antioxidants and Risk of Major CVD Outcomes

Trial/Author, Country	Population/Sex	N	Age (years)	Follow-Up (years)	Exposure (Plasma/Dietary/Supplements)	Outcomes, RR (Highest vs. Lowest) and (95% CI), p-Value
Vitamin E						
Ascherio et al. 1999, USA (Ascherio et al. 1999)	Male health professionals who did not have CVD or diabetes	43,748	40–75	8	Total vitamin E intake Supplemental vitamin E	Stroke, 1.25 (0.88–1.78), >0.2 Stroke, 1.13 (0.84–1.52), >0.2
ATBC, Finland 2000 (Hirvonen et al. 2000)	Male smokers	26,593	50–69	6.1	Dietary vitamin E	CI, 0.86 (0.70–1.06), 0.25 SH, 0.81 (0.44–1.50), 0.55 IH, 0.64 (0.36–1.15), 0.15
Muntwyler et al. 2002, USA (Muntwyler et al. 2002)	Male physicians	83,639	40–84	5.5	Supplemental vitamin E	CVD mortality, 0.92 (0.70–1.21), 0.52 CHD mortality, 0.88 (0.61–1.27), 0.47
Muntwyler et al. 2004, USA (Genkinger et al. 2004)	Men and women	6151	30–93	1989–2002	Dietary vitamin E	CVD mortality, 1.07 (0.79–1.46), 0.69
CLUE, Europe 2008 (Buijsse et al. 2008)	Men free of chronic diseases	559	65–84	15	Dietary α-tocopherol Dietary γ-tocopherol	CVD mortality, 0.96 (0.82–1.12), NS CVD mortality, 0.94 (0.79–1.12), NS
Vitamin C						
HPFS, USA 1993 (Rimm et al. 1993)	Male health professionals	39,910	40–75	4	Total vitamin C intake	CHD, 1.25 (0.91–1.71), 0.98
Knekt et al. 1994, Finland (Knekt et al. 1994)	Men and women	5133	30–69	14 (Mean)	Dietary vitamin C	M: CHD mortality, 1.00 (0.68–1.45), 0.94; F: CHD mortality, 0.49 (0.24–0.98), 0.06

(Continued)

TABLE 8.2 (CONTINUED)

Observational Studies on Intake of Antioxidants and Risk of Major CVD Outcomes

Trial/Author, Country	Population/Sex	N	Age (years)	Follow-Up (years)	Exposure (Plasma/ Dietary/Supplements)	Outcomes, RR (Highest vs. Lowest) and (95% CI), *p*-Value
			Vitamin C			
Sahyoun et al. 1996, USA (Sahyoun et al. 1996)	Noninstitutionalized Massachusetts residents, men and women	725	≥60	9–12	Vitamin C intake	Mortality from HD, 0.38 (0.19–0.75), 0.22
Kushi et al. 1996, USA (Kushi et al. 1996)	Postmenopausal women with no CVD	34,486	55–69	7	Total vitamin E intake / Dietary vitamin E / Supplemental vitamin E	CHD mortality, 1.49 (0.96–2.30), 0.02 / CHD mortality, 1.43 (0.75–2.70), 0.47 / CHD mortality, 0.74 (0.30–1.83), 0.60
Daviglus et al. 1997, USA (Daviglus et al. 1997)	Middle-aged men	1843		30	Vitamin C intake	Stroke, 0.71 (0.47–1.05), 0.17
Rotterdam study, Netherlands 1999 (Klipstein-Grobusch et al. 1999)	Free of MI at baseline	4802	55–95	4 (Mean)	Dietary vitamin C	Risk of MI, 1.05 (0.65–1.67), 0.856
HPFS, USA 1999 (Ascherio et al. 1999)	Male health professionals who did not have CVD or diabetes	43,748	40–75	8	Total vitamin C intake / Supplemental vitamin C	Stroke, 0.95 (0.66–1.35), >0.2 / Stroke, 0.85 (0.59–1.24), >0.2
ATBC, Finland 2000 (Hirvonen et al. 2000)	Male smokers	26,593	50–69	6.1	Dietary vitamin C	CI, 0.89 (0.72–1.09), 0.20 / SH, 1.16 (0.62–2.18), 0.61 / IH, 0.39 (0.21–0.74), 0.02
Muntwyler et al. 2002, USA (Muntwyler et al. 2002)	Male physicians	83,639	40–84	5.5	Supplemental vitamin C	CVD mortality, 0.88 (0.70–1.12), 0.29 / CHD mortality, 0.86 (0.63–1.18), 0.34

(Continued)

TABLE 8.2 (CONTINUED)
Observational Studies on Intake of Antioxidants and Risk of Major CVD Outcomes

Trial/Author, Country	Population/Sex	N	Age (years)	Follow-Up (years)	Exposure (Plasma/ Dietary/Supplements)	Outcomes, RR (Highest vs. Lowest) and (95% CI), p-Value
Vitamin C						
NHS, USA 2003 (Osganian et al. 2003)	Female nurses	85,118	30–55	16	Total vitamin C intake	CHD, 0.73 (0.57–0.94), 0.005
					Dietary vitamin C	CHD, 0.86 (0.59–1.26), 0.52
					Supplemental vitamin C	CHD, 0.72 (0.61–0.86), S
CLUE, Europe 2008 (Buijsse et al. 2008)	Men free of chronic diseases	559	65–84	15	Dietary vitamin C	CVD mortality, 1.02 (0.85–1.23), NS
Carotenoids						
HPFS, USA 1993 (Rimm et al. 1993)	Men	39,910	40–75	4	Dietary carotene	CHD (former smokers), 0.60 (0.38–0.94), <0.05; CHD (current smokers), 0.30 (0.11–0.82), <0.05
Morris et al. 1994, USA (Morris et al. 1994)	Men	1883	40–59	13	Total carotenoids	CHD, 0.64 (0.44–0.92), 0.01
Knekt et al. 1994, Finland (Knekt et al. 1994)	Men and women	5133	30–69	14 (Mean)	Dietary carotenoids	M: CHD mortality, 1.02 (0.70–1.48), 0.36; F: CHD mortality, 0.62 (0.30–1.29), 0.60
Kushi et al. 1996, USA (Kushi et al. 1996)	Postmenopausal women with no CVD	34,486	55–69	7	Total carotenoids intake	CHD mortality, 1.03 (0.63–1.70), 0.71
					Total vitamin A	CHD mortality, 1.22 (0.76–1.96), 0.89
					Dietary carotenoids	CHD mortality, 1.19 (0.67–2.12), 0.89
					Dietary vitamin A	CHD mortality, 1.25 (0.57–2.31), 0.83
					Supplemental vitamin A	CHD mortality, 1.29 (0.70–2.39), 0.22

(Continued)

TABLE 8.2 (CONTINUED)
Observational Studies on Intake of Antioxidants and Risk of Major CVD Outcomes

Trial/Author, Country	Population/Sex	N	Age (years)	Follow-Up (years)	Exposure (Plasma/Dietary/Supplements)	Outcomes, RR (Highest vs. Lowest) and (95% CI), *p*-Value
			Carotenoids			
Sayoun et al. 1996, USA (Sahyoun et al. 1996)	Noninstitutionalized Massachusetts residents, men and women	725	≥60	9–12	Carotenoid intake	Mortality from HD, 0.64 (0.33–1.27), 0.14
Daviglus et al. 1997, USA (Daviglus et al. 1997)	Middle-aged men	1843		30	β-Carotene	Stroke, 0.84 (0.57–1.24), 0.59
HPFS, USA 1999 (Ascherio et al. 1999)	Male health professionals who did not have CVD or diabetes	43,748	40–75	8	Total β-carotene intake	Stroke, 0.77 (0.54–1.08), >0.2
					Supplemental β-carotene	Stroke, 1.18 (0.68–2.07), >0.2
					Total α-carotene	Stroke, 0.94 (0.66–1.34), >0.2
					Total lutein	Stroke, 0.70 (0.49–1.01), >0.06
					Total lycopene	Stroke, 0.96 (0.68–1.36), >0.2
Rotterdam study, Netherlands 1999 (Klipstein-Grobusch et al. 1999)	Free of MI at baseline	4802	55–95	4 (Mean)	Dietary β-carotene	Risk of MI, 0.55 (0.34–0.83), 0.013
ATBC, Finland 2000 (Hirvonen et al. 2000)	Male smokers	26,593	50–69	6.1	Dietary β-carotene	CI, 0.74 (0.60–0.91), 0.0009; SH, 0.67 (0.35–1.28), 0.77; IH, 0.66 (0.36–1.19), 0.19
					Dietary lutein and zeaxanthin	CI, 0.81 (0.66–1.00), 0.10; SH, 0.47 (0.24–0.93), 0.03; IH, 0.81 (0.46–1.43), 0.86
					Dietary lycopene	CI, 0.74 (0.59–0.92), 0.02; SH, 0.63 (0.33–1.20), 0.13; IH, 0.45 (0.24–0.86), 0.01

(Continued)

TABLE 8.2 (CONTINUED)
Observational Studies on Intake of Antioxidants and Risk of Major CVD Outcomes

Trial/Author, Country	Population/Sex	N	Age (years)	Follow-Up (years)	Exposure (Plasma/Dietary/Supplements)	Outcomes, RR (Highest vs. Lowest) and (95% CI), p-Value
Carotenoids						
NHS, USA 2003 (Osganian et al. 2003)	Female nurses	73,286	30–55	12	Dietary α-carotene	CAD, 0.80 (0.65–0.99), 0.04
					Dietary β-carotene	CAD, 0.74 (0.59–0.93), 0.05
					Dietary lutein and zeaxanthin	CAD, 0.90 (0.72–1.12), 0.42
					Dietary lycopene	CAD, 0.93 (0.77–1.14), 0.74
					Dietary β-cryptoxanthin	CAD, 1.17 (0.94–1.44), 0.21
CLUE, Europe 2008 (Buijsse et al. 2008)	Men free of chronic diseases	559	65–84	15	Dietary total carotenoids	CVD mortality, 0.82 (0.69–0.98)
					Dietary α-carotene	CVD mortality, 0.81 (0.66–0.99), S
					Dietary β-carotene	CVD mortality, 0.80 (0.66–0.97), S
					Dietary lutein	CVD mortality, 0.95 (0.81–1.12)
					Dietary lycopene	CVD mortality, 0.91 (0.76–1.08)
					Dietary β-cryptoxanthin	CVD mortality, 0.86 (0.72–1.03)
					Dietary zeaxanthin	CVD mortality, 0.88 (0.70–1.10)
Polyphenols						
Zutphen Elderly Study, 1993, Netherlands (Hertog et al. 1993)	Men	805	65–84	5	Flavonols, flavones	CAD, 0.32 (0.15–0.71), 0.003
Knekt et al. 1996, Finland (Knekt et al. 1996)	Men and women free of known heart disease	5133	30–69	26	Flavonols, flavones	CAD (F), 0.73 (0.41–1.32), 0.21; CAD (M), 0.67 (0.44–1.00), 0.12

(Continued)

TABLE 8.2 (CONTINUED)
Observational Studies on Intake of Antioxidants and Risk of Major CVD Outcomes

Trial/Author, Country	Population/Sex	N	Age (years)	Follow-Up (years)	Exposure (Plasma/Dietary/Supplements)	Outcomes, RR (Highest vs. Lowest) and (95% CI), p-Value
Polyphenols						
HPFS, USA, 1996 (Rimm et al. 1996)	Male health professionals	34,789	40–75	6	Flavonols, flavones	Nonfatal MI, 1.08 (0.81–1.43), NS; CAD, 0.77 (0.45–1.35), NS
ZEN, Netherlands 1996 (Keli et al. 1996)	Men	552	50–69	15	Dietary flavonoids	Incident stroke, 0.27 (0.11–0.70), 0.004
Hertog et al. 1997, Netherlands (Hertog et al. 1997a)	Men	804		10	Flavonols, flavones	CAD, 0.47 (0.27, 0.82), 0.01
Hertog et al. 1997, UK (Hertog et al. 1997b)	Men	1900	45–59	14	Dietary flavonol	IHD, 1.6 (0.9, 2.9), 0.119
Yochum et al. 1999, USA (Yochum et al. 1999)	Postmenopausal women	34,492	55–69	10	Dietary flavonoids	Death from CHD, 0.62 (0.44, 0.87), 0.11; stroke, 1.18 (0.70–2.00), 0.83
Vanharanta et al. 1999, Finland (Vanharanta et al. 1999)	Men	2005	50–69	10	Enterolactone	Incident CAD, 0.35 (0.14–0.88), 0.01
ATBC, Finland 2000 (Hirvonen et al. 2000)	Men	26,593	50–69	6.1	Flavonols, flavones	Incident stroke, 0.98 (0.8–1.21), 0.81
Arts et al. 2001, USA (Arts et al. 2001)	Postmenopausal women	32,857		13	Catechins	CAD, 0.85 (0.67, 1.07), NS
ZEN, Netherlands 2001	Men	806	65–84	10	Dietary catechin intake	IHD, 0.49 (0.27, 0.88), 0.02; MI, 0.70 (0.39, 1.26), 0.23; incident stroke, 0.92 (0.51, 1.68), 0.75

(Continued)

TABLE 8.2 (CONTINUED)
Observational Studies on Intake of Antioxidants and Risk of Major CVD Outcomes

Trial/Author, Country	Population/Sex	N	Age (years)	Follow-Up (years)	Exposure (Plasma/Dietary/Supplements)	Outcomes, RR (Highest vs. Lowest) and (95% CI), p-Value
ATBC, Finland 2001 (Hirvonen et al. 2000)	Men	25,372	50–69	6.1	Flavonols, flavones	Nonfatal MI, 0.77 (0.64, 093), NS; CAD, 0.89 (0.71, 1.11), NS
Rotterdam study, Netherlands 2002 (Geleijnse et al. 2002)	Men and women, independently living	4807	≥55	5.6	Dietary flavonoids	Nonfatal MI, 0.93 (0.57, 1.52), NS; fatal MI, 0.35 (0.13, 0.98), NS
Finland 2002 (Knekt et al. 2002)	Men and women	9131		28	Dietary flavonoids	Ischemic HD, 0.93 (0.74, 1.17), 0.30
WHS, USA 2003 (Sesso et al. 2003)	Female health professionals free of CVD and cancer	38,445	≥45	6.9 (Mean)	Dietary flavonoids	Total CVD, 0.80 (0.59, 1.09), 0.8
Vanharanta et al. 2003, Finland (Vanharanta et al. 2003)	Men	1889	42–60	12.2	Enterolactone	CVD, 0.55 (0.29–1.01), 0.04; CAD, 0.44 (0.20–0.96), 0.03
NHS, USA 2007 (Lin et al. 2007)	Female nurses	66,360	30–55	12	Flavones, flavonoids	Nonfatal MI, 1.05 (0.85–1.29), 0.55; fatal CHD, 0.81 (0.57–1.16), 0.29
IWHS, USA 2007 (Mink et al. 2007)	Postmenopausal women free of CVD	34,492	55–69	16	Total flavonoids	Total mortality, 0.94 (0.69–1.29), 0.796; CHD mortality, 0.94 (0.78–1.13), 0.980; CVD mortality, 0.93 (0.81–1.07), 0.628
KIHD, Finland 2008 (Mursu et al. 2008)	Men free of CHD or stroke	1950	42–60	15.2	Flavonoid intake	Ischemic stroke, 0.71 (0.37–1.37), 0.137; CVD mortality, 1.25 (0.74–2.11), 0.730
CPS-II, USA, 2012 (McCullough et al. 2012)	Men and women	38,180 (M), 60,289 (F)	70 (M), 69 (F)	7	Total flavonoids	CVD mortality, 0.82 (0.73–0.92), 0.01

Note: ATBC, Alpha-Tocopherol Beta-Carotene Cancer Prevention Study; CAD, coronary artery disease; CHD, coronary heart disease; CI, cerebral infarction; CPS-II, Cancer Prevention Study II; CVD, cardiovascular disease; EPESE, Established Populations for Epidemiologic Studies of the Elderly; F, female; HD, heart disease; HPFS, Health Professionals' Follow-up Study; IH, intracerebral hemorrhage; M, male; MI, myocardial infarction; NHS, Nurses' Health Study; SH, subarachnoid hemorrhage.

CHD events in the pooled population not taking vitamin supplements; after adjustment for confounding factors, only lutein was significantly and inversely associated with CHD incidence. However, because the associations observed with lutein disappeared after further exclusion of cases during the first 2 years of follow-up, the authors concluded that none of the carotenoids, when consumed in usual dietary quantities, can predict reduced incidence of CHD. These conclusions are further replicated in a more recent meta-analysis of 15 prospective cohort studies that examined the effect of β-carotene on CHD (Ye and Song 2008), whereas an earlier meta-analysis of RCTs suggested that β-carotene supplementation should be actively discouraged as it was found to be associated with a small but significant excess of all-cause and CVD mortality (Vivekananthan et al. 2003).

Table 8.1 presents the available randomized controlled trials that examine the effect of β-carotene, either alone or in combination with other antioxidants, on major CVD outcomes. The vast majority of studies produced nonsignificant results. The study that showed a significant association was the ATBC (Alpha-Tocopherol Beta-Carotene) trial in which a population of male smokers was examined (Rapola et al. 1997, Virtamo et al. 1998, Leppala et al. 2000). In fact, a meta-analysis of RCTs concluded that there is no evidence to support antioxidant vitamin supplements (including β-carotene supplements) for the primary or secondary prevention of various diseases (Bjelakovic et al. 2012), and this finding has also been replicated in more recent meta-analyses of RCTs (Myung et al. 2013, Ye et al. 2013). In addition, a meta-analysis of RCTs concluded that there was no evidence of a protective effect of β-carotene on the progression of atherosclerosis (Bleys et al. 2006).

In conclusion, there is no evidence to support a role of carotenoid supplementation for the prevention or treatment of CVD.

SELENIUM

Selenium is an essential trace element that is involved in the protection against oxidative damage (Rayman 2000). The main sources of selenium include plant foods, meat, and seafood; however, the selenium content of foods varies according to the soil, water concentrations, and selenium-containing fertilizers (Flores-Mateo et al. 2006), and this is the reason why dietary assessment methods are irrelevant in the study of selenium status; instead, toenail, blood, erythrocyte, or serum and plasma selenium concentrations are used (Longnecker et al. 1996, Satia et al. 2006). Observational studies investigating the association between low selenium concentration with CVD outcomes and RCTs investigating supplemental selenium and CHD have been inconclusive.

Flores-Mateo et al. (2006) appraised the evidence with regard to the association of selenium and CHD, and the meta-analysis suggests that there is a statistically significant inverse association between selenium concentration in several tissues and CHD outcomes in observational studies; a 50% increase was associated with 24% reduced risk of coronary events. However, given the experience from observational studies of other antioxidants, this validity is uncertain, as RCTs might show a different result. RCTs examining selenium supplementation are few, and selenium has been administered in combination with other antioxidants (Table 8.1). Another meta-analysis of RCTs that examined vitamin–mineral supplementation and the progression of atherosclerosis reached a similar conclusion (Bleys et al. 2006).

In addition, a Cochrane collaboration review by Rees et al. (2013), which included 19,715 participants, found no statistically significant effects of selenium supplementation on all-cause mortality, CVD mortality, nonfatal CVD events, and all CVD events, and therefore suggests that selenium supplements do not prevent the occurrence of major CVDs. They also suggest that taking selenium supplements is neither beneficial nor harmful for CVD, but is probably unnecessary for those who are already well nourished and who take their selenium from natural foods.

POLYPHENOLS

A vast number of molecules has a polyphenol structure; thousands have been identified in higher plants and several hundred in edible plants, and they can be classified according to the number of phenol rings that they contain as well as the structural rings that bind these rings together (Manach et al. 2004). Polyphenols can be found in a wide range of fruits and vegetables, as well as in other foods/beverages (e.g., tea, wine, and soy milk), and include phenolic acids, flavonoids, stilbenes and lignans, and flavonoids, which may be further subdivided to six subclasses: flavonols, flavones, isoflavones, flavanones, anthocyanidins, and flavanols (Manach et al. 2004). Polyphenols in plants act as a defense system against infection and protect against ultraviolet radiation, pathogens, and physical damage (Davidson and Duchen 2007).

During the last few decades, researchers became interested in polyphenols, and the main reason for this was the recognition of the antioxidant properties of polyphenols (Manach et al. 2004). Apart from their antioxidant properties, polyphenols also have several other specific biological actions that are yet poorly understood (Manach et al. 2004). With regard to *in vivo* studies, one can find many experimental studies in the literature that show that polyphenols have many effects in animal models; they act as free radical scavengers, regulate nitric oxide, decrease leukocyte immobilization, induce apoptosis, inhibit cell proliferation and angiogenesis, and exhibit phytoestrogenic activity (Arts and Hollman 2005). However, results from animal studies cannot be extrapolated to humans as the bioavailability and metabolism of polyphenols vary between animals; consequently, human studies are needed before moving on to making recommendations (Chong et al. 2010).

As noted earlier, for other antioxidants, increased fruit and vegetable consumption has been associated with beneficial effects on CVD. However, fruits and vegetables contain an array of antioxidant substances, such as vitamins and nonnutrient phytochemicals like carotenoids and polyphenols, and the contribution of each of these substances in cardioprotection is not very clear (Chong et al. 2010). Although no information on causality can be obtained, researchers have suggested that polyphenols may explain part of the beneficial effect of fruit and vegetable consumption on CVD (Arts and Hollman 2005).

Up to date, most studies in humans have explored the associations of polyphenolic-rich beverages like tea, cocoa, and red wine, and intervention studies examining fruits are few (Chong-Han 2010). In addition, there is lack of studies examining hard outcomes. In a review by Chong-Han (2010) where fruit polyphenols were examined in relation to CVD risk (platelet function, hypertension, lipid metabolism, and vascular function), it was concluded that there is some supportive evidence for the beneficial effects of fruit polyphenols on CVD risk; however, the literature is limited and the study design often varies.

Table 8.2 provides an overview of observational studies that have examined the effects of polyphenols on CVD risk. As Wang et al. (2013) noted, accurate estimation of polyphenol intake is critical for the investigation of their association with CVD outcomes, and it was only after 2003 that the U.S. Department of Agriculture released the first flavonoids databases, which included 26 flavonoids. This database was also updated in 2013. In addition, another database of polyphenol content of foods was recently published (Neveu et al. 2010). Owing to the limitation mentioned with regard to the availability of nutrition data on polyphenol content of foods, studies conducted after the release of the databases have shown a significant inverse association with CVD outcomes (Wang et al. 2013).

A meta-analysis of six prospective cohort studies that examined the association between flavonol intake and stroke risk concluded that a high intake of dietary flavonols compared with a low intake is associated with 20% lower stroke incidence (Hollman et al. 2010). However, the authors also note that owing to the small number of studies and an indication for publication bias, results should be interpreted with caution. Similar findings have also been reported in a meta-analysis that examined the relationship between flavonol intake and CHD mortality (Huxley and Neil 2003).

Currently, there is no clinical trial available examining the effects of polyphenols on major CVD outcomes; however, observational studies suggest a beneficial association. Some researchers have even suggested that polyphenols could be expected to have a "pleiotropic effect" similar to that of statins in the prevention of atherosclerosis (Kishimoto et al. 2013).

RESVERATROL

Resveratrol is a polyphenol found in grape skin/seed, a variety of berries, peanuts, red wine, and the root of *Polygonum cuspidatum*, a traditional Chinese and Japanese medicinal material (Smoliga et al. 2011, Wang et al. 2012). Owing to red wine's rich resveratrol content, it has been hypothesized to be an important factor in the French paradox (Liu et al. 2007). Cross-sectional evidence shows that 69.8% of women and 64.1% of men that are long-term consumers of multiple dietary supplements take supplemental resveratrol (Block et al. 2007).

A number of studies have proposed that it has many properties that can confer, among others, CVD benefit (Wang et al. 2012). *In vivo* evidence suggests that resveratrol has some beneficial effects in rodent models of stress and disease (Baur and Sinclair 2006). Moreover, the effects of resveratrol on isolated tissues or organs, many of which are associated with oxidative stress, are well documented (Opie and Lecour 2007).

Resveratrol can act as a radical-scavenging antioxidant and an anti-inflammatory agent, has been shown to induce platelet apoptosis, activate antiaging genes and facilitate extending lifespan in organisms like yeasts and worms, prevent the proliferation and differentiation of preadipocytes, promote fat mobilization in white adipocytes, trigger lipolysis, and protect mice against diet-induced obesity (Wang et al. 2012). *In vivo* studies also suggest that dietary resveratrol is hypolipidemic, with a tendency for antitumor growth and antimetastasis effects observed in hepatoma-bearing rats (Miura et al. 2003). In addition, resveratrol has some beneficial anti-oxidant activity related to LDL oxidation (Fremont et al. 1999). Other metabolic roles of resveratrol include statin-like effects; furthermore, resveratrol treatment has been observed to elevate high-density lipoprotein (HDL) levels as well as promote the capacity of HDL to mediate cholesterol efflux (Wang et al. 2012). Moreover, it has been suggested that resveratrol has beneficial effects on glucose metabolism and insulin sensitivity, endothelial function, and cardiovascular remodeling (Wang et al. 2012). It also seems that resveratrol directly improves the function of a failing heart (Wang et al. 2012).

In contrast to the above, the complexity of resveratrol's effects *in vivo* presents a major challenge in human studies (Smoliga et al. 2011). Although resveratrol seems to have many potential beneficial effects on CVD, its effects *in vivo* as well as its effective dose in animals cannot be generalized to humans (Reagan-Shaw et al. 2008). Many clinical trials that aim to decipher the safety, effective dose, and the effects of resveratrol are currently ongoing (Wang et al. 2012). Some skepticism exists with regard to resveratrol's very low bioavailability (Smoliga et al. 2011), as effects seen *in vivo* may not be replicated in humans because of its rapid metabolism (Goldberg et al. 2003). In addition, resveratrol's bioavailability from supplements is highly variable (Smoliga et al. 2011).

Lycopene

Lycopene is a carotenoid and is the pigment that gives tomatoes their distinctive red color (Ried and Fakler 2011). In addition, owing to its chemical structure, lyco-pene is a powerful antioxidant and free radical scavenger; however, it has also been hypothesized to reduce cholesterol levels and increase LDL degradation (Ried and Fakler 2011). *In vitro* evidence suggests that lycopene protects against oxidation, and it is considered to be the most effective quencher of LDL and human lymphoid cells; however, evidence in humans is limited (Chen et al. 2013b).

Observational studies have suggested that increased consumption of foods rich in lycopene has an inverse relationship with CVD and cancer (Rao and Agarwal 2000). However, lycopene metabolism is not yet fully understood, and, as with other anti-oxidants, its effects *in vitro* might differ from its effects *in vivo* (Chen et al. 2013b).

There is a lack of RCTs examining the relationship between long-term lyco-pene intake/supplementation and major CVD outcomes. However, a meta-analysis by Chen et al. (2013b) that pooled results from 13 RCTs revealed no statistically significant difference in the LDL lag time between the lycopene treatment group and the control group. In contrast, a meta-analysis of another three trials within the same publication suggests that lycopene significantly increases DNA tail length. The authors conclude that the effect of lycopene supplementation remains unconfirmed and its efficiency as an antioxidant *in vivo* needs further investigation. They also report that consumption of natural carotenoid-rich fruits and vegetables is preferable to lycopene supplementation. Another recent meta-analysis suggests that lycopene taken in doses of ≥25 mg daily is effective in reducing LDL cholesterol by approximately 10% in patients with slightly elevated cholesterol levels.

A meta-analysis by Ried and Fakler (2011) suggests that lycopene is effective in reducing LDL and total serum cholesterol if taken in doses of >25 mg daily, and in reducing systolic blood pressure in individuals with hypertension.

CONCLUSION

In contrast to the observational evidence showing that increased consumption of fruits and vegetables is inversely associated with reduced CVD risk, prospective studies and RCTs of antioxidants have failed to show a consistent effect on CVD outcomes. Therefore, antioxidant supplement administration is not advisable for reducing the risk of developing CHD or stroke. In addition, there are no guidelines with regard to which fruits and vegetables contribute most to the risk reduction and, therefore, consuming a variety would be advisable. Further studies that examine which fruits and vegetables contribute more to the CVD risk reduction, as well as other chronic diseases, seen in observational studies are needed to make more specific recommendations.

REFERENCES

AHA (2013a). *Coronary Artery Disease—Coronary Heart Disease*. Available at: http://www .heart.org/HEARTORG/Conditions/More/MyHeartandStrokeNews/Coronary-Artery -Disease---Coronary-Heart-Disease_UCM_436416_Article.jsp.

AHA (2013b). *What Is Cardiovascular Disease (Heart Disease)?* Available at: http://www .heart.org/HEARTORG/Caregiver/Resources/WhatisCardiovascularDisease/What-is -Cardiovascular-Disease_UCM_301852_Article.jsp.

Allender, S. S., P. Peto, V. et al. (2008). *European Cardiovascular Disease Statistics 2008*, 3rd edition. London: European Health Network.

Arts, I. C. and P. C. Hollman (2005). "Polyphenols and disease risk in epidemiologic studies." *Am J Clin Nutr* **81**(1 Suppl): 317S–325S.

Arts, I. C., D. R. Jacobs, Jr., L. J. Harnack, M. Gross and A. R. Folsom (2001). "Dietary catechins in relation to coronary heart disease death among postmenopausal women." *Epidemiology* **12**(6): 668–675.

Ascherio, A., E. B. Rimm, M. A. Hernan, E. Giovannucci, I. Kawachi, M. J. Stampfer and W. C. Willett (1999). "Relation of consumption of vitamin E, vitamin C, and carotenoids to risk for stroke among men in the United States." *Ann Intern Med* **130**(12): 963–970.

Baur, J. A. and D. A. Sinclair (2006). "Therapeutic potential of resveratrol: The *in vivo* evidence." *Nat Rev Drug Discov* **5**(6): 493–506.

Bhupathiraju, S. N. and K. L. Tucker (2011). "Coronary heart disease prevention: Nutrients, foods, and dietary patterns." *Clin Chim Acta* **412**(17–18): 1493–1514.

Bin, Q., X. Hu, Y. Cao and F. Gao (2011). "The role of vitamin E (tocopherol) supplementation in the prevention of stroke. A meta-analysis of 13 randomised controlled trials." *Thromb Haemost* **105**(4): 579–585.

Bjelakovic, G., D. Nikolova, L. L. Gluud, R. G. Simonetti and C. Gluud (2012). "Antioxidant supplements for prevention of mortality in healthy participants and patients with various diseases." *Cochrane Database Syst Rev* **3**: Cd007176.

Bleys, J., E. R. Miller, 3rd, R. Pastor-Barriuso, L. J. Appel and E. Guallar (2006). "Vitamin– mineral supplementation and the progression of atherosclerosis: A meta-analysis of randomized controlled trials." *Am J Clin Nutr* **84**(4): 880–887; quiz 954–955.

Block, G., C. D. Jensen, E. P. Norkus, T. B. Dalvi, L. G. Wong, J. F. McManus and M. L. Hudes (2007). "Usage patterns, health, and nutritional status of long-term multiple dietary supplement users: A cross-sectional study." *Nutr J* **6**: 30.

Boaz, M., S. Smetana, T. Weinstein, Z. Matas, U. Gafter, A. Iaina, A. Knecht, Y. Weissgarten, D. Brunner, M. Fainaru and M. S. Green (2000). "Secondary prevention with antioxidants of cardiovascular disease in endstage renal disease (SPACE): Randomised placebo-controlled trial." *Lancet* **356**(9237): 1213–1218.

Brown, B. G., X. Q. Zhao, A. Chait, L. D. Fisher, M. C. Cheung, J. S. Morse, A. A. Dowdy, E. K. Marino, E. L. Bolson, P. Alaupovic, J. Frohlich and J. J. Albers (2001). "Simvastatin and niacin, antioxidant vitamins, or the combination for the prevention of coronary disease." *N Engl J Med* **345**(22): 1583–1592.

Buijsse, B., E. J. Feskens, L. Kwape, F. J. Kok and D. Kromhout (2008). "Both alpha- and beta-carotene, but not tocopherols and vitamin C, are inversely related to 15-year cardiovascular mortality in Dutch elderly men." *J Nutr* **138**(2): 344–350.

Chen, G. C., D. B. Lu, Z. Pang and Q. F. Liu (2013a). "Vitamin C intake, circulating vitamin C and risk of stroke: A meta-analysis of prospective studies." *J Am Heart Assoc* **2**(6): e000329.

Chen, J., Y. Song and L. Zhang (2013b). "Effect of lycopene supplementation on oxidative stress: An exploratory systematic review and meta-analysis of randomized controlled trials." *J Med Food* **16**(5): 361–374.

Chen, K., J. Suh, A. C. Carr, J. D. Morrow, J. Zeind and B. Frei (2000). "Vitamin C suppresses oxidative lipid damage *in vivo*, even in the presence of iron overload." *Am J Physiol Endocrinol Metab* **279**(6): E1406–E1412.

Chong, M. F., R. Macdonald and J. A. Lovegrove (2010). "Fruit polyphenols and CVD risk: A review of human intervention studies." *Br J Nutr* **104 Suppl 3**: S28–S39.

Chong-Han, K. (2010). "Dietary lipophilic antioxidants: Implications and significance in the aging process." *Crit Rev Food Sci Nutr* **50**(10): 931–937.

Cook, N. R., C. M. Albert, J. M. Gaziano, E. Zaharris, J. MacFadyen, E. Danielson, J. E. Buring and J. E. Manson (2007). "A randomized factorial trial of vitamins C and E and beta carotene in the secondary prevention of cardiovascular events in women: Results from the Women's Antioxidant Cardiovascular Study." *Arch Intern Med* **167**(15): 1610–1618.

Dauchet, L., P. Amouyel and J. Dallongeville (2009). "Fruits, vegetables and coronary heart disease." *Nat Rev Cardiol* **6**(9): 599–608.

Davidson, S. M. and M. R. Duchen (2007). "Endothelial mitochondria: Contributing to vascular function and disease." *Circ Res* **100**(8): 1128–1141.

Daviglus, M. L., A. J. Orencia, A. R. Dyer, K. Liu, D. K. Morris, V. Persky, N. Chavez, J. Goldberg, M. Drum, R. B. Shekelle and J. Stamler (1997). "Dietary vitamin C, beta-carotene and 30-year risk of stroke: Results from the Western Electric Study." *Neuroepidemiology* **16**(2): 69–77.

de Gaetano, G. (2001). "Low-dose aspirin and vitamin E in people at cardiovascular risk: A randomised trial in general practice. Collaborative Group of the Primary Prevention Project." *Lancet* **357**(9250): 89–95.

Eidelman, R. S., D. Hollar, P. R. Hebert, G. A. Lamas and C. H. Hennekens (2004). "Randomized trials of vitamin E in the treatment and prevention of cardiovascular disease." *Arch Intern Med* **164**(14): 1552–1556.

Flores-Mateo, G., A. Navas-Acien, R. Pastor-Barriuso and E. Guallar (2006). "Selenium and coronary heart disease: A meta-analysis." *Am J Clin Nutr* **84**(4): 762–773.

Fremont, L., L. Belguendouz and S. Delpal (1999). "Antioxidant activity of resveratrol and alcohol-free wine polyphenols related to LDL oxidation and polyunsaturated fatty acids." *Life Sci* **64**(26): 2511–2521.

Geleijnse, J. M., L. J. Launer, D. A. Van der Kuip, A. Hofman and J. C. Witteman (2002). "Inverse association of tea and flavonoid intakes with incident myocardial infarction: The Rotterdam Study." *Am J Clin Nutr* **75**(5): 880–886.

Genkinger, J. M., E. A. Platz, S. C. Hoffman, G. W. Comstock and K. J. Helzlsouer (2004). "Fruit, vegetable, and antioxidant intake and all-cause, cancer, and cardiovascular disease mortality in a community-dwelling population in Washington County, Maryland." *Am J Epidemiol* **160**(12): 1223–1233.

Gey, K. F., P. Puska, P. Jordan and U. K. Moser (1991). "Inverse correlation between plasma vitamin E and mortality from ischemic heart disease in cross-cultural epidemiology." *Am J Clin Nutr* **53**(1 Suppl): 326S–334S.

Go, A. S., D. Mozaffarian, V. L. Roger, E. J. Benjamin, J. D. Berry, W. B. Borden, D. M. Bravata, S. Dai, E. S. Ford, C. S. Fox, S. Franco, H. J. Fullerton, C. Gillespie, S. M. Hailpern, J. A. Heit, V. J. Howard, M. D. Huffman, B. M. Kissela, S. J. Kittner, D. T. Lackland, J. H. Lichtman, L. D. Lisabeth, D. Magid, G. M. Marcus, A. Marelli, D. B. Matchar, D. K. McGuire, E. R. Mohler, C. S. Moy, M. E. Mussolino, G. Nichol, N. P. Paynter, P. J. Schreiner, P. D. Sorlie, J. Stein, T. N. Turan, S. S. Virani, N. D. Wong, D. Woo, M. B. Turner, C.; American Heart Association Statistics Committee and Stroke Statistics Subcommittee (2013). "Heart disease and stroke statistics—2013 update: A report from the American Heart Association." *Circulation* **127**(1): e6–e245.

Goldberg, D. M., J. Yan and G. J. Soleas (2003). "Absorption of three wine-related polyphenols in three different matrices by healthy subjects." *Clin Biochem* **36**(1): 79–87.

Griendling, K. K. and G. A. FitzGerald (2003a). "Oxidative stress and cardiovascular injury: Part I: Basic mechanisms and *in vivo* monitoring of ROS." *Circulation* **108**(16): 1912–1916.

Griendling, K. K. and G. A. FitzGerald (2003b). "Oxidative stress and cardiovascular injury: Part II: Animal and human studies." *Circulation* **108**(17): 2034–2040.

Gruppo Italiano per lo Studio della Sopravvivenza nell'Infarto Miocardico (1999). "Dietary supplementation with n-3 polyunsaturated fatty acids and vitamin E after myocardial infarction: Results of the GISSI-Prevenzione trial. Gruppo Italiano per lo Studio della Sopravvivenza nell'Infarto Miocardico." *Lancet* **354**(9177): 447–455.

He, F. J., C. A. Nowson and G. A. MacGregor (2006). "Fruit and vegetable consumption and stroke: Meta-analysis of cohort studies." *Lancet* **367**(9507): 320–326.

Hennekens, C. H., J. E. Buring, J. E. Manson, M. Stampfer, B. Rosner, N. R. Cook, C. Belanger, F. LaMotte, J. M. Gaziano, P. M. Ridker, W. Willett and R. Peto (1996). "Lack of effect of long-term supplementation with beta carotene on the incidence of malignant neoplasms and cardiovascular disease." *N Engl J Med* **334**(18): 1145–1149.

Hercberg, S., P. Galan, P. Preziosi, S. Bertrais, L. Mennen, D. Malvy, A. M. Roussel, A. Favier and S. Briancon (2004). "The SU.VI.MAX Study: A randomized, placebo-controlled trial of the health effects of antioxidant vitamins and minerals." *Arch Intern Med* **164**(21): 2335–2342.

Hertog, M. G., E. J. Feskens, P. C. Hollman, M. B. Katan and D. Kromhout (1993). "Dietary antioxidant flavonoids and risk of coronary heart disease: The Zutphen Elderly Study." *Lancet* **342**(8878): 1007–1011.

Hertog, M. G., E. J. Feskens and D. Kromhout (1997a). "Antioxidant flavonols and coronary heart disease risk." *Lancet* **349**(9053): 699.

Hertog, M. G., P. M. Sweetnam, A. M. Fehily, P. C. Elwood and D. Kromhout (1997b). "Antioxidant flavonols and ischemic heart disease in a Welsh population of men: The Caerphilly Study." *Am J Clin Nutr* **65**(5): 1489–1494.

Hirvonen, T., J. Virtamo, P. Korhonen, D. Albanes and P. Pietinen (2000). "Intake of flavonoids, carotenoids, vitamins C and E, and risk of stroke in male smokers." *Stroke* **31**(10): 2301–2306.

Hollman, P. C., A. Geelen and D. Kromhout (2010). "Dietary flavonol intake may lower stroke risk in men and women." *J Nutr* **140**(3): 600–604.

Hu, F. B. and W. C. Willett (2002). "Optimal diets for prevention of coronary heart disease." *JAMA* **288**(20): 2569–2578.

Huxley, R. R. and H. A. Neil (2003). "The relation between dietary flavonol intake and coro-
nary heart disease mortality: A meta-analysis of prospective cohort studies." *Eur J Clin
Nutr* **57**(8): 904–908.
Juraschek, S. P., E. Guallar, L. J. Appel and E. R. Miller, 3rd (2012). "Effects of vitamin C
supplementation on blood pressure: A meta-analysis of randomized controlled trials."
Am J Clin Nutr **95**(5): 1079–1088.
Keli, S. O., M. G. Hertog, E. J. Feskens and D. Kromhout (1996). "Dietary flavonoids, anti-
oxidant vitamins, and incidence of stroke: The Zutphen study." *Arch Intern Med* **156**(6):
637–642.
Kishimoto, Y., M. Tani and K. Kondo (2013). "Pleiotropic preventive effects of dietary poly-
phenols in cardiovascular diseases." *Eur J Clin Nutr* **67**(5): 532–535.
Klipstein-Grobusch, K., J. M. Geleijnse, J. H. den Breeijen, H. Boeing, A. Hofman, D. E.
Grobbee and J. C. Witteman (1999). "Dietary antioxidants and risk of myocardial
infarction in the elderly: The Rotterdam Study." *Am J Clin Nutr* **69**(2): 261–266.
Knekt, P., A. Reunanen, R. Jarvinen, R. Seppanen, M. Heliovaara and A. Aromaa (1994).
"Antioxidant vitamin intake and coronary mortality in a longitudinal population study."
Am J Epidemiol **139**(12): 1180–1189.
Knekt, P., R. Jarvinen, A. Reunanen and J. Maatela (1996). "Flavonoid intake and coronary
mortality in Finland: A cohort study." *BMJ* **312**(7029): 478–481.
Knekt, P., J. Kumpulainen, R. Jarvinen, H. Rissanen, M. Heliovaara, A. Reunanen, T.
Hakulinen and A. Aromaa (2002). "Flavonoid intake and risk of chronic diseases." *Am
J Clin Nutr* **76**(3): 560–568.
Knekt, P., J. Ritz, M. A. Pereira, E. J. O'Reilly, K. Augustsson, G. E. Fraser, U. Goldbourt,
B. L. Heitmann, G. Hallmans, S. Liu, P. Pietinen, D. Spiegelman, J. Stevens, J. Virtamo,
W. C. Willett, E. B. Rimm and A. Ascherio (2004). "Antioxidant vitamins and coronary
heart disease risk: A pooled analysis of 9 cohorts." *Am J Clin Nutr* **80**(6): 1508–1520.
Kushi, L. H., A. R. Folsom, R. J. Prineas, P. J. Mink, Y. Wu and R. M. Bostick (1996). "Dietary
antioxidant vitamins and death from coronary heart disease in postmenopausal women."
N Engl J Med **334**(18): 1156–1162.
Lee, I. M., N. R. Cook, J. E. Manson, J. E. Buring and C. H. Hennekens (1999). "Beta-
carotene supplementation and incidence of cancer and cardiovascular disease: The
Women's Health Study." *J Natl Cancer Inst* **91**(24): 2102–2106.
Lee, I. M., N. R. Cook, J. M. Gaziano, D. Gordon, P. M. Ridker, J. E. Manson, C. H. Hennekens
and J. E. Buring (2005). "Vitamin E in the primary prevention of cardiovascular disease and
cancer. The Women's Health Study: A randomized controlled trial." *JAMA* **294**(1): 56–65.
Leppala, J. M., J. Virtamo, R. Fogelholm, J. K. Huttunen, D. Albanes, P. R. Taylor and O. P.
Heinonen (2000). "Controlled trial of alpha-tocopherol and beta-carotene supplements
on stroke incidence and mortality in male smokers." *Arterioscler Thromb Vasc Biol*
20(1): 230–235.
Lin, J., K. M. Rexrode, F. Hu, C. M. Albert, C. U. Chae, E. B. Rimm, M. J. Stampfer and J. E.
Manson (2007). "Dietary intakes of flavonols and flavones and coronary heart disease in
US women." *Am J Epidemiol* **165**(11): 1305–1313.
Liu, B. L., X. Zhang, W. Zhang and H. N. Zhen (2007). "New enlightenment of French
Paradox: Resveratrol's potential for cancer chemoprevention and anti-cancer therapy."
Cancer Biol Ther **6**(12): 1833–1836.
Lock, K., J. Pomerleau, L. Causer, D. R. Altmann and M. McKee (2005). "The global burden
of disease attributable to low consumption of fruit and vegetables: Implications for the
global strategy on diet." *Bull World Health Organ* **83**(2): 100–108.
Longnecker, M. P., D. O. Stram, P. R. Taylor, O. A. Levander, M. Howe, C. Veillon, P. A.
McAdam, K. Y. Patterson, J. M. Holden, J. S. Morris, C. A. Swanson and W. C. Willett
(1996). "Use of selenium concentration in whole blood, serum, toenails, or urine as a
surrogate measure of selenium intake." *Epidemiology* **7**(4): 384–390.

Lonn, E., J. Bosch, S. Yusuf, P. Sheridan, J. Pogue, J. M. Arnold, C. Ross, A. Arnold, P. Sleight, J. Probstfield, G. R. Dagenais; HOPE and HOPE-TOO Trial Investigators (2005). "Effects of long-term vitamin E supplementation on cardiovascular events and cancer: A randomized controlled trial." *JAMA* **293**(11): 1338–1347.

Losonczy, K. G., T. B. Harris and R. J. Havlik (1996). "Vitamin E and vitamin C supplement use and risk of all-cause and coronary heart disease mortality in older persons: The Established Populations for Epidemiologic Studies of the Elderly." *Am J Clin Nutr* **64**(2): 190–196.

Maiolino, G., G. Rossitto, P. Caielli, V. Bisogni, G. P. Rossi and L. A. Calo (2013). "The role of oxidized low-density lipoproteins in atherosclerosis: The myths and the facts." *Mediators Inflamm* **2013**: 1–13. Article ID 714653.

Manach, C., A. Scalbert, C. Morand, C. Remesy and L. Jimenez (2004). "Polyphenols: Food sources and bioavailability." *Am J Clin Nutr* **79**(5): 727–747.

McCullough, M. L., J. J. Peterson, R. Patel, P. F. Jacques, R. Shah and J. T. Dwyer (2012). "Flavonoid intake and cardiovascular disease mortality in a prospective cohort of US adults." *Am J Clin Nutr* **95**(2): 454–464.

Milman, U., S. Blum, C. Shapira, D. Aronson, R. Miller-Lotan, Y. Anbinder, J. Alshiek, L. Bennett, M. Kostenko, M. Landau, S. Keidar, Y. Levy, A. Khemlin, A. Radan and A. P. Levy (2008). "Vitamin E supplementation reduces cardiovascular events in a subgroup of middle-aged individuals with both type 2 diabetes mellitus and the haptoglobin 2-2 genotype: A prospective double-blinded clinical trial." *Arterioscler Thromb Vasc Biol* **28**(2): 341–347.

Mink, P. J., C. G. Scrafford, L. M. Barraj, L. Harnack, C. P. Hong, J. A. Nettleton and D. R. Jacobs, Jr. (2007). "Flavonoid intake and cardiovascular disease mortality: A prospective study in postmenopausal women." *Am J Clin Nutr* **85**(3): 895–909.

Miura, D., Y. Miura and K. Yagasaki (2003). "Hypolipidemic action of dietary resveratrol, a phytoalexin in grapes and red wine, in hepatoma-bearing rats." *Life Sci* **73**(11): 1393–1400.

Morris, D. L., S. B. Kritchevsky and C. E. Davis (1994). "Serum carotenoids and coronary heart disease. The Lipid Research Clinics Coronary Primary Prevention Trial and Follow-up Study." *JAMA* **272**(18): 1439–1441.

Muntwyler, J., C. H. Hennekens, J. E. Manson, J. E. Buring and J. M. Gaziano (2002). "Vitamin supplement use in a low-risk population of US male physicians and subsequent cardiovascular mortality." *Arch Intern Med* **162**: 1472–1476.

Mursu, J., S. Voutilainen, T. Nurmi, T. P. Tuomainen, S. Kurl and J. T. Salonen (2008). "Flavonoid intake and the risk of ischaemic stroke and CVD mortality in middle-aged Finnish men: The Kuopio Ischaemic Heart Disease Risk Factor Study." *Br J Nutr* **100**(4): 890–895.

Myung, S. K., W. Ju, B. Cho, S. W. Oh, S. M. Park, B. K. Koo, B. J. Park and Korean Meta-Analysis Study Group (2013). "Efficacy of vitamin and antioxidant supplements in prevention of cardiovascular disease: Systematic review and meta-analysis of randomised controlled trials." *BMJ* **346**: f10.

National Cancer Institute (2013). *Antioxidants and Cancer Prevention*. Available at: http://www.cancer.gov/cancertopics/factsheet/prevention/antioxidants.

National Institutes of Health (2013). *What is Atherosclerosis?* Available at: http://www.nhlbi.nih.gov/health/health-topics/topics/atherosclerosis.

Neveu, V., J. Perez-Jimenez, F. Vos, V. Crespy, L. du Chaffaut, L. Mennen, C. Knox, R. Eisner, J. Cruz, D. Wishart and A. Scalbert (2010). "Phenol-explorer: An online comprehensive database on polyphenol contents in foods." *Database (Oxford)* **2010**: bap024.

Omenn, G. S., G. E. Goodman, M. D. Thornquist, J. Balmes, M. R. Cullen, A. Glass, J. P. Keogh, F. L. Meyskens, B. Valanis, J. H. Williams, S. Barnhart and S. Hammar (1996). "Effects of a combination of beta carotene and vitamin A on lung cancer and cardiovascular disease." *N Engl J Med* **334**(18): 1150–1155.

Opie, L. H. and S. Lecour (2007). "The red wine hypothesis: From concepts to protective signalling molecules." *Eur Heart J* **28**(14): 1683–1693.

Osganian, S. K., M. J. Stampfer, E. Rimm, D. Spiegelman, F. B. Hu, J. E. Manson and W. C. Willett (2003a). "Vitamin C and risk of coronary heart disease in women." *J Am Coll Cardiol* **42**(2): 246–252.

Osganian, S. K., M. J. Stampfer, E. Rimm, D. Spiegelman, J. E. Manson and W. C. Willett (2003b). "Dietary carotenoids and risk of coronary artery disease in women." *Am J Clin Nutr* **77**(6): 1390–1399.

Ozkanlar, S. and F. Akcay (2012). "Antioxidant vitamins in atherosclerosis—Animal experiments and clinical studies." *Adv Clin Exp Med* **21**(1): 115–123.

Rao, A. V. and S. Agarwal (2000). "Role of antioxidant lycopene in cancer and heart disease." *J Am Coll Nutr* **19**(5): 563–569.

Rapola, J. M., J. Virtamo, S. Ripatti, J. K. Huttunen, D. Albanes, P. R. Taylor and O. P. Heinonen (1997). "Randomised trial of alpha-tocopherol and beta-carotene supplements on incidence of major coronary events in men with previous myocardial infarction." *Lancet* **349**(9067): 1715–1720.

Rayman, M. P. (2000). "The importance of selenium to human health." *Lancet* **356**(9225): 233–241.

Reagan-Shaw, S., M. Nihal and N. Ahmad (2008). "Dose translation from animal to human studies revisited." *FASEB J* **22**(3): 659–661.

Rees, K., L. Hartley, C. Day, N. Flowers, A. Clarke and S. Stranges (2013). "Selenium supplementation for the primary prevention of cardiovascular disease." *Cochrane Database Syst Rev* **1**: CD009671.

Ried, K. and P. Fakler (2011). "Protective effect of lycopene on serum cholesterol and blood pressure: Meta-analyses of intervention trials." *Maturitas* **68**(4): 299–310.

Rimm, E. B., M. J. Stampfer, A. Ascherio, E. Giovannucci, G. A. Colditz and W. C. Willett (1993). "Vitamin E consumption and the risk of coronary heart disease in men." *N Engl J Med* **328**(20): 1450–1456.

Rimm, E. B., M. B. Katan, A. Ascherio, M. J. Stampfer and W. C. Willett (1996). "Relation between intake of flavonoids and risk for coronary heart disease in male health professionals." *Ann Intern Med* **125**(5): 384–389.

Sahyoun, N. R., P. F. Jacques and R. M. Russell (1996). "Carotenoids, vitamins C and E, and mortality in an elderly population." *Am J Epidemiol* **144**(5): 501–511.

Satia, J. A., I. B. King, J. S. Morris, K. Stratton and E. White (2006). "Toenail and plasma levels as biomarkers of selenium exposure." *Ann Epidemiol* **16**(1): 53–58.

Schurks, M., R. J. Glynn, P. M. Rist, C. Tzourio and T. Kurth (2010). "Effects of vitamin E on stroke subtypes: Meta-analysis of randomised controlled trials." *BMJ* **341**: c5702.

Sesso, H. D., J. M. Gaziano, S. Liu and J. E. Buring (2003). "Flavonoid intake and the risk of cardiovascular disease in women." *Am J Clin Nutr* **77**(6): 1400–1408.

Sesso, H. D., J. E. Buring, W. G. Christen, T. Kurth, C. Belanger, J. MacFadyen, V. Bubes, J. E. Manson, R. J. Glynn and J. M. Gaziano (2008). "Vitamins E and C in the prevention of cardiovascular disease in men: The Physicians' Health Study II randomized controlled trial." *JAMA* **300**(18): 2123–2133.

Shekelle, P. G., S. C. Morton, L. K. Jungvig, J. Udani, M. Spar, W. Tu, M. J. Suttorp, I. Coulter, S. J. Newberry and M. Hardy (2004). "Effect of supplemental vitamin E for the prevention and treatment of cardiovascular disease." *J Gen Intern Med* **19**(4): 380–389.

Singh, U., S. Devaraj and I. Jialal (2005). "Vitamin E, oxidative stress, and inflammation." *Annu Rev Nutr* **25**: 151–174.

Smoliga, J. M., J. A. Baur and H. A. Hausenblas (2011). "Resveratrol and health—A comprehensive review of human clinical trials." *Mol Nutr Food Res* **55**(8): 1129–1141.

Stampfer, M. J. and E. B. Rimm (1995). "Epidemiologic evidence for vitamin E in prevention of cardiovascular disease." *Am J Clin Nutr* **62**(6 Suppl): 1365S–1369S.

Stampfer, M. J., C. H. Hennekens, J. E. Manson, G. A. Colditz, B. Rosner and W. C. Willett (1993). "Vitamin E consumption and the risk of coronary disease in women." *N Engl J Med* **328**(20): 1444–1449.

Stanner, S. A., J. Hughes, C. N. Kelly and J. Buttriss (2004). "A review of the epidemiological evidence for the 'antioxidant hypothesis'." *Public Health Nutr* **7**(3): 407–422.

Stephens, N. G., A. Parsons, P. M. Schofield, F. Kelly, K. Cheeseman and M. J. Mitchinson (1996). "Randomised controlled trial of vitamin E in patients with coronary disease: Cambridge Heart Antioxidant Study (CHAOS)." *Lancet* **347**(9004): 781–786.

Stranges, S., J. R. Marshall, M. Trevisan, R. Natarajan, R. P. Donahue, G. F. Combs, E. Farinaro, L. C. Clark and M. E. Reid (2006). "Effects of selenium supplementation on cardiovascular disease incidence and mortality: Secondary analyses in a randomized clinical trial." *Am J Epidemiol* **163**(8): 694–699.

Taverne, Y. J., A. J. Bogers, D. J. Duncker and D. Merkus (2013). "Reactive oxygen species and the cardiovascular system." *Oxid Med Cell Longev* **2013**: 862423.

Traber, M. G. (2007). "Heart disease and single-vitamin supplementation." *Am J Clin Nutr* **85**(1): 293S–299S.

Vanharanta, M., S. Voutilainen, T. A. Lakka, M. van der Lee, H. Adlercreutz and J. T. Salonen (1999). "Risk of acute coronary events according to serum concentrations of enterolactone: A prospective population-based case–control study." *Lancet* **354**(9196): 2112–2115.

Vanharanta, M., S. Voutilainen, T. H. Rissanen, H. Adlercreutz and J. T. Salonen (2003). "Risk of cardiovascular disease-related and all-cause death according to serum concentrations of enterolactone: Kuopio Ischaemic Heart Disease Risk Factor Study." *Arch Intern Med* **163**(9): 1099–1104.

Virtamo, J., J. M. Rapola, S. Ripatti, O. P. Heinonen, P. R. Taylor, D. Albanes and J. K. Huttunen (1998). "Effect of vitamin E and beta carotene on the incidence of primary nonfatal myocardial infarction and fatal coronary heart disease." *Arch Intern Med* **158**(6): 668–675.

Vivekananthan, D. P., M. S. Penn, S. K. Sapp, A. Hsu and E. J. Topol (2003). "Use of antioxidant vitamins for the prevention of cardiovascular disease: Meta-analysis of randomised trials." *Lancet* **361**(9374): 2017–2023.

Wang, H., Y. J. Yang, H. Y. Qian, Q. Zhang, H. Xu and J. J. Li (2012). "Resveratrol in cardiovascular disease: What is known from current research?" *Heart Fail Rev* **17**(3): 437–448.

Wang, Y., O. K. Chun and W. O. Song (2013). "Plasma and dietary antioxidant status as cardiovascular disease risk factors: A review of human studies." *Nutrients* **5**(8): 2969–3004.

World Health Organization (2011a). "Global atlas on cardiovascular disease prevention and control." Available at: http://www.who.int/cardiovascular_diseases/publications/atlas_cvd/en/.

World Health Organization (2011b). "Global status report on noncommunicable diseases 2010." Available at: http://www.who.int/nmh/publications/ncd_report_full_en.pdf.

World Health Organization (2013a). "10 Facts on noncommunicable diseases." Available at: http://www.who.int/features/factfiles/noncommunicable_diseases/en/.

World Health Organization (2013b). "Cardiovascular diseases (CVDs)." Available at: http://www.who.int/cardiovascular_diseases/en/.

World Heart Federation (2013). "Cardiovascular disease risk factors." Available at: http://www.world-heart-federation.org/cardiovascular-health/cardiovascular-disease-risk-factors/.

Ye, Y., J. Li and Z. Yuan (2013). "Effect of antioxidant vitamin supplementation on cardiovascular outcomes: A meta-analysis of randomized controlled trials." *PLoS One* **8**(2): e56803.

Ye, Z. and H. Song (2008). "Antioxidant vitamins intake and the risk of coronary heart disease: Meta-analysis of cohort studies." *Eur J Cardiovasc Prev Rehabil* **15**(1): 26–34.

Yochum, L., L. H. Kushi, K. Meyer and A. R. Folsom (1999). "Dietary flavonoid intake and risk of cardiovascular disease in postmenopausal women." *Am J Epidemiol* **149**(10): 943–949.

9 Diabetes

*Vaia Lambadiari, Foteini Kousathana,
and George Dimitriadis*

CONTENTS

Introduction.. 151
Antioxidants and Diabetes 152
    Vitamin E 153
    Vitamin C 153
    Carotenoids 154
    Serum Retinol.. 154
    Lycopene 154
    Selenium... 155
    Polyphenols 155
Diet versus Pills: And the Winner Is.. 157
Conclusion 157
References.. 158

INTRODUCTION

Diabetes mellitus—a noncommunicable disease that has reached the dimensions of an epidemic—affects more than 370 million people nowadays, mainly due to a worldwide explosion of obesity [1].

For many years, the pathophysiology of type 2 diabetes remained obscure, and insulin resistance was thought to be the leading cause of metabolic dysregulation. However, in recent years, a feedback loop that operates to ensure integration of glucose homeostasis and maintenance of glucose concentration in a narrow range has been recognized [2]. This feedback loop relies on a crosstalk between β-cells and peripheral tissues. Insulin released following β-cell stimulation mediates uptake of substrates—glucose, amino acids, and fatty acids—by insulin-sensitive tissues. In turn, peripheral tissues signal to islet cells according to their insulin needs. The whole process probably includes interaction between the brain and the humoral system. When insulin resistance is present, as in people with obesity and a sedentary lifestyle, β-cells increase insulin secretion to maintain euglycemia. However, if β-cells are defective, dysglycemia develops [3].

The combination of genes and environmental factors mediates insulin resistance and β-cell dysfunction. Even the *in utero* environment could result in epigenetic and gene expression changes that increase the risk of development of obesity and type 2 diabetes for the offspring later in life [4]. Diabetes mellitus is a complex and multifactorial disease presenting with dysregulation in glucose homeostasis, and lipid and protein metabolism.

The metabolic derangement associated with diabetes causes secondary pathophysiologic changes in multiple organ systems that impose a heavy burden of morbidity and mortality from macrovascular and microvascular complications [5]. Moreover, metabolic syndrome and type 2 diabetes are related to chronic systemic inflammation and increased oxidative stress. Prolonged hyperglycemia alters intracellular metabolism and induces cumulative long-term changes in the structure and function of macromolecules like lipids, carbohydrates, proteins, and nucleic acids [6]. Oxidative stress also plays an important role in chronic diabetic complications and is considered to be associated with increased lipid peroxidation [7].

Under normal physiological conditions, there is a critical balance in the generation of oxygen free radicals and antioxidant defense systems used by organisms to deactivate the former and protect themselves against free radical toxicity [8]. Impairment in this equilibrium increases oxidative stress. Formation of lipid peroxides by the action of free radicals on unsaturated fatty acids has been implicated in the pathogenesis of atherosclerosis [9]. Other mechanisms that contribute to increased oxidative stress in diabetes may include increased advanced glycation and autoxidative glycosylation, metabolic stress resulting from changes in energy metabolism, alterations in the sorbitol pathway, increased inflammatory mediators, disturbed status of antioxidant defense systems, and localized tissue damage as a result of hypoxia and ischemic reperfusion injury. Advanced oxidation protein products accelerate atherosclerosis through promoting oxidative stress and inflammation [7,10,11].

Antioxidants are reducing agents that, by being oxidized themselves, stop the oxidation reaction that can lead to the creation of free radicals, and provoke oxidative stress and the damage and even the death of cells [12]. Hyperglycemia causes the generation of reactive oxygen species (ROS), which, in case endogenous antioxidants such as vitamins C and E, catalase, glutathione, and superoxide dismutase are missing, can lead to the generation of DNA alterations whose gene products can damage cells and tissues [13,14]. Oxidative stress, in turn, elevates the level of glycosylated hemoglobin (HbA1c) [15], increases insulin resistance, and decreases β-cell secretory capacity [16,17]. As a result, the idea that antioxidants can contribute to glycemic control in diabetes mellitus type 2 is reasonable but under question.

ANTIOXIDANTS AND DIABETES

Antioxidants can be provided through food or may be synthesized within the body [18] and are divided into two categories: hydrophilic antioxidants such as ascorbic acid (vitamin C), glutathione, lipoic acid, uric acid, and bilirubin, and lipophilic ones such as carotenes, oxy-carotenoid (vitamin A), tocopherol (vitamin E), and ubiquinol (coenzyme Q) [12].

Antioxidants act in three ways to prevent oxidant-induced cell damages. They can limit the generation of ROS, scavenge them, or eliminate and correct the damage that they can induce [19].

VITAMIN E

Tocopherol (vitamin E) is a lipophilic reducing agent that scavenges ROS and thus prevents oxidant-induced cell damage [20]. The intake of vitamin E, which can be through fruits, vegetable oils, green vegetables, and nuts [21], is inversely related to the risk of type 2 diabetes, according to a 23-year population-based study involving 4304 middle-aged individuals from Finland [22]. Approximately 12.7% of the adult population in the United States take vitamin E as a dietary supplement [23]. Many studies have tried to describe exactly the way vitamin E acts to control the levels of plasma glucose and decrease oxidative stress [24]. Vitamin E inhibits the formation of advanced glycosylation end products, and interrupts glycosylation at an early step in the Maillard reaction [25], thus decreasing the glucosylation of hemoglobin [26]. On the other hand, it limits the apoptosis of pancreatic β-cells [27,28] and decreases, as the majority of antioxidants do, the creation of ROS and their disposal on β-cells [14]. It is also found that vitamin E is beneficial for nonalcoholic steatohepatitis, although in particularly high doses [29]. According to observational cohorts, high serum vitamin E level corresponds to a lower risk of diabetes. Case–control trials demonstrated that vitamin E supplementation improves glycemic control and reduces fasting glucose [30] and fasting insulin [31] in diabetic subjects. However, some RCTs [32] and other studies [33] showed no association between the risk of type 2 diabetes and vitamin E supplementation. Future large-scale, randomized trials are needed to demonstrate the actual effect of vitamin E supplementation on glycemic control [34], as the findings are controversial thus far.

VITAMIN C

Ascorbic acid (vitamin C) is a hydrophilic antioxidant that resets tocopherol in the phase it was in before being oxidized [35]. It is a cofactor in several enzymatic reactions whose deficiency causes symptoms of scurvy. In healthy people, ascorbate blood levels range from 61 to 80 μmol/L; however, in people who have increased oxidative stress, these levels are lower than 45 μmol/L [36]. The levels of vitamin C are related in a larger extent to the consumption of fruits and vegetables than do vitamin E or carotenoids [37]. According to previous findings, people with diabetes have lower levels of vitamin C in their blood [38]. Thus, in persons with diabetes, this deficiency may lead to an increased risk of oxidative tissue damage. This may be explained by the fact that in diabetic individuals, (i) hyperglycemia may reduce renal reabsorption of vitamin C, (ii) blood glucose may compete with vitamin C for uptake into several cells and tissues, and (iii) increased oxidative stress may result in consumption antioxidant vitamin C. However, other studies sustain that although higher intake of antioxidants such as vitamin E, α-tocopherol, γ-tocopherol, δ-tocopherol, β-tocotrienol, and β-cryptoxanthin was inversely related to the risk for type 2 diabetes, intake of vitamin C as a supplement indicated no association to that risk [22].

CAROTENOIDS

Carotenoids are lipophilic antioxidants that exist in chloroplasts and chromoplasts of plants and some photosynthetic bacteria and fungi. They exist in fruits and vegetables [39–41] and are responsible for their color (orange, red, and yellow). In nature, more than 600 carotenoids exist, 40 of which can be provided through diet; 90% of these are represented by α-carotene, β-carotene, lycopene, lutein, and cryptoxanthin [42]. Particularly, α-carotene and β-carotene exist in fruits; yellow–orange vegetables provide α-cryptoxanthin, tomatoes provide lycopene [39,43], whereas lutein can be found in egg yolks [40]. Despite the general belief that serum retinol and carotenoids may battle chronic disease pathogenesis through their antioxidative properties [41,42], randomized controlled trials have not indicated any relation between β-carotene supplements and the risk of type 2 diabetes [43–46]. In addition, observational studies have shown ambiguous results [47–56].

SERUM RETINOL

Levels of serum retinol may positively relate to impaired glucose metabolism [57–59]. In two National Health and Nutrition Examination Surveys (NHANES) analyses—NHANES III (1988–1994) [56] and NHANES 2001–2006 [47]—hyperglycemia and insulin resistance did not relate to serum retinol, despite its association to the metabolic syndrome. The BioCycle Study (2005–2007), a prospective cohort of 259 healthy premenopausal women, indicated that retinol was positively associated with HOMA-IR (homeostasis model assessment of insulin resistance), and that this relationship was driven by insulin. Retinol was inversely associated with sex hormone–binding globulin (SHBG); the relation between serum carotenoids and HOMA-IR was not significant; whereas β-carotene was positively related to SHBG and β-cryptoxanthin was inversely associated with fasting glucose [60]. This is also in agreement with recent findings indicating a positive association of retinol-binding protein-4 with the presence and severity of coronary artery disease in people with or without overt diabetes [61].

LYCOPENE

Lycopene is the most efficient biological carotenoid singlet in oxygen quenching [62]. With reference to its relation to the risk of type 2 diabetes, the results remain controversial. In the first phase of NHANES, Ford et al. [47] found that type 2 diabetic subjects and people with glucose intolerance had lower serum lycopene than the healthy population and a negative relation to fasting plasma insulin. Coyne et al. [52] described a reduction of serum lycopene as age or physical inactivity increased.

According to a cohort of the women's health study conducted by Wang et al. [63], no relation between type 2 diabetes and lycopene intake was found. The CARDIA cohort study showed that people who had several risk factors for diabetes had higher concentration of lycopene in their blood [64]. Case–control studies also found decreased lycopene levels in persons with diabetes [65].

SELENIUM

In 1957, selenium was recognized as an essential nutrient for animals and 15 years later cellular glutathione peroxidase (GPX1) was identified to be the first selenium-dependent enzyme [66]. Although GPX1 was shown to induce type 2 diabetes in mice, human studies have shown that low selenium intake increases the risk of type 2 diabetes, and there seems to be an association between low whole-blood GPx activity and higher measures of general and central adiposity [67,68].

A number of correlative epidemiological studies showed that in serious chronic diseases such as diabetes, there is a deficiency in serum levels of selenium [69]. On the contrary, in randomized, blinded, controlled prospective trials in humans, and a meta-analysis, the supplementation of selenium has not indicated a reduction in the incidence of diabetes and did not decrease mortality [70].

Gao et al. [71], through a recently published cohort study of 1925 Swedish men who were 50 years old and did not have diabetes, showed that dietary selenium does not play a role in glucose values, metabolism, or diabetes risk. On the other hand, Sarmento et al. [72], in a systematic review, indicated that although in patients with diabetes type 2, selenium levels lower than 14.1 μmol/L were associated with an increased risk for cardiovascular disease (RR 1.70; 95% CI 1.21–2.38), further prospective studies are needed to prove the proliferative role of selenium supplementation in cardiovascular disease in patients with diabetes.

POLYPHENOLS

Polyphenols are the most abundant antioxidants in the diet. Their dietary intake is 1 g/day, which is much higher than intake of other dietary antioxidants [73,74]. Polyphenols can be found in fruits and vegetables, green tea, coffee, red wine, chocolate, olives, herbs, spices, nuts, and extra olive virgin oil [75]. They include two main classes: hydroxybenzoic acid derivatives (gallic acid, p-hydroxybenzoic acid, and protocatechuic acid) and hydroxycinnamic acid derivatives (chlorogenic acid, coumaric acid, caffeic acid, ferulic acid, and sinapic acid) [75]. Flavonoids are the most abundant polyphenols in the human diet. There exist six subclasses of flavonoids: anthocyanins (in red wine, black grape, strawberry), flavonols (in onions, blueberries, and broccoli), flavanols, flavanones, flavones, and isoflavones (in soybeans, soy products). Dietary polyphenols are found to have antiallergic, anticarcinogenic, anti-inflammatory, free radical scavenging, antiviral, and antimicrobial properties, through their modulation of important signaling cell pathways, such as the activator protein-1 DNA binding, phosphoinositide 3 kinase/protein kinase B, nuclear factor-κB, mitogen-activated protein kinases, nuclear factor erythroid 2 related factor 2, and extracellular signal-regulated protein kinase [76].

Studies *in vitro*, animal models, and clinical trials have been conducted to determine the impact of polyphenols on glucose metabolism and homeostasis [77]. Polyphenols inhibit α-glucosidase and α-amylase, which are responsible for the transformation of dietary carbohydrates to glucose [78–80]. Some polyphenols, such as ferulic, chlorogenic, caffeic, and tannic acids, can inhibit glucose absorption by interacting with sodium-dependent glucose cotransporters, SGLT1 and SGLT2, in the gut [81,82].

Some studies have shown that polyphenols reduce insulin resistance and induce the production of glucose-dependent insulinotropic polypeptide GIP and glucagon-like polypeptide-1 (GLP-1), both known for their beneficial role on glucose metabolism [83,84]. Studies in mice also indicated that ferulic acid induces glucokinase activity and hepatic production of glycogen and increased insulin sensitivity [85]. They also showed that hesperidin and naringin, except for inducing gluconeogenesis in the liver, also decrease the activity of glucose-6-phosphatase and phosphoenolpyruvate carboxykinase, and in that way improve glycemic control [86,87]. *In vitro* studies showed that polyphenolic compounds such as resveratrol or quercetin promote glucose translocation in adipose and muscle cells through GLUT4 transporters, and through inducing the AMP-activated protein kinase pathway [88,89]. They may also induce phosphatidylinositide 3-kinase, which can lead to increase in glucose uptake [90].

Some polyphenolic compounds protect β-cells from glucotoxicity and oxidative stress (Figure 9.1) [91]. Resveratrol is also found to improve glucose tolerance, reduce oxidative stress in β-cells, and inhibit their apoptosis [92,93]. As a conclusion, polyphenols have a good impact on carbohydrate metabolism, insulin secretion, insulin resistance, and glucose homeostasis [94].

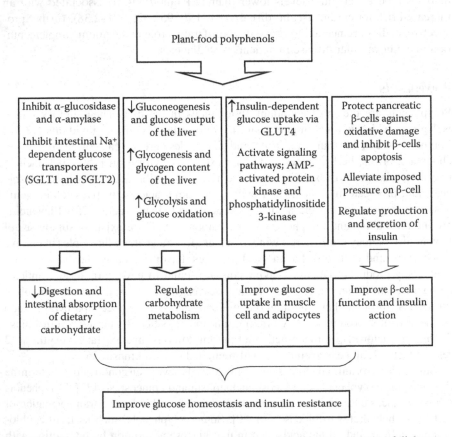

FIGURE 9.1 Dietary polyphenols as potential nutraceuticals in management of diabetes: a review. (From Bahadoran Z et al., *J Diabetes Metab Disord*, 12, 43, 2013.)

DIET VERSUS PILLS: AND THE WINNER IS...

Numerous studies have assessed the dilemma of whether the supplementation of antioxidants is noninferior to the ingestion of natural antioxidants through diet. The market share of supplements is tremendous, and the actual effectiveness or safety of a long-term supranutritional supplementation of antioxidants remains obscure. For instance, a number of studies suggest a neutral or a negative effect of supplements on metabolism. Wang et al. [95] recently demonstrated that selenium supplementation to a mouse model of type 2 diabetes exhibited conflicting actions on glucose regulation. On the one hand, it increased β-cell mass and insulin secretion, thus lowering blood glucose; on the other hand, subsequent hyperinsulinemia reduced antioxidant defense capacity and exacerbated fatty liver degeneration, inducing insulin resistance.

A systematic review and meta-analysis of randomized control trials showed that vitamin E and/or C supplementation improved endothelial function in nonobese diabetic patients but had no impact in obese or overweight ones [96]. Another systematic review assessing the effect of supplement consumption of vitamin E, vitamin C, coenzyme Q10, α-lipoic acid, L-carnitine, ruboxistaurin, and diabetes management concluded there is no established benefit for antioxidant use in the management of diabetic complications [97].

More specifically, in biological systems, vitamin C may exert antioxidant, anti-inflammatory, enzyme cofactor, or prooxidant activity, depending on the specific tissue context. Commonly in clinical trials, vitamin C is assumed to act as an anti-oxidant or an anti-inflammatory factor without actual measurements of antioxidant capacity or oxidative stress to prove the latter [98].

Suksomboon et al. [99], in another systematic review for vitamin E supplementation, suggests no actual benefit for glycemic control in diabetic subjects in general, but implies a positive effect in a subgroup with low serum levels of the antioxidant component. The latter again points out the need for an individual approach.

De Leeuw et al. [100] has shown that intensive supplementation of magnesium in Mg-depleted patients with type 1 diabetes did not improve antioxidant capacity or the rate of LDL oxidation, although it increased magnesium concentration within erythrocytes.

Study designs and potential residual confounding with diet and lifestyle patterns may account for the conflicting results. For example, individuals who use nutrient supplements are also more likely to eat sophisticated or healthier diets, exercise more, and smoke fewer cigarettes. Although nutritional supplements are at the peak of dietetic therapies, the consumption of several specific foods (fatty fish, vegetables and fruits, nuts, etc.) with bioactive components within a balanced diet is a promising approach to manage dysmetabolic manifestations.

CONCLUSION

It is now well established that the risk of the development of diabetes and its complications, as well as the management of the metabolic disorder itself, are highly ameliorated when the ingestion of antioxidants through a diet rich in fruits and vegetables is increased. The same has not been proven concerning the consumption of supplements. The results in the literature are highly controversial, indicating that even serum levels of antioxidants might represent a marker of the derangement and not a direct causative effect. On the other hand, supplementation of antioxidants present with either beneficial or detrimental effects on metabolism, which in turn might have controversial effects on target tissues and clinical implications. Antioxidant supplements should be considered as medicinal products and undergo sufficient evaluation before marketing. Until there is enough evidence for their safety and efficacy, it is advisable that people with diabetes and related disorders should follow the European Association for the Study of Diabetes/American Diabetes Association and American Association of Clinical Endocrinologists nutritional guidelines and consume a diet rich in a variety of natural antioxidants in combination with an overall healthy lifestyle.

REFERENCES

1. International Diabetes Federation. *IDF Diabetes Atlas*, update 2012, 5th edn. International Diabetes Federation, Brussels, Belgium.
2. Kahn SE, Cooper ME, Del Prato S. Pathophysiology and treatment of type 2 diabetes: Perspectives on the past, present, and future. *Lancet*, 2014.383:1068–83.
3. Stancakova A, Javorsky M, Kuulasmaa T, Haffner SM, Kuusisto J, Laakso M. Changes in insulin sensitivity and insulin release in relation to glycemia and glucose tolerance in 6414 Finnish men. *Diabetes*, 2009.58:1212–21.
4. Guenard F, Deshaies Y, Cianflone K, Kral JG, Marceau P, Vohl M-C. Differential methylation in glucoregulatory genes of off spring born before vs. after maternal gastrointestinal bypass surgery. *Proc Natl Acad Sci U S A*, 2013.110:11439–44.
5. American Diabetes Association. Diagnosis and classification of diabetes mellitus. *Diabetes Care*, 2005.28:37–42.
6. Sheetz MJ, King GL. Molecular understanding of hyperglycemia's adverse effects for diabetic complications. *JAMA*, 2002.288:2579–88.
7. Pasupathi P, Chandrasekar V, Kumar US. Evaluation of oxidative stress, enzymatic and non-enzymatic antioxidants and metabolic thyroid hormone status in patients with diabetes mellitus. *Diab Metab Syndr Clin Res Rev*, 2009.3:160–5.
8. Halliwell B, Whiteman M. Measuring reactive species and oxidative damage *in vivo* and in cell culture: How should you do it and what do the results mean? *Br J Pharmacol*, 2004.142:231–55.
9. Donald DH. Oxidative stress and vascular disease. *Arterioscler Thromb Vasc Biol*, 2005.26:689–95.
10. Mahboob M, Rahman MF, Grover P. Serum lipid peroxidation and antioxidant enzyme levels in male and female diabetic patients. *Singapore Med J*, 2005.46:322–4.
11. Xi LS, Fan HF, Jian GZ et al. Advanced oxidation protein products accelerate atherosclerosis through promoting oxidative stress and inflammation. *Arterioscler Thromb Vasc Biol*, 2006.26:1156–62.
12. Sies H. Oxidative stress: Oxidants and antioxidants. *Exp Physiol*, 2007.82(2):291–5.
13. Fardoun RZ. The use of vitamin E in type 2 diabetes mellitus. *Clin Exp Hypertens*, 2007.29(3):135–48.
14. Paolisso G, Esposito R, D'Alessio MA, Barbieri M. Primary and secondary prevention of atherosclerosis: Is there a role for antioxidants? *Diabetes Metab*, 1999.25:298–306.
15. Madian AG, Myracle AD, Diaz-Maldonado N, Rochelle NS, Janle EM, Regnier FE. Differential carbonylation of proteins as a function of *in vivo* oxidative stress. *J Proteome Res*, 2011.10:3959–72.

16. Robertson RP. Chronic oxidative stress as a central mechanism for glucose toxicity in pancreatic islet beta cells in diabetes. *J Biol Chem*, 2004.279:42351–4.
17. Robertson RP, Harmon JS. Diabetes, glucose toxicity, and oxidative stress: A case of double jeopardy for the pancreatic islet beta cell. *Free Radic Biol Med*, 2006.41:177–84.
18. Vertuani S, Angusti A, Manfredini S. The antioxidants and pro-antioxidants network: An overview. *Curr Pharm Des*, 2004.10(14):1677–94.
19. Vassort G, Turan B. Protective role of antioxidants in diabetes-induced cardiac dysfunction. *Cardiovasc Toxicol*, 2010.10(2):73–86.
20. Schurks M, Glynn RJ, Rist PM, Tzourio C, Kurth T. Effects of vitamin E on stroke subtypes: Meta-analysis of randomised controlled trials. *BMJ*, 2010.341:c5702.
21. Clarke MW, Burnett JR, Croft KD. Vitamin E in human health and disease. *Crit Rev Clin Lab Sci*, 2008.45:417–50.
22. Montonen J, Knekt P, Järvinen R, Reunanen A. Dietary antioxidant intake and risk of type 2 diabetes. *Diabetes Care*, 2004.27(2):362–6.
23. Radimer K, Bindewald B, Hughes J, Ervin B, Swanson C, Picciano MF. Dietary supplement use by US adults: Data from the National Health and Nutrition Examination Survey 1999–2000. *Am J Epidemiol*, 2004.160(4):339–49.
24. Paolisso G, D'Amore A, Galzerano D et al. Daily vitamin E supplements improve metabolic control but not insulin secretion in elderly type II diabetic patients. *Diabetes Care*, 2003.16:1433–7.
25. Xu R, Zhang S, Tao A, Chen G, Zhang M. Influence of vitamin E supplementation on glycaemic control: A meta-analysis of randomised controlled trial. *PLoS One*, 2014.9(4):e95008.
26. Minamiyama Y, Takemura S, Bito Y et al. Supplementation of alpha-tocopherol improves cardiovascular risk factors via the insulin signalling pathway and reduction of mitochondrial reactive oxygen species in type II diabetic rats. *Free Radic Res*, 2008. 42:261–71.
27. Pazdro R, Burgess JR. The role of vitamin E and oxidative stress in diabetes complications. *Mech Ageing Dev*, 2010.131:276–86.
28. Jin L, Xue HY, Jin LJ, Li SY, Xu YP. Antioxidant and pancreas-protective effect of aucubin on rats with streptozotocin-induced diabetes. *Eur J Pharmacol*, 2008.582:162–7.
29. Bell LN, Wang J, Muralidharan S et al. Relationship between adipose tissue insulin resistance and liver histology in nonalcoholic steatohepatitis: A pioglitazone versus vitamin E versus placebo for the treatment of nondiabetic patients with nonalcoholic steatohepatitis trial follow-up study. *Hepatology*, 2012.56(4):1311–8.
30. Tütüncü NB, Bayraktar M, Varli K. Reversal of defective nerve conduction with vitamin E supplementation in type 2 diabetes: A preliminary study. *Diabetes Care*, 1998.21(11):1915–8.
31. Paolisso G, Tagliamonte MR, Barbieri M et al. Chronic vitamin E administration improves brachial reactivity and increases intracellular magnesium concentration in type II diabetic patients. *J Clin Endocrinol Metab*, 2000.85(1):109–15.
32. Manzella D, Barbieri M, Ragno E, Paolisso G. Chronic administration of pharmacologic doses of vitamin E improves the cardiac autonomic nervous system in patients with type 2 diabetes. *Am J Clin Nutr*, 2001.73(6):1052–7.
33. Liu S, Lee IM, Song Y et al. Vitamin E and risk of type 2 diabetes in the women's health study randomized controlled trial. *Diabetes*, 2006.55(10):2856–62.
34. Economides PA, Khaodhiar L, Caselli A et al. The effect of vitamin E on endothelial function of micro- and macrocirculation and left ventricular function in type 1 and type 2 diabetic patients. *Diabetes*, 2005.54(1):204–11.
35. Chen K, Suh J, Carr AC, Morrow JD, Zeind J, Frei B. Vitamin C suppresses oxidative lipid damage *in vivo*, even in the presence of iron overload. *Am J Physiol Endocrinol Metab*, 2000.279(6):E1406–12.

36. Schorah CJ, Downing C, Piripitsi A et al. Total vitamin C, ascorbic acid, and dehy-droascorbic acid concentrations in plasma of critically ill patients. *Am J Clin Nutr*, 1996.63(5):760–5.
37. Block G, Norkus E, Hudes M, Mandel S, Helzlsouer K. Which plasma antioxidants are most related to fruit and vegetable consumption? *Am J Epidemiol*, 2001.154(12):1113–8.
38. Will JC, Byers T. Does diabetes mellitus increase the requirement for vitamin C? *Nutr Rev*, 1996.54:193–202.
39. Mangels AR, Holden JM, Beecher GR, Forman MR, Lanza E. Carotenoid contents of fruits and vegetables: An evaluation of analytical data. *J Am Diet Assoc*, 1993.93:284–96.
40. Johnson EJ. The role of carotenoids in human health. *Nutr Clin Care*, 2002.5(2):47–9.
41. Agarwal S, Rao AV. Carotenoids and chronic diseases. *Drug Metab Drug Interact*, 2000.17(1–4):189–210.
42. Gerster H. The potential role of lycopene for human health. *J Am Coll Nutr*, 1997.16:109–26.
43. Ong ASH, Tee ES. Natural sources of carotenoids from plants and oils. *Methods Enzymol*, 1992.213:142–67.
44. Liu S, Ajani U, Chae C, Hennekens C, Buring JE, Manson JE. Long-term β-carotene supplementation and risk of type 2 diabetes mellitus: A randomized controlled trial. *J Am Med Assoc*, 1999.282(11):1073–5.
45. Czernichow S, Couthouis A, Bertrais S et al. Antioxidant supplementation does not affect fasting plasma glucose in the Supplementation with Antioxidant Vitamins and Minerals (SU.VI.MAX) study in France: Association with dietary intake and plasma concentrations. *Am J Clin Nutr*, 2006.84(2):395–9.
46. Kataja-Tuomola M, Sundell JR, Männistö S et al. Effect of α-tocopherol and β-carotene supplementation on the incidence of type 2 diabetes. *Diabetologia*, 2008.51(1):47–53.
47. Ford ES, Will JC, Bowman BA, Narayan KMV. Diabetes mellitus and serum carot-enoids: Findings from the Third National Health and Nutrition Examination Survey. *Am J Epidemiol*, 1999.149(2):168–76.
48. Beydoun MA, Shroff MR, Chen X, Beydoun HA, Wang Y, Zonderman AB. Serum antioxidant status is associated with metabolic syndrome among U.S. adults in recent national surveys. *J Nutr*, 2011.141(5):903–13.
49. Wang L, Liu S, Pradhan AD et al. Plasma lycopene, other carotenoids, and the risk of type 2 diabetes in women. *Am J Epidemiol*, 2006.164(6):576–85.
50. Ylönen K, Alfthan G, Groop L, Saloranta C, Aro A, Virtanen SM. Dietary intakes and plasma concentrations of carotenoids and tocopherols in relation to glucose metabolism in subjects at high risk of type 2 diabetes: The Botnia Dietary Study. *Am J Clin Nutr*, 2003.77(6):1434–41.
51. Coyne T, Ibiebele TI, Baade PD, McClintock CS, Shaw JE. Metabolic syndrome and serum carotenoids: Findings of a cross-sectional study in Queensland, Australia. *Br J Nutr*, 2009.102(11):1668–77.
52. Coyne T, Ibiebele TI, Baade PD et al. Diabetes mellitus and serum carotenoids: Findings of a population-based study in Queensland, Australia. *Am J Clin Nutr*, 2005.82(3):685–93.
53. Czernichow S, Vergnaud AC, Galan P et al. Effects of long-term antioxidant supple-mentation and association of serum antioxidant concentrations with risk of metabolic syndrome in adults. *Am J Clin Nutr*, 2009.90(2):329–35.
54. Suzuki K, Ito Y, Nakamura S, Ochiai J, Aoki K. Relationship between serum carot-enoids and hyperglycemia: A population-based cross–sectional study. *J Epidemiol*, 2002.12(5):357–66.
55. Suzuki K, Ito Y, Inoue T, Hamajima N. Inverse association of serum carotenoids with prevalence of metabolic syndrome among Japanese. *Clin Nutr*, 2011.30(3):369–75.

56. Ford ES, Mokdad AH, Giles WH, Brown DW. The metabolic syndrome and antioxidant concentrations: Findings from the Third National Health and Nutrition Examination Survey. *Diabetes*, 2003.52(9):2346–52.

57. Graham TE, Yang Q, Blüher M et al. Retinol-binding protein 4 and insulin resistance in lean, obese, and diabetic subjects. *N Engl J Med*, 2006.354(24):2552–63.

58. Yang Q, Graham TE, Mody N et al. Serum retinol binding protein 4 contributes to insulin resistance in obesity and type 2 diabetes. *Nature*, 2005.436(7049):356–62.

59. Kowalska I, Straczkowski M, Adamska A et al. Serum retinol binding protein 4 is related to insulin resistance and nonoxidative glucose metabolism in lean and obese women with normal glucose tolerance. *J Clin Endocrinol Metab*, 2008.93(7):2786–9.

60. Blondin SA, Yeung EH, Mumford SL et al. Serum retinol and carotenoids in association with biomarkers of insulin resistance among premenopausal women. *ISRN Nutr*, 2013.2013:619516.

61. Lambadiari V, Kadoglou NP, Stasinos V et al. Serum levels of retinol-binding protein-4 are associated with the presence and severity of coronary artery disease. *Cardiovasc Diabetol*, 2014.13(1):121.

62. Di Mascio P, Kaiser S, Sies H. Lycopene as the most efficient biological carotenoid singlet oxygen quencher. *Arch Biochem Biophys*, 1989.274(2):532–8.

63. Wang L, Liu S, Manson JE, Gaziano JM, Buring JE, Sesso HD. The consumption of lycopene and tomato-based food products is not associated with the risk of type 2 diabetes mellitus in women. *J Nutr*, 2006.136:620–5.

64. Hozawa A, Jacobs DR, Steffes MW, Gross MD, Steffen LM, Lee DH. Associations of serum carotenoid concentrations with the development of diabetes and with insulin concentration: Interaction with smoking. The Coronary Artery Risk Development in Young Adults (CARDIA) study. *Am J Epidemiol*, 2006.163:929–37.

65. Polidori MC, Mecocci P, Stahl W et al. Plasma levels of lipophilic antioxidants in very old patients with type 2 diabetes. *Diabetes Metab Res Rev*, 2000.16:15–9

66. McClung JP, Roneker CA, Mu W et al. Development of insulin resistance and obesity in mice overexpressing cellular glutathione peroxidase. *Proc Natl Acad Sci U S A*, 2004.101:8852–7.

67. Pepper MP, Vatamaniuk MZ, Yan X, Roneker CA, Lei XG. Impacts of dietary selenium deficiency on metabolic phenotypes of diet-restricted GPX1-overexpressing mice. *Antioxid Redox Signal*, 2011.14:383–90.

68. Wang X, Vatamaniuk MZ, Roneker CA et al. Knockouts of SOD1 and GPX1 exert different impacts on murine islet function and pancreatic integrity. *Antioxid Redox Signal*, 2011.14:391–401.

69. Stranges S, Marshall JR, Natarajan R et al. Effects of long-term selenium supplementation on the incidence of type 2 diabetes: A randomized trial. *Ann Intern Med*, 2007.147:217–23.

70. Bjelakovic G, Nikolova D, Gluud LL, Simonetti RG, Gluud C. Antioxidant supplements for prevention of mortality in healthy participants and patients with various disease. *Cochrane Database Syst Rev*, 2012.3:CD007176. doi:10.1002/14651858.CD007176.pub2.

71. Gao H, Hägg S, Sjögren P, Lambert PC, Ingelsson E, van Dam RM. Serum selenium in relation to measures of glucose metabolism and incidence of type 2 diabetes in an older Swedish population. *Diabet Med*, 2014.31(7):787–93.

72. Sarmento RA, Silva FM, Sbruzzi G, Schaan BD, Almeida JC. Antioxidant micronutrients and cardiovascular risk in patients with diabetes: A systematic review. *Arq Bras Cardiol*, 2013.101(3):240–8.

73. Scalbert A, Williamson G. Dietary intake and bioavailability of polyphenols. *J Nutr*, 2000.130:2073S–85S.

74. D'Archivio M, Filesi C, Varì R, Scazzocchio B, Masella R. Bioavailability of the poly-phenols: Status and controversies. *Int J Mol Sci*, 2010.11(4):1321–42.
75. Am Manach C, Scalbert A, Morand C, Rémésy C, Jiménez L. Polyphenols: Food sources and bioavailability. *Am J Clin Nutr*, 2004.12:727–47.
76. Han X, Loa T. Dietary polyphenols and their biological significance. *Int J Mol Sci*, 2007.12:950–88.
77. Hanhineva K, Törrönen R, Bondia-Pons I et al. Impact of dietary polyphenols on carbo-hydrate metabolism. *Int J Mol Sci*, 2010.12:1365–402.
78. Iwai K. Antidiabetic and antioxidant effects of polyphenols in brown alga *Ecklonia sto-lonifera* in genetically diabetic KK-A(y) mice. *Plant Foods Hum Nutr*, 2008.12:163–9.
79. Cabrera C, Artacho R, Giménez R. Beneficial effects of green tea—A review. *J Am Coll Nutr*, 2006.12:79–99.
80. Tadera K, Minami Y, Takamatsu K, Matsuoka T. Inhibition of alpha-glucosidase and alpha-amylase by flavonoids. *J Nutr Sci Vitaminol (Tokyo)*, 2006.12:149–53.
81. Kobayashi Y, Suzuki M, Satsu H et al. Green tea polyphenols inhibit the sodium-dependent glucose transporter of intestinal epithelial cells by a competitive mechanism. *J Agric Food Chem*, 2000.12:5618–23.
82. Johnston K, Sharp P, Clifford M, Morgan L. Dietary polyphenols decrease glucose uptake by human intestinal Caco-2 cells. *FEBS Lett*, 2005.12:1653–7.
83. Johnston KL, Clifford MN, Morgan LM. Coffee acutely modifies gastrointestinal hor-mone secretion and glucose tolerance in humans: Glycemic effects of chlorogenic acid and caffeine. *Am J Clin Nutr*, 2003.2:728–33.
84. Dao TM, Waget A, Klopp P et al. Resveratrol increases glucose induced GLP-1 secre-tion in mice: A mechanism which contributes to the glycemic control. *PLoS One*, 2011.12:e20700.
85. Jung EH, Kim SR, Hwang IK, Ha TY. Hypoglycemic effects of a phenolic acid frac-tion of rice bran and ferulic acid in C57BL/KsJ-db/db mice. *J Agric Food Chem*, 2007.12:9800–4.
86. Jung UJ, Lee MK, Jeong KS, Choi MS. The hypoglycemic effects of hesperidin and naringin are partly mediated by hepatic glucose-regulating enzymes in C57BL/KsJ-db/db mice. *J Nutr*, 2004.12:2499–503.
87. Jung UJ, Lee MK, Park YB, Kang MA, Choi MS. Effect of citrus flavonoids on lipid metabolism and glucose-regulating enzyme mRNA levels in type-2 diabetic mice. *Int J Biochem Cell Biol*, 2006.12:1134–45.
88. Zhang B, Kang M, Xie Q et al. Anthocyanins from Chinese bayberry extract protect β-cells from oxidative stress-mediated injury via HO-1 upregulation. *J Agric Food Chem*, 2011.12:537–45.
89. Park CE, Kim MJ, Lee JH et al. Resveratrol stimulates glucose transport in C2C12 myo-tubes by activating AMP-activated protein kinase. *Mol Med*, 2007.12:222–9.
90. Kumar R, Balaji S, Uma TS, Sehgal PK. Fruit extracts of *Momordica charantia* potenti-ate glucose uptake and up-regulate Glut-4, PPAR gamma and PI3K. *J Ethnopharmacol*, 2009.12:533–7.
91. Yin P, Zhao S, Chen S et al. Hypoglycemic and hypolipidemic effects of polyphenols from burs of *Castanea mollissima* Blume. *Molecules*, 2011.12:9764–74.
92. Szkudelski T, Szkudelska K. Anti-diabetic effects of resveratrol. *Ann N Y Acad Sci*, 2011.12:34–9.
93. Szkudelski T. Resveratrol inhibits insulin secretion from rat pancreatic islets. *Eur J Pharmacol*, 2006.12:176–81.
94. Bahadoran Z, Mirmiran P, Azizi F. Dietary polyphenols as potential nutraceuticals in management of diabetes: A review. *J Diabetes Metab Disord*, 2013.12:43.

95. Wang C, Yang S, Zhang N et al. Long-term supranutritional supplementation with selenate decreases hyperglycemia and promotes fatty liver degeneration by inducing hyperinsulinemia in diabetic db/db mice. *PLoS One*, 2014.9:e101315.

96. Montero D, Walther G, Stehouwer CD, Houben AJ, Beckman JA, Vinet A. Effect of antioxidant vitamin supplementation on endothelial function in type 2 diabetes mellitus: A systematic review and meta-analysis of randomized controlled trials. *Obes Rev*, 2014.15:107–16.

97. Golbidi S, Ebadi SA, Laher I. Antioxidants in the treatment of diabetes. *Curr Diabetes Rev*, 2011.7:106–25.

98. Michels AJ, Frei B. Myths, artifacts, and fatal flaws: Identifying limitations and opportunities in vitamin C research. *Nutrients*, 2013.5:5161–92.

99. Suksomboon N, Poolsup N, Sinprasert S. Effects of vitamin E supplementation on glycaemic control in type 2 diabetes: Systematic review of randomized controlled trials. *J Clin Pharm Ther*, 2011.36:53–63.

100. De Leeuw I, Engelen W, Aerts P, Schrans S. Effect of intensive magnesium supplementation on the *in vitro* oxidizability of LDL and VLDL in Mg-depleted type 1 diabetic patients. *Magnes Res*, 1998.11:179–82.

10 Cancer

Eleni Andreou

CONTENTS

Introduction 166
Free Radicals and Their Contribution to Cancer Development 166
Antioxidants 166
    Cancer and Folic Acid 167
    Cancer and Selenium 170
    Cancer and Vitamin C 172
    Antioxidant Supplementation and Prevention of Cancer 174
    Dilemma of Taking Antioxidant Supplements while Having Cancer 177
    Foods Rich in Antioxidants 179
Prevention 179
    Cancer and Fruits and Vegetables 179
        Intake Recommendations 181
    Cruciferous Vegetables 181
    Iodine and Thyroid Function and Cruciferous Vegetables 182
        Intake Recommendations 182
    Cancer and Legumes 182
        Dry Beans, Peas, and Lentils 182
        Prostate Cancer 182
    Cancer and Soy 183
        Prostate Cancer 183
        Breast Cancer 183
        Intake Recommendations 183
    Cancer and Whole Grains 184
        Intake Recommendations 184
    Cancer and Carotenoids 184
        Food Sources 184
        β-Carotene and α-Carotene 185
        β-Cryptoxanthin 185
        Lycopene 185
        Lutein and Zeaxanthin 186
        Curcumin 186
    Cancer and Curcumin 187
    Colorectal Cancer and Fiber 188

Breast Cancer 188
    Intake Recommendations 189
Cancer and Flavonoids.. 190
    Food Sources 190
References.. 192

INTRODUCTION

Antioxidants are chemicals that obstruct the action of other chemicals known as free radicals. Free radicals are highly reactive and have the potential to cause damage to cells, including damage that may lead to cancer. Free radicals are produced naturally in the body. Additionally, some environmental toxins may contain high levels of free radicals or encourage the body's cells to produce more free radicals (Higdon, 2007).

Although some antioxidants are made naturally by the body, others can only be obtained by external (exogenous) sources, including the diet and dietary supplements. Laboratory and animal research has shown that exogenous antioxidants can help prevent the free radical damage associated with the development of cancer (Higdon and Drake, 2011).

FREE RADICALS AND THEIR CONTRIBUTION TO CANCER DEVELOPMENT

Free radicals are produced when an atom or a molecule either gains or losses an electron. Free radicals are formed naturally in the body and play an important role in many normal cellular processes. Nevertheless, at high concentrations, free radicals can be harmful to the body and hurt all major components of cells, including DNA, proteins, and cell membranes. The damage to cells caused by free radicals may cause the progression of cancer and other health conditions (Diplock et al., 1998; Valko et al., 2007).

Unusually high concentrations of free radicals in the body can be caused by exposure to ionizing radiation and other environmental toxins. When ionizing radiation hits an atom or a molecule in a cell, an electron may be misplaced, resulting to the formation of a free radical. The fabrication of oddly high levels of free radicals is the mechanism by which ionizing radiation kills cells. Furthermore, some environmental toxins (i.e., cigarette) may include large amounts of free radicals or encourage the cells to produce more free radicals.

Free radicals that contain the element oxygen are the most common type of free radicals produced in living tissue, also called reactive oxygen species (ROS) (Diplock et al., 1998; Valko et al., 2007).

ANTIOXIDANTS

Antioxidants ("free radical scavengers") are chemicals that work together with and neutralize free radicals, hence preventing them from causing damage.

The body makes some of the antioxidants it uses to neutralize free radicals, known as endogenous antioxidants. Nevertheless, the body relies on external (exogenous) sources, primarily the diet, to obtain the rest of the antioxidants it needs, known as dietary antioxidants. Fruits, vegetables, and grains are rich sources of dietary antioxidants (Bouayed and Bohn, 2010). Examples of dietary antioxidants include folic acid, β-carotene, lycopene, and vitamins A, C, and E (α-tocopherol). The mineral element selenium is often thought to be a dietary antioxidant, the antioxidant effects of selenium are most likely due to the antioxidant activity of proteins in which it is an essential component, and not to selenium itself (Davis et al., 2012).

CANCER AND FOLIC ACID

Cancer is thought to arise from DNA damage in excess of ongoing DNA repair and/or the inappropriate expression of critical genes. Because of the important roles played by folate in DNA and RNA synthesis and methylation, it is possible for folate intake to affect both DNA repair and gene expression with the consumption of at least five servings of fruits and vegetables per day, which it is associated with a diminished incidence of cancer. Fruits and vegetables are excellent sources of folate and contribute positively to the anticarcinogenic effect. Observational studies have found that a decreased folate status in human nutrition is associated with cancers of the cervix, colon and rectum, lung, esophagus, brain, pancreas, and breast. Intervention trials in humans have been conducted mainly with respect to cervical and colorectal cancer. The results in cervical cancer have been inconsistent (Choi and Mason, 2000), but with more relevant randomized intervention trials regarding colorectal cancer there is a different point of view (Gravo et al., 1998; Kim et al., 2001).

- *Colorectal cancer*: The role of folate in preventing colorectal cancer provides an example of the complexity of the interactions between genetics and the nutritional environment. In general, observational studies have found relatively low folate intake and high alcohol intake to be associated with increased incidence of colorectal cancer (Food and Nutrition Board, Institute of Medicine, 1998; Su and Arab, 2001; Terry et al., 2002). Alcohol interferes with the absorption and metabolism of folate (Herbert, 1999). In a prospective study of more than 45,000 male health professionals, an intake of more than two alcoholic drinks per day doubled the risk of colon cancer. The combination of high alcohol and low folate intake yielded an even greater risk of colon cancer. However, increased alcohol intake in individuals who consumed 650 μg or more of folate per day was not associated with an increased risk of colon cancer (Giovannucci et al., 1995). In some studies, individuals who are homozygous for the C677T MTHFR polymorphism (T/T) have been found to be at decreased risk for colon cancer when folate intake is adequate. However, when folate intake is low and/or alcohol intake is high, individuals with the (T/T) genotype have been found to be at an increased risk of colorectal cancer (Ma et al., 1997; Slattery et al., 1999).

- *Breast cancer*: A number of prospective studies have found that even moderate alcohol intake is associated with an increased risk of breast cancer in women. Recently, the results of three prospective studies suggested that increased folate intake may reduce the risk of breast cancer in women who regularly consume alcohol (Zhang et al., 1999b; Rohan et al., 2000; Sellers et al., 2001). A prospective study of more than 88,000 nurses found no relationship between folic acid intake and breast cancer in women who consumed less than one alcoholic drink per day. However, in those women consuming at least one alcoholic drink per day, folic acid intake of at least 600 μg daily resulted in about half the risk of breast cancer compared with women who consumed less than 300 μg of folic acid daily (Zhang et al., 1999b).

Table 10.1 presents the current recommended dietary allowance (RDA) for folate as micrograms (μg) of dietary folate equivalents (DFEs). The Food and Nutrition Board (FNB) developed DFEs to reflect the higher bioavailability of folic acid than that of food folate. At least 85% of folic acid is estimated to be bioavailable when taken with food, whereas only about 50% of folate naturally present in food is bioavailable. On the basis of these values, the FNB defined DFE as follows:

- 1 μg DFE = 1 μg food folate
- 1 μg DFE = 0.6 μg folic acid from fortified foods or dietary supplements consumed with foods
- 1 μg DFE = 0.5 μg folic acid from dietary supplements taken on an empty stomach

According to the Dietary Guidelines for Americans, moderate alcohol consumption is defined as having up to one drink per day for women and up to two drinks per day for men. This definition is referring to the amount consumed on any single day and is not intended as an average over several days. The Dietary Guidelines also state that it is not recommended that anyone begin drinking or drink more frequently on the basis of potential health benefits because moderate alcohol intake is also associated with increased risk of breast cancer, violence, drowning, and injuries from falls and motor vehicle crashes. For men, heavy drinking is typically defined as consuming 15 drinks or more per week; significant alcohol intake is considered >140 g/week in men and >70 g/week in women. For women, heavy drinking is typically defined as consuming eight drinks or more per week (U.S. Department of Agriculture [USDA] and U.S. Department of Health and Human Services, 2010).

A standard drink in the United States is equal to 14.0 g (0.6 oz) of pure alcohol. Generally, this amount of pure alcohol is found in

- 12 oz of beer (5% alcohol content)
- 8 oz of malt liquor (7% alcohol content)
- 5 oz of wine (12% alcohol content)
- 1.5 oz or a "shot" of 80-proof (40% alcohol content) distilled spirits or liquor (e.g., gin, rum, vodka, and whiskey)

TABLE 10.1
Food Sources of Folate and Folic Acid

Food	µg DFE per Serving	% DVª
Beef liver, braised, 3 oz	215	54
Spinach, boiled, 1/2 cup	131	33
Black-eyed peas (cowpeas), boiled, 1/2 cup	105	26
Breakfast cereals, fortified with 25% of the DVᵇ	100	25
Rice, white, medium-grain, cooked, 1/2 cupᵇ	90	23
Asparagus, boiled, 4 spears	89	22
Spaghetti, cooked, enriched, 1/2 cupᵇ	83	21
Brussels sprouts, frozen, boiled, 1/2 cup	78	20
Lettuce, romaine, shredded, 1 cup	64	16
Avocado, raw, sliced, 1/2 cup	59	15
Spinach, raw, 1 cup	58	15
Broccoli, chopped, frozen, cooked, 1/2 cup	52	13
Mustard greens, chopped, frozen, boiled, 1/2 cup	52	13
Green peas, frozen, boiled, 1/2 cup	47	12
Kidney beans, canned, 1/2 cup	46	12
Bread, white, 1 sliceᵇ	43	11
Peanuts, dry roasted, 1 oz	41	10
Wheat germ, 2 tablespoons	40	10
Tomato juice, canned, 3/4 cup	36	9
Crab, Dungeness, 3 oz	36	9
Orange juice, 3/4 cup	35	9
Turnip greens, frozen, boiled, 1/2 cup	32	8
Orange, fresh, 1 small	29	7
Papaya, raw, cubed, 1/2 cup	27	7
Banana, 1 medium	24	6
Yeast, baker's, 1/4 teaspoon	23	6
Egg, whole, hard-boiled, 1 large	22	6
Vegetarian baked beans, canned, 1/2 cup	15	4
Cantaloupe, raw, 1 wedge	14	4
Fish, halibut, cooked, 3 oz	12	3
Milk, 1% fat, 1 cup	12	3
Ground beef, 85% lean, cooked, 3 oz	7	2
Chicken breast, roasted, 1/2 breast	3	1

Source: U.S. Department of Agriculture, Agricultural Research Service. 2012. USDA National Nutrient Database for Standard Reference, Release 25. Available at: http://www.nal .usda.gov/fnic/foodcomp/search/.

ª DV = daily value. The Food and Drug Administration (FDA) developed DVs to help consumers compare the nutrient contents of products within the context of a total diet. The DV for folate is 400 µg for adults and children aged 4 years and older. However, the FDA does not require food labels to list folate content unless a food has been fortified with this nutrient. Foods providing 20% or more of the DV are considered to be high sources of a nutrient.

ᵇ Fortified with folic acid as part of the folate fortification program.

CANCER AND SELENIUM

There is a lot of evidence that selenium supplementation at high levels reduces the incidence of cancer in animals. In fact, in animal models of spontaneous, viral, and chemically induced cancers, selenium supplementation greatly reduced tumor incidence (Rayman and Clark, 2000). The evidence indicated that the methylated forms of selenium were the active species against tumors, and these methylated selenium compounds were produced at the greatest amounts with excess selenium intakes. Selenium deficiency did not appear to make animals more susceptible to developing cancerous tumors (Combs and Gray, 1998).

Various studies have shown a tendency for population that reside in areas with low soil selenium and have relatively low selenium intakes to have higher cancer mortality rates. Food sources of selenium depends from the soil content of selenium (Table 10.2). Results of epidemiologic studies of cancer incidence in groups with less variable selenium intakes have been less consistent, but also show a trend for individuals with lower selenium levels (blood and nails) to have a higher incidence of several different types of cancer. This trend is less pronounced in women. Chronic infection with viral hepatitis B or C significantly increases the risk of liver cancer. In a study of Taiwanese men with chronic viral hepatitis B or C, decreased plasma selenium concentrations were associated with an even greater risk of liver cancer (Yu et al., 1999). A case–control study within a prospective study of more than 9000 Finnish men and women examined serum selenium levels in 95 individuals consequently found to have lung cancer and 190 matched controls (Knckt et al., 1998). Lower serum selenium levels were related with an enlarged risk of lung cancer, and the association was more prominent in smokers. Additionally, a case–control study within a prospective study of more than 50,000 male health professionals in the United States found a significant inverse relationship between toenail selenium content and risk of prostate cancer in 181 men with advanced prostate cancer and 181 matched controls (Yoshizawa et al., 1998).

Toenail selenium concentration has been proposed as a long-term (6–12 months) indicator of human selenium status. In the analysis of covariance, the best predictors of toenail selenium concentration were selenium intake from supplements and food, and among supplement users also dietary β-carotene (Ovaskaimen et al., 1993). In persons whose toenail selenium substance was consistent with an average intake of 159 µg/day, the possibility of progressive prostate cancer was only 35% of those whose toenail selenium content was consistent with an intake of 86 µg/day. In a prospective study of more than 9000 Japanese–American men, a case–control study that examined 249 established cases of prostate cancer and 249 matched controls found the risk of developing prostate cancer to be 50% lower in men with serum selenium levels in the highest quartile paralleled with those in the lowest quartile (Nomura et al., 2000). Moreover, another case–control study found that men with prediagnostic plasma selenium levels in the lowest quartile were four to five times more prone to progress to prostate cancer than those in the highest quartile (Brooks et al., 2001). On the other hand, a case–control study indicated an important inverse association between toenail selenium and the risk of colon cancer, but found no

TABLE 10.2
Food Sources of Selenium

Food	Micrograms (μg) per Serving	Percent DV[a]
Brazil nuts, 1 oz (6–8 nuts)	544	777
Tuna, yellowfin, cooked, dry heat, 3 oz	92	131
Halibut, cooked, dry heat, 3 oz	47	67
Sardines, canned in oil, drained solids with bone, 3 oz	45	64
Ham, roasted, 3 oz	42	60
Shrimp, canned, 3 oz	40	57
Macaroni, enriched, cooked, 1 cup	37	53
Beef steak, bottom round, roasted, 3 oz	33	47
Turkey, boneless, roasted, 3 oz	31	44
Beef liver, pan fried, 3 oz	28	40
Chicken, light meat, roasted, 3 oz	22	31
Cottage cheese, 1% milk fat, 1 cup	20	29
Rice, brown, long-grain, cooked, 1 cup	19	27
Beef, ground, 25% fat, broiled, 3 oz	18	26
Egg, hard-boiled, 1 large	15	21
Puffed wheat ready-to-eat cereal, fortified, 1 cup	15	21
Bread, whole-wheat, 1 slice	13	19
Baked beans, canned, plain or vegetarian, 1 cup	13	19
Oatmeal, regular and quick, unenriched, cooked with water, 1 cup	13	19
Spinach, frozen, boiled, 1 cup	11	16
Milk, 1% fat, 1 cup	8	11
Yogurt, plain, low fat, 1 cup	8	11
Lentils, boiled, 1 cup	6	9
Bread, white, 1 slice	6	9
Spaghetti sauce, marinara, 1 cup	4	6
Cashew nuts, dry roasted, 1 oz	3	4
Corn flakes, 1 cup	2	3
Green peas, frozen, boiled, 1 cup	2	3
Bananas, sliced, 1 cup	2	3
Potato, baked, flesh and skin, 1 potato	1	1
Peaches, canned in water, solids and liquids, 1 cup	1	1
Carrots, raw, 1 cup	0	0
Lettuce, iceberg, raw, 1 cup	0	0

Source: U.S. Department of Agriculture, Agricultural Research Service. 2010. USDA Database for the Oxygen Radical Absorbance Capacity (ORAC) of Selected Foods, Release 2. Available at: http://www.orac-info-portal.de/download/ORAC_R2.pdf.

[a] DV = daily value. DVs were developed by the FDA to help consumers compare the nutrient contents of products within the context of a total diet. The DV for selenium is 70 μg for adults and children aged 4 years and older. Foods providing 20% or more of the DV are considered to be high sources of a nutrient. 1 oz = 28.350 g.

associations between toenail selenium and the risk of breast cancer or prostate cancer (Ghadirian et al., 2000).

An intervention trial commenced among a general population of more than 130,000 individuals in five townships of Qidong, China, a high-risk area for viral hepatitis B infection and liver cancer, which provided table salt enriched with sodium selenite to the population of one township (almost 21,000 people), with the other four areas designated as controls. Throughout an 8-year follow-up period, the average frequency of liver cancer was condensed by 35% in the selenium-enhanced population, while no decline was uncovered in the control populations. In a clinical trial in the identical area, 226 persons with sign of chronic hepatitis B infection were supplemented with either 200 μg of selenium in the form of selenium-enhanced yeast tablet or a placebo yeast tablet daily. Throughout the 4-year follow-up period, 7 of 113 individuals receiving placebo advanced to primary liver cancer, while none of the 113 subjects supplemented with selenium presented liver cancer (Yu et al., 1997).

Furthermore, a double-blind, placebo-controlled study in the United States of 1250 older people with a history of skin cancer discovered that 200 μg/day of selenium-enhanced yeast for an average of 7.4 years did not influence the reappearance of skin cancers (Clark et al., 1996). Nevertheless, selenium supplementation was related to a 52% reduction in prostate cancer frequency and a 33% reduction in total cancer in men. The protective outcome of selenium supplementation was highest in those with lesser pretreatment plasma selenium levels. Selenium supplementation did not decrease the probability of cancer in women, who were 25% of the participants (Rayman and Clark, 2000).

The mechanisms for the protective effect of selenium are the maximized activity of antioxidant selenoenzymes and improved antioxidant status, improved immune system function, distressed metabolism of carcinogens, and increased levels of selenium metabolites that prevent tumor cell growth. The nutritional quantity of 40–100 μg/day selenium in adults maximizes antioxidant selenoenzyme activity and probably enhances immune system function and carcinogen metabolism. At supranutritional levels of 200–300 μg/day selenium in adults, the formation of selenium metabolites, especially methylated forms of selenium, may also exert anticarcinogenic effects (Combs and Gray, 1998).

CANCER AND VITAMIN C

A large number of studies have shown that increased consumption of fresh fruits and vegetables is associated with a reduced risk for most types of cancer (Steinmetz and Potter, 1996) (Table 10.3). These studies are the core for dietary guidelines recognized by the USDA and the National Cancer Institute, which endorse at least five servings of fruits and vegetables per day. A number of case–control studies have investigated the role of vitamin C in cancer prevention. Most have shown that higher intakes of vitamin C are associated with decreased incidence of cancers of the mouth, throat and vocal chords, esophagus, stomach, colon–rectum, and lung (Carr and Frei, 1999). Because the possibility of bias is greater in case–control studies, prospective studies are generally given more weight in the evaluation of the effect of nutrient intake on disease. In general, prospective studies in which the lowest intake

TABLE 10.3
Food Sources of Vitamin C

Food	Milligrams (mg) per Serving	Percent (%) DV[a]
Red pepper, sweet, raw, 1/2 cup	95	158
Orange juice, 3/4 cup	93	155
Orange, 1 medium	70	117
Grapefruit juice, 3/4 cup	70	117
Kiwifruit, 1 medium	64	107
Green pepper, sweet, raw, 1/2 cup	60	100
Broccoli, cooked, 1/2 cup	51	85
Strawberries, fresh, sliced, 1/2 cup	49	82
Brussels sprouts, cooked, 1/2 cup	48	80
Grapefruit, 1/2 medium	39	65
Broccoli, raw, 1/2 cup	39	65
Tomato juice, 3/4 cup	33	55
Cantaloupe, 1/2 cup	29	48
Cabbage, cooked, 1/2 cup	28	47
Cauliflower, raw, 1/2 cup	26	43
Potato, baked, 1 medium	17	28
Tomato, raw, 1 medium	17	28
Spinach, cooked, 1/2 cup	9	15
Green peas, frozen, cooked, 1/2 cup	8	13

Source: U.S. Department of Agriculture, Agricultural Research Service. 2011. USDA National Nutrient Database for Standard Reference, Release 24. Available at: http://www.ars.usda.gov/ba/bhnrc/ndl.

[a] DV = daily value. DVs were developed by the FDA to help consumers compare the nutrient contents of products within the context of a total diet. The DV for vitamin C is 60 mg for adults and children aged 4 years and older. The FDA requires all food labels to list the percent DV for vitamin C. Foods providing 20% or more of the DV are considered to be high sources of a nutrient.

group consumed more than 86 mg of vitamin C daily have not found differences in cancer risk, while studies finding significant cancer risk reductions found them in people consuming at least 80–110 mg of vitamin C daily (Carr and Frei, 1999).

A prospective study of 870 men for a period of 25 years established that those who had an intake of more than 83 mg of vitamin C daily had a 64% reduction in lung cancer compared with those who received less than 63 mg/day (Kromhout, 1987). Although most large prospective studies found no association between breast cancer and vitamin C intake, two studies found dietary vitamin C intake to be inversely associated with breast cancer risk in certain subgroups. In the Nurses' Health Study, premenopausal women with a family history of breast cancer who consumed an average of 205 mg/day of vitamin C from foods had a 63% lower risk of breast cancer than those who consumed an average of 70 mg/day (Zhang et al., 1999a). In the Swedish Mammography Cohort, women who were overweight and consumed an average of 110 mg/day of vitamin C had a 39% lower risk of breast cancer compared with overweight women who consumed an average of 31 mg/day (Michels et al., 2001). A number of observational studies have found increased dietary vitamin C intake to be associated with decreased risk of stomach cancer, and laboratory experiments indicate that vitamin C inhibits the formation of carcinogenic compounds in the stomach. Infection with the bacterium *Helicobacter pylori* is known to increase the risk of stomach cancer and also appears to lower the vitamin C content of stomach secretions. Although two intervention studies did not find a decrease in the occurrence of stomach cancer with vitamin C supplementation, more recent research suggests that vitamin C supplementation may be a useful addition to standard *H. pylori* eradication therapy in reducing the risk of gastric cancer (Feiz and Mobarhan, 2002).

ANTIOXIDANT SUPPLEMENTATION AND PREVENTION OF CANCER

In laboratory and animal studies, the presence of increased levels of exogenous antioxidants has been shown to prevent the types of free radical damage that have been associated with cancer development. Therefore, researchers have investigated whether taking dietary antioxidant supplements can help lower the risk of developing or dying from cancer in humans.

Many observational studies, including case–control studies and cohort studies, have been conducted to investigate whether the use of dietary antioxidant supplements is associated with reduced risks of cancer in humans. Overall, these studies have yielded mixed results (Patterson et al., 1997). Because observational studies cannot adequately control for biases that might influence study outcomes, the results of any individual observational study must be viewed with caution.

Randomized controlled clinical trials, on the other hand, lack most of the biases that limit the reliability of observational studies. As a result, randomized trials are deemed to present the most powerful and reliable evidence of the benefit and/or harm of a health-related intervention. To date, nine randomized controlled trials of dietary antioxidant supplements for cancer prevention have been conducted worldwide. Many of the trials were sponsored by the National Cancer Institute, and some of them are presented below.

- *α-Tocopherol/β-Carotene Cancer Prevention Study (ATBC)*: This trial investigated whether the use of α-tocopherol and/or β-carotene supplements for 5–8 years could help reduce the incidence of lung and other cancers in middle-aged male smokers in Finland. Initial results of the trial, reported in 1994, showed an increase in the incidence of lung cancer among the participants who took β-carotene supplements (20 mg/day); in contrast, α-tocopherol supplementation (50 mg/day) had no effect on lung cancer incidence (The Alpha-Tocopherol, Beta Carotene Cancer Prevention Study Group, 1994). Later results showed no effect of β-carotene or α-tocopherol supplementation on the incidence of urothelial (bladder, ureter, or renal pelvis), pancreatic, colorectal, renal cell (kidney), or upper aerodigestive tract (oral/pharyngeal, esophageal, or laryngeal) cancers (Rautalahti et al., 1999; Albanes et al., 2000; Virtamo et al., 2000; Wright et al., 2007).

- *Carotene and Retinol Efficacy Trial (CARET)*: This U.S. trial examined the effects of daily supplementation with β-carotene and retinol (vitamin A) on the incidence of lung cancer, other cancers, and death among people who were at high risk of lung cancer because of a history of smoking or exposure to asbestos. The trial began in 1983 and ended in late 1995, 2 years earlier than originally planned. Results reported in 1996 showed that daily supplementation with both 15 mg β-carotene and 25,000 international units (IU) retinol was associated with increased lung cancer and increased death from all causes (all-cause mortality) (Omenn et al., 1996). A 2004 report showed that these adverse effects persisted up to 6 years after supplementation ended, although the elevated risks of lung cancer and all-cause mortality were no longer statistically significant (Goodman et al., 2004). Additional results, reported in 2009, showed that β-carotene and retinol supplementation had no effect on the incidence of prostate cancer (Neuhouser et al., 2009).
- *Women's Health Study (WHS)*: This trial investigated the effects of β-carotene supplementation (50 mg every other day), vitamin E supplementation (600 IU every other day), and aspirin (100 mg every other day) on the incidence of cancer and cardiovascular disease in U.S. women ages 45 years and older. The results, reported in 1999, showed no benefit or harm associated with 2 years of β-carotene supplementation (Lee et al., 1999). In 2005, similar results were reported for vitamin E supplementation (Lee et al., 2005).
- *Heart Outcomes Prevention Evaluation—The Ongoing Outcomes (HOPE-TOO) Study*: This international trial examined the effects of α-tocopherol supplementation on cancer incidence, death from cancer, and the incidence of major cardiovascular events (heart attack, stroke, or death from heart disease) in people with cardiovascular disease or diabetes. The results, reported in 2005, showed no effect of daily supplementation with α-tocopherol (400 IU) for a median of 7 years on any of the outcomes (Lonn et al., 2005).
- *Selenium and Vitamin E Cancer Prevention Trial (SELECT)*: This U.S. trial investigated whether daily supplementation with selenium (200 µg), vitamin E (400 IU), or both would reduce the incidence of prostate cancer in men ages 50 years and older. The study began in 2001 and was stopped in 2008, approximately 5 years earlier than originally planned. Results reported in late 2008 showed that the use of these supplements for a median duration of 5.5 years did not reduce the incidence of prostate or other cancers (Lippman et al., 2009). Updated findings from the study, reported in 2011, showed that, after an average of 7 years (5.5 years on supplements and 1.5 years off supplements), there were 17% more cases of prostate cancer among men taking vitamin E alone than among men taking a placebo (Klein et al., 2011). No increase in prostate risk was observed for men assigned to take selenium alone or vitamin E plus selenium compared with men assigned to take a placebo (Lippman et al., 2009).
- *Physicians' Health Study II (PHS II)*: This trial examined whether supplementation with vitamin E, vitamin C, or both would reduce the incidence of cancer in male U.S. physicians ages 50 years and older. The results, reported in 2009, showed that the use of these supplements (400 IU vitamin

E every other day, 500 mg vitamin C every day, or a combination of the two) for a median of 7.6 years did not reduce the incidence of prostate cancer or other cancers, including lymphoma, leukemia, melanoma, and cancers of the lung, bladder, pancreas, and colon and rectum (Gaziano et al., 2009).

Overall, the nine randomized controlled clinical trials did not provide evidence that dietary antioxidant supplements are beneficial in primary cancer prevention. In addition, a systematic review of the available evidence regarding the use of vitamin and mineral supplements for the prevention of chronic diseases, including cancer, conducted for the U.S. Preventive Services Task Force likewise found no clear evidence of a benefit in preventing cancer (Fortmann et al., 2013). A review of almost 80 randomized clinical studies on antioxidant use (vitamins A, C, E; β-carotene; and selenium) for preventing disease-related death provides evidence that further challenges the widely claimed benefits of antioxidants. Collectively, the studies included a total of almost 300,000 men and women (described as both "healthy" and with diseases in a "stable phase"). Significantly more deaths were observed in men and women taking vitamin E, β-carotene, or doses of vitamin A that exceed the RDA, which are 700 µg for women and 900 µg for men. These findings led the authors to caution against the use of antioxidant supplements for both the general population and in those with various diseases (Bjelakovic et al., 2012).

The lack of benefit in clinical studies can be explained by differences in the effects of the tested antioxidants when they are consumed as purified chemicals as opposed to when they are consumed in foods, which contain complex mixtures of antioxidants, vitamins, and minerals (Bouayed and Bohn, 2010). Therefore, obtaining a more inclusive information of the antioxidant content of individual foods, how the various antioxidants and other substances in foods interact with one another, and factors that influence the uptake and distribution of food-derived antioxidants in the body are active areas of ongoing cancer prevention research.

The measure of antioxidant capacity (AC) considers the cumulative action of all the antioxidants present in plasma and body fluids, thus providing an integrated parameter rather than the simple sum of measurable antioxidants. The capacity of known and unknown antioxidants and their synergistic interaction is therefore assessed, giving an insight into the delicate balance *in vivo* between oxidants and antioxidants. Measuring plasma AC may help in the evaluation of physiological, environmental, and nutritional factors of the redox status in humans. Determining plasma AC may help identify conditions affecting oxidative status *in vivo* (e.g., exposure to reactive oxygen species and antioxidant supplementation) (Ghiselli, 2000). The term "antioxidant" refers mainly to nonnutrient compounds in foods, such as polyphenols, which have AC *in vitro* and so provide an artificial index of antioxidant strength—the ORAC measurement. Oxygen radical absorbance capacity (ORAC) is a method of measuring antioxidant capacities in biological samples *in vitro*. Values are expressed as the sum of the lipid-soluble (e.g., carotenoid) and water-soluble (e.g., phenolic) antioxidant fractions (i.e., "total ORAC") reported as in micromoles Trolox equivalents per 100 g sample, and are compared with assessments of total polyphenol content in the samples. These values are considered biologically irrelevant by the European Food Safety Authority (EFSA) and USDA (EFSA Panel on Dietetic Products, Nutrition and Allergies, 2010).

Many common foods are good sources of antioxidants. In the list of foods given below, "rich in antioxidants" usually means at least an ORAC rating of 1000 per 100 g. A typical apple or pear weighs around 200 g, and hence 200 g can be considered as the serving size.

Spices, herbs, and essential oils are rich in antioxidant properties in the plant itself and *in vitro*; however, the serving size is too small to supply antioxidants via the diet. Typical spices high in antioxidants (confirmed *in vitro*) are clove, cinnamon, oregano, turmeric, cumin, parsley, basil, curry powder, mustard seed, ginger, pepper, chili powder, paprika, garlic, coriander, onion, and cardamom. Typical herbs are sage, thyme, marjoram, tarragon, peppermint, oregano, savory, basil, and dill weed.

Dried fruits are a good source of antioxidants by weight/serving size as the water has been removed, making the ratio of antioxidants higher. Typical dried fruits are pears, apples, plums, peaches, raisins, figs, and dates. Dried raisins are high in polyphenol. Red wine is high in total polyphenol, which supplies antioxidant quality that is unlikely to be conserved following digestion (see the next section).

Deeply pigmented fruits like cranberries, blueberries, plums, blackberries, raspberries, strawberries, blackcurrants, figs, cherries, guava, oranges, mango, grape juice, and pomegranate juice also have significant ORAC scores (Table 10.4) (USDA, 2012).

With nearly all vegetables, conventional boiling can reduce the ORAC value by up to 90%, while steaming retains more of the antioxidants.

DILEMMA OF TAKING ANTIOXIDANT SUPPLEMENTS WHILE HAVING CANCER

Several randomized controlled trials, some including only small numbers of patients, have investigated whether taking antioxidant supplements during cancer treatment alters the effectiveness or reduces the toxicity of specific therapies (Lawenda et al., 2008). Although these trials had mixed results, some found that people who took antioxidant supplements during cancer therapy had worse outcomes, especially if they were smokers.

Additional large randomized controlled trials are needed to provide clear scientific evidence about the potential benefits or harms of taking antioxidant supplements during cancer treatment. Until more is known about the effects of antioxidant supplements in cancer patients, these supplements should be used with caution.

Antioxidants prevent the chemical process of oxidation. However, oxidation helps the body kill off bad cells like cancer cells, as well as healthy cells. Different parts of the body have their own unique ways of developing cancer. Similarly, one organ responds differently to nutrients than another; thus, the supplement that helps lower your risk for one cancer could raise your risk of another.

Studies also suggest that taking antioxidant supplements such as vitamin C during chemotherapy may not be a good idea. In one study, large doses of vitamin C supplements reduced the effectiveness of several anticancer drugs including methotrexate, doxorubicin, and imatinib, resulting in 30–70% fewer cancer cells killed. The authors concluded that vitamin C may actually be helping cancer cells survive by protecting the cells' power source (Heaney et al., 2008). In another study, the antioxidants vitamin C and *N*-acetylcysteine (often sold under the name "NAC") significantly reduced the effectiveness of anticancer drugs vinblastine and cisplatin (Fukumura et al., 2012).

TABLE 10.4
Food ORAC Scores

Rank	Food Item	Serving Size	Total Antioxidant Capacity per Serving Size
1	Small red bean (dried)	Half cup	13,727
2	Wild blueberry	1 cup	13,427
3	Red kidney bean (dried)	Half cup	13,259
4	Pinto bean	Half cup	11,864
5	Blueberry (cultivated)	1 cup	9019
6	Cranberry	1 cup (whole)	8983
7	Artichoke (cooked)	1 cup (hearts)	7904
8	Blackberry	1 cup	7701
9	Prune	Half cup	7291
10	Raspberry	1 cup	6058
11	Strawberry	1 cup	5938
12	Red delicious apple	1 whole	5900
13	Granny Smith apple	1 whole	5381
14	Pecan	1 oz	5095
15	Sweet cherry	1 cup	4873
16	Black plum	1 whole	4844
17	Russet potato (cooked)	1 whole	4649
18	Black bean (dried)	Half cup	4181
19	Plum	1 whole	4118
20	Gala apple	1 whole	3903

Source: U.S. Department of Agriculture, Agricultural Research Service. 2010. USDA Database for the Oxygen Radical Absorbance Capacity (ORAC) of Selected Foods, Release 2. Available at: http://www.orac-info-portal.de/download/ORAC_R2.pdf

Antioxidant supplements have not been found to diminish the risk of cancer in most studies. In effect, for people with a higher than normal risk of cancer (smokers and people who have already survived one cancer) and those being treated for cancer with chemotherapy, antioxidant supplements were found to be destructive. Dietary supplements are intended to be used when the body is not receiving certain nutrients in the right amounts; however, like drugs, they can have unplanned adverse effects and therefore should only be taken as recommended.

Consequently, some established strategies that can help reduce the risk of cancer are as follows:

- Maintain a healthy weight by limiting the high-calorie foods you eat and getting regular physical activity.
- Eat foods rich in antioxidants (rather than use supplements).
- Eat plenty of fruits and vegetables every day (fruits and vegetables should cover half of the plate).

- Limit the amount of red meat and processed meat (hot dogs, sausages, bologna, etc.) eaten.
- Eat foods made of whole grains.

FOODS RICH IN ANTIOXIDANTS

Antioxidants are plentiful in fruits and vegetables, nuts, grains, and some meats, poultry, and fish. The list below describes food sources of common antioxidants.

- *β-Carotene* is found in many foods that are orange in color, including sweet potatoes, carrots, cantaloupe, squash, apricots, pumpkin, and mangoes. Some green leafy vegetables, including collard greens, spinach, and kale, are also rich in β-carotene.
- *Lutein*, best known for its association with healthy eyes, is abundant in green, leafy vegetables such as collard greens, spinach, and kale.
- *Lycopene* is a potent antioxidant found in tomatoes, watermelon, guava, papaya, apricots, pink grapefruit, blood oranges, and other foods. Estimates suggest that 85% of the American dietary intake of lycopene comes from tomatoes and tomato products.
- *Selenium* is a mineral, not an antioxidant nutrient. However, it is a component of antioxidant enzymes. Plant foods like rice and wheat are the major dietary sources of selenium in most countries. The amount of selenium in soil, which varies by region, determines the amount of selenium in the foods grown in that soil. Animals that eat grains or plants grown in selenium-rich soil have higher levels of selenium in their muscle. In the United States, meats and bread are common sources of dietary selenium. Brazil nuts also contain large quantities of selenium.
- *Vitamin A* is found in three main forms: retinol (vitamin A1), 3,4-didehydro-retinol (vitamin A2), and 3-hydroxy-retinol (vitamin A3). Foods rich in vitamin A include liver, sweet potatoes, carrots, milk, egg yolks, and mozzarella cheese.
- *Vitamin C* is also called ascorbic acid, and can be found in high abundance in many fruits and vegetables and is also found in cereals, beef, poultry, and fish.
- *Vitamin E*, also known as α-tocopherol, is found in almonds; in many oils including wheat germ, safflower, corn, and soybean oils; and also in mangoes, nuts, broccoli, and other foods.

PREVENTION

CANCER AND FRUITS AND VEGETABLES

Many studies discovered a physically powerful link between eating fruits and vegetables and protection against cancer. The results of the case–control studies indicate that eating a diet rich in fruits and vegetables decreases the risk of developing several different types of cancer, particularly cancers of the digestive tract (oropharynx, esophagus, stomach, colon, and rectum) and lung (Block et al., 1992; World Cancer Research Fund, 1997). The balanced combinations of fruits and vegetables decreases the risk of cancer (Ohigashi and Murakami, 2004). The results of these studies are the foundation for the National Cancer Institute's "five-a-day" program, which is aimed at increasing the fruit and vegetable consumption of the American public to a minimum of five servings daily. In contrast to the results of case–control studies, many prospective cohort studies have found little or no association between total fruit and vegetable intake and the risk of various cancers (Michels et al., 2000; Smith-Warner et al., 2001, 2003; Flood et al., 2002; Michaud et al., 2002; McCullough et al., 2003; Hung et al., 2004; Key et al., 2004; Lin et al., 2005; Sato et al., 2005; Tsubono et al., 2005; Van Gils et al., 2005). There is some reasoning for this. Case–control studies, in which the past diets of people with a particular type of cancer are compared with the diets of those without cancer, are more susceptible to bias in the selection of participants and dietary recall than prospective cohort studies, which collect information on the diets of large cohorts of patients over time. Although prospective cohort studies provide weak support for an association between total fruit and vegetable consumption and cancer risk, they provide some evidence that high intakes of certain classes of fruits or vegetables are associated with a reduced risk of individual cancers. Higher intakes of fruits were associated with modest but significant reductions in lung cancer risk in a pooled analysis of eight prospective cohort studies (Smith-Warner et al., 2003). In men, higher intakes of cruciferous vegetables were associated with significant reductions in the risk of bladder cancer, and higher intakes of tomato products were associated with significant reductions in the risk of prostate cancer (Higdon, 2007).

Cohort studies, which follow large groups of initially healthy individuals for years, generally provide more reliable information than case–control studies because they do not rely on information from the past. Furthermore, data from cohort studies have not consistently shown that a diet rich in fruits and vegetables prevents cancer in general. For example, in the Nurses' Health Study and the Health Professionals Follow-up Study, during a 14-year period, men and women with the highest intake of fruits and vegetables (8+ servings a day) were just as likely to have developed cancer as those who ate the fewest daily servings (<1.5) (Hung et al., 2004).

A more likely possibility is that some types of fruits and vegetables may protect against certain cancers. A massive report by the World Cancer Research Fund and the American Institute for Cancer Research suggests that nonstarchy vegetables— such as lettuce and other leafy greens, broccoli, bok choy, cabbage, as well as garlic, onions, and the like—and fruits "probably" protect against several types of cancers, including those of the mouth, throat, voice box, esophagus, and stomach; fruits probably also protect against lung cancer (World Cancer Research Fund, 2007).

Specific components of fruits and vegetables may also be protective against cancer. For example, a line of research stemming from a finding from the Health Professionals Follow-up Study suggests that tomatoes may help protect men against prostate cancer, especially aggressive forms of it (Giovannucci et al., 2007). One of the pigments that give tomatoes their red hue, lycopene, could be involved in this protective effect. Although several studies other than the Health Professionals

Study have also demonstrated a link between tomatoes or lycopene and prostate cancer, others have not or have found only a weak connection (Kavanaugh et al., 2007). Taken as a whole, however, these studies suggest that increased consumption of tomato-based products (especially cooked tomato products) and other lycopene-containing foods may reduce the occurrence of prostate cancer (World Cancer Research Fund, 2007). Lycopene is one of several carotenoids (compounds that the body can turn into vitamin A) found in brightly colored fruits and vegetables, and research suggests that foods containing carotenoids may protect against lung, mouth, and throat cancer (World Cancer Research Fund, 2007). However, more research is needed before we know the exact relationship between fruits and vegetables, carotenoids, and cancer.

Intake Recommendations

The National Cancer Institute recommends a range of five to nine servings of fruits and vegetables daily. Specifically, adolescent and adult women should aim for seven daily servings, whereas adolescent and adult men should aim for nine daily servings. The 2010 Dietary Guidelines for Americans are similar with respect to fruit and vegetable intake recommendations; however, they are tied to energy (caloric) intake rather than age and sex. Daily consumption of 2 cups (4 servings) of fruit and 2.5 cups (5 servings) of vegetables are recommended for people who consume 8368 kJ/day (2000 kcal/day), whereas 1.5 cups of fruit (3 servings) and 2 cups (4 servings) of vegetables are recommended for people who consume 6693.4 kJ/day (1600 kcal/day). In both cases, consumption of a variety of different fruits and vegetables is recommended, including dark green, red, orange, yellow, blue, and purple fruits and vegetables, as well as legumes (peas and beans), onions, and garlic (Higdon, 2007).

CRUCIFEROUS VEGETABLES

Cruciferous or *Brassica* vegetables are plants in the family known as *Cruciferae* (*Brassicaceae*). Many commonly consumed cruciferous vegetables come from the *Brassica* genus, including broccoli, Brussels sprouts, cabbage, cauliflower, collard greens, kale, kohlrabi, mustard, rutabaga, turnips, bok choy, and Chinese cabbage (Kristal and Lampe, 2002). Arugula, horseradish, radish, wasabi, and watercress are also cruciferous vegetables. Cruciferous vegetables are exceptional as they are good sources of glucosinolates, sulfur-containing compounds that are responsible for their pungent aromas and spicy (or bitter) taste. The hydrolysis (breakdown) of glucosinolates by a class of plant enzymes called myrosinase results in the formation of biologically active compounds, such as indoles and isothiocyanates. Myrosinase is physically separated from glucosinolates in intact plant cells. However, when cruciferous vegetables are chopped or chewed, myrosinase comes in contract with glucosinolates and catalyzes their hydrolysis. Scientists are currently investigating the potential for high intakes of cruciferous vegetables and several glucosinolate hydrolysis products to prevent cancer.

Akin to most other vegetables, cruciferous vegetables are good sources of a variety of nutrients and phytochemicals that may work synergistically to help prevent cancer. One challenge in studying the relationships between cruciferous vegetable intakes and cancer risk in humans is sorting out the benefits of diets that are generally rich in vegetables from those that are specifically rich in cruciferous vegetables. One characteristic that sets cruciferous vegetables apart from other vegetables is their high glucosinolate content. Glucosinolate hydrolysis products could help prevent cancer by enhancing the elimination of carcinogens before they can damage DNA or by altering cell signaling pathways in ways that help prevent normal cells from being transformed into cancerous cells. Some glucosinolate hydrolysis products may alter the metabolism or activity of hormones like estrogen in ways that inhibit the development of hormone-sensitive cancers (Higdon, 2007).

IODINE AND THYROID FUNCTION AND CRUCIFEROUS VEGETABLES

Very high intakes of cruciferous vegetables, such as cabbage and turnips, have been found to cause hypothyroidism in animals (Fenwick et al., 1983). Two mechanisms have been identified to explain this effect. The hydrolysis of some glucosinolates found in cruciferous vegetables (e.g., progoitrin) may yield a compound known as goitrin, which has been found to interfere with thyroid hormone synthesis. The hydrolysis of another class of glucosinolates, known as indole glucosinolates, results in the release of thiocyanate ions, which can compete with iodine for uptake by the thyroid gland. Increased exposure to thiocyanate ions from cruciferous vegetable consumption or, more commonly, cigarette smoking does not appear to increase the risk of hypothyroidism unless accompanied by iodine deficiency. One study in humans found that the consumption of 150 g/day (5 oz/day) of cooked Brussels sprouts for 4 weeks had no adverse effects on thyroid function (Higdon, 2007).

Intake Recommendations

Although many organizations, including the National Cancer Institute, recommend the consumption of five to nine servings (2.5–4.5 cups) of fruits and vegetables daily, separate recommendations for cruciferous vegetables have not been established. Much remains to be learned regarding cruciferous vegetable consumption and cancer prevention; however, the results of some prospective cohort studies suggest that adults should aim for at least five weekly servings of cruciferous vegetables (Michaud et al., 1999).

CANCER AND LEGUMES

Dry Beans, Peas, and Lentils

Dry beans, peas, and lentils are rich in several compounds that could decrease the risk of certain cancers (Mathers, 2002).

Prostate Cancer

There is limited evidence from observational studies that legume intake is inversely related to the risk of prostate cancer. In a 6-year prospective study of more than 14,000 Seventh Day Adventist men living in the United States, those with the highest intakes of legumes (beans, lentils, or split peas) had a significantly lower risk of prostate cancer (Mills et al., 1989). A prospective study of more than 58,000 men in the Netherlands found that those with the highest intakes of legumes had a risk of prostate cancer that was 29% lower than those with the lowest intakes. Similarly, in a case–control study of 1619 North American men with prostate cancer and 1618 healthy men matched for age and ethnicity, those with the highest legume intakes had a risk of prostate cancer that was 38% lower than those with the lowest intakes (Kolonel et al., 2000). Excluding the intake of soy foods from the analysis did not weaken the inverse association between legume intake and prostate cancer, suggesting that soy was not the only legume that conferred protection against prostate cancer.

CANCER AND SOY

Prostate Cancer

Although there is substantial scientific interest in the possibility for soy products to prevent prostate cancer, evidence that higher intakes of soy foods can reduce the risk of prostate cancer in humans is limited. Only two out of six case–control studies found that higher intakes of soy products were associated with significantly lower prostate cancer risk. In the largest case–control study, North American men who consumed an average of at least 1.4 oz of soy foods daily were 38% less likely to have prostate cancer than men who did not consume soy foods. A much smaller case–control study of Chinese men found that men who consumed at least 4 oz of soy foods daily were only half as likely to have prostate cancer as those who consumed less than 1 oz daily. A 6-year prospective cohort study of more than 12,000 Seventh Day Adventist men in the United States found that those who drank soy milk more than once daily had a risk of prostate cancer that was 70% lower than those who never dark soy milk; however, a 23-year study of more than 5000 Japanese American men found no association between tofu consumption and prostate cancer risk (Nomura et al., 2004).

Breast Cancer

At least 15 epidemiological studies have assessed the relationship between soy food intake and the risk of breast cancer. One out of four prospective studies found that higher intakes of soy food were associated with a significant reduction in breast cancer risk. In that 9-year study of more than 21,000 Japanese women, higher intakes of miso soup (no other soy foods) were inversely associated with breast cancer risk. Most case–control studies did not find that women with higher soy intakes were at lower risk of breast cancer, except for women who had higher soy intakes during adolescence (Shannon et al., 2005). Two case–control studies, one of Chinese women and one of Asian American women, found that women with higher soy intakes during adolescence were significantly less likely to develop breast cancer later in life (Higdon, 2007).

Intake Recommendations

Substituting beans, peas, and lentils for foods that are high in saturated fat or refined carbohydrates is likely to help lower the risk of type 2 diabetes mellitus (DM) and cardiovascular disease. Soybeans and foods made from soybeans (soy foods) are excellent sources of protein. In fact, soy protein is a complete protein, meaning it provides all of the essential amino acids in adequate amounts for human health (Messina, 1999). As with beans, peas, and lentils, soy foods are also excellent substitutes for protein sources that are high in saturated fat like red meat or cheese. In the 2010 Dietary Guidelines of Americans, an intake of three cups (six servings) of legumes weekly is recommended for people who consume 8368 kJ/2000 kcal/day. A serving of legumes is equal to one-half cup of cooked beans, peas, lentils, or tofu.

CANCER AND WHOLE GRAINS

Even if the protecting effects of whole grains against various types of cancer are not as well known as those against diabetes and cardiovascular disease, numerous case–control studies have found inverse associations between various measures of whole-grain intake and cancer risk (La Vecchia et al., 2003). A meta-analysis of 40 case–control studies examining 20 different types of cancer found that those with high whole-grain intakes had an overall risk of cancer that was 34% lower than those with low whole-grain intakes. Elevated intakes of whole grain were most constantly associated with decreased risk of gastrointestinal tract cancers, including cancers of the mouth, throat, stomach, colon, and rectum. A prospective cohort study that followed more than 61,000 Swedish women for 15 years found that those who consumed more than 4.5 servings of whole grain daily had a risk of colon cancer that was 35% lower than those who consumed less than 1.5 servings of whole grain daily. Higher fiber intakes are known to speed up the passage of stool through the colon, allowing less time for potentially carcinogenic compounds to stay in contact with cells that line the inner surface of the colon. Lignans in whole grains are phytoestrogens and may affect the development of hormone-dependent cancers.

Phenolic compounds in whole grains may modify signal transduction pathways that promote the development of cancer or bind potentially damaging free metal ions in the gastrointestinal tract (Higdon, 2007).

Intake Recommendations

Whole-grain intakes approaching three servings daily are associated with significant reductions in chronic disease risk in populations with relatively low whole-grain intakes. The 2010 Dietary Guidelines for Americans recommend consuming three or more servings of whole-grain products daily (U.S. Department of Agriculture and U.S. Department of Health and Human Services, 2010). Whole-grain foods should be substituted for refined carbohydrates whenever possible.

CANCER AND CAROTENOIDS

Food Sources

The most common dietary carotenoids in typical Western diets are β-carotene, α-carotene, β-cryptoxanthin, lycopene, lutein, and zeaxanthin. Carotenoids in foods are mainly in the all-*trans* form, although cooking may result in the formation of other isomers. The relatively low bioavailability of carotenoids from most foods compared with supplements is partly because they are associated with proteins in the plant matrix. Chopping, homogenizing, and cooking disrupt the plant matrix, increasing the bioavailability of carotenoids. The bioavailability of lycopene from tomatoes is substantially improved by heating tomatoes in oil (Gartner et al., 1997).

β-Carotene and α-Carotene

β-Carotene and α-carotene are provitamin A carotenoids; that is, they can be converted by the body to vitamin A. The vitamin A activity of β-carotene in foods is 1/12 that of retinol (preformed vitamin A). Thus, it would take 12 µg of β-carotene from foods to provide the equivalent of 1 µg of retinol. The vitamin A activity of α-carotene from foods is 1/24 that of retinol, so it would take 24 µg of α-carotene from foods to provide the equivalent of 1 µg of retinol. Orange and yellow vegetables like carrots and winter squash are rich sources of β- and α-carotene. Spinach is also a rich source of β-carotene, although the chlorophyll in spinach leaves hides the yellow–orange pigment. Some foods that are good sources of α-carotene and β-carotene are listed in Tables 10.5 and 10.6, respectively.

β-Cryptoxanthin

Like β- and α-carotene, β-cryptoxanthin is a provitamin A carotenoid. The vitamin A activity of β-cryptoxanthin from foods is 1/24 that of retinol, so it would take 24 µg of β-cryptoxanthin from food to provide the equivalent of 1 µg of retinol. Orange and red fruits and vegetables, like sweet red peppers and oranges, are particularly rich sources of β-cryptoxanthin.

Lycopene

Lycopene gives tomatoes, pink grapefruit, watermelon, and guava their red color. It has been estimated that 80% of the lycopene in the diet of the U.S. population

TABLE 10.5
α-Carotene Content of Selected Foods

Food	Serving	α-Carotene (mg)
Pumpkin, canned	1 cup	11.7
Carrot juice, canned	1 cup (8 fl oz)	10.2
Carrots, cooked	1 cup	5.9
Carrots, raw	1 medium	2.0
Mixed vegetables, frozen cooked	1 cup	1.8
Winter squash, baked	1 cup	1.4
Plantains, raw	1 medium	0.8
Pumpkin pie	1 piece	0.7
Collards, frozen cooked	1 cup	0.2
Tomatoes, raw	1 medium	0.1
Tangerines, raw	1 medium	0.08
Peas, frozen, cooked	1 cup	0.08

TABLE 10.6
β-Carotene Content of Selected Foods

Food	Serving	β-Carotene (mg)
Carrot juice, canned	1 cup (8 fl oz)	22.0
Pumpkin, canned	1 cup	17.0
Sweet potato, baked	1 medium	16.8
Spinach, frozen, cooked	1 cup	13.7
Carrots, cooked	1 cup	13.0
Collards, frozen, cooked	1 cup	11.6
Kale, frozen, cooked	1 cup	11.5
Turnip greens, frozen, cooked	1 cup	10.6
Pumpkin pie	1 piece	7.4
Dandelion greens, cooked	1 cup	6.2
Winter squash, cooked	1 cup	5.7
Cantaloupe, raw	1 cup	3.2

comes from tomatoes and tomato products like tomato sauce, tomato paste, and catsup (ketchup) (Clinton, 1998). Lycopene is not a provitamin A carotenoid, meaning the body cannot convert lycopene to vitamin A.

Lutein and Zeaxanthin

Although lutein and zeaxanthin are different compounds, they are both from the class of carotenoids known as xanthophylls. They are not provitamin A carotenoids. Some methods used to quantify lutein and zeaxanthin in foods do not separate the two compounds, so they are typically reported as lutein and zeaxanthin or lutein + zeaxanthin. Lutein and zeaxanthin are present in a variety of fruits and vegetables. Dark green leafy vegetables like spinach and kale are particularly rich sources of lutein and zeaxanthin. Some foods that are good sources of lutein and zeaxanthin are listed in Table 10.7.

Curcumin

Turmeric is a spice derived from the rhizomes of *Curcuma longa*, which is a member of the ginger family (*Zingiberaceae*) (Aggarwal et al., 2005). Curcumin is the principal curcuminoid found in turmeric and is generally considered its most active constituent (Sharma et al., 2005).

The ability of curcumin to induce apoptosis in cultured cancer cells by several different mechanisms has generated scientific interest in the potential for curcumin to prevent some types of cancer (Sharma et al., 2005). Oral curcumin administration has been found to inhibit the development of chemically induced cancer in animal models of oral (Krishnaswamy et al., 1998; Li et al., 2002), stomach (Huang et al., 1994; Ikezaki et al., 2001), liver (Chuang et al., 2000), and colon cancer (Rao et al., 1995; Pereira et al., 1996; Kawamori et al., 1999). Apc[Min/+] mice have a mutation in the *adenomatous polyposis coli* (*Apc*) gene similar to that in humans with familial adenomatous polyposis, a genetic condition that is characterized by the development

TABLE 10.7

Lutein + Zeaxanthin Content of Foods

Food	Serving	Lutein + Zeaxanthin (mg)
Spinach, frozen, cooked	1 cup	29.8
Kale, frozen, cooked	1 cup	25.6
Turnip greens, frozen cooked	1 cup	19.5
Collards, frozen, cooked	1 cup	18.5
Mustard greens, cooked	1 cup	8.3
Dandelion greens, cooked	1 cup	4.9
Summer squash, cooked	1 cup	4.0
Peas, frozen, cooked	1 cup	3.8
Winter squash, baked	1 cup	2.9
Broccoli, frozen, cooked	1 cup	2.8
Pumpkin, cooked	1 cup	2.5
Brussels sprouts, frozen, cooked	1 cup	2.4
Sweet yellow corn, boiled	1 cup	1.6

of numerous colorectal adenomas (polyps) and a high risk for colorectal cancer. Oral curcumin administration has been found to inhibit the development of intestinal adenomas in $Apc^{Min/+}$ mice (Mahmoud et al., 2000; Perkins et al., 2002).

CANCER AND CURCUMIN

The ability of curcumin to induce apoptosis in a variety of cancer cell lines in culture and its low toxicity have led to scientific interest in its potential for cancer therapy as well as cancer prevention (Karunagaran et al., 2005). To date, most of the controlled clinical trials of curcumin supplementation in cancer patients have been phase I trials. Phase I trials are clinical trials in small groups of people, aimed at determining bioavailability, optimal dose, safety, and early evidence of the efficacy of a new therapy (National Institutes of Health, 2005). A phase I clinical trial in patients with advanced colorectal cancer found that doses up to 3.6 g/day for 4 months were well tolerated, although the systemic availability of oral curcumin was low (Sharma et al., 2004). When colorectal cancer patients with liver metastases took 3.6 g/day of curcumin orally for 7 days, trace levels of curcumin metabolites were measured in liver tissue; however, curcumin itself was not detected (Garcea et al., 2004). In contrast, curcumin was measured in normal and malignant colorectal tissue after patients with advanced colorectal cancer took 3.6 g/day of curcumin orally for 7 days (Garcea et al., 2005). These findings suggest that oral curcumin is more likely to be effective as a therapeutic agent in cancers of the gastrointestinal tract than other tissues. Phase II trials are clinical trials designed to investigate the effectiveness of a new therapy in larger numbers of people and to further evaluate the short-term adverse effects and safety of the new therapy. Phase II clinical trials of curcumin in patients with advanced pancreatic cancer are currently under way, and phase II trials of curcumin for colorectal cancer have been recommended (Sharma et al., 2005).

Colorectal Cancer and Fiber

Most case–control studies conducted before 1990 found the incidence of colorectal cancer to be lower in people with higher fiber intakes. In contrast, most prospective cohort studies conducted more recently have not found significant associations between measures of dietary fiber intake and colorectal cancer risk. Three controlled clinical trials also failed to demonstrate a protective effect of fiber consumption on the recurrence of colorectal adenomas (precancerous polyps). The rate of recurrence of colorectal adenomas during a 4-year period was not significantly different between those who consumed 33 g/day of fiber from a fruit- and vegetable-rich, low-fat diet and those in a control group who consumed 19 g/day. In another trial, there was no significant difference in the rate of colorectal adenoma recurrence during a 3-year period between those supplemented with 13.5 g/day of wheat bran fiber and those supplemented with 2 g/day. Surprisingly, supplementation with 3.5 g/day of psyllium for 3 years resulted in a significant increase in adenoma recurrence compared with placebo (Bonithon-Kopp et al., 2000).

The reasons for the discrepancies between the findings of early case–control studies with those of most prospective cohort studies and recent interventions trials have generated considerable debate among scientists. Potential reasons for the lack of a protective effect by dietary fiber observed in these studies include the possibility that the type or the amount of fiber consumed by most people in these studies was inadequate to prevent colorectal cancer, or that other dietary factors like fat may interact with fiber, influencing its effects on colorectal cancer (Higdon, 2007).

Breast Cancer

Although several early case–control studies found significant inverse associations between dietary fiber intake and breast cancer incidence, most prospective cohort studies have not found dietary fiber intake to be associated with significant reduction in breast cancer risk. The only exception was a prospective cohort study in Sweden, which found that women with the highest fiber intakes (averaging 26 g/day) had a risk of breast cancer that was 40% lower than women with the lowest fiber intakes (averaging 13 g/day) (Mattisson et al., 2004). Those women with the highest fiber and lowest fat intakes had the very lowest risk of breast cancer. The results of small short-term intervention trials in premenopausal and postmenopausal women suggest that low-fat (10–25% of energy), high-fiber (25–40 g/day) diets could decrease circulating estrogen levels by increasing the excretion of estrogens and promoting the metabolism of estrogens to less estrogenic forms. Nevertheless, it is not known whether fiber-associated effects on endogenous estrogen levels have a clinically significant impact on breast cancer risk (Institute of Medicine, 2002). At present, the available evidence does not support the idea that high-fiber intakes significantly decrease the risk of breast cancer in women (Higdon, 2007).

Intake Recommendations

Adequate Intake

In light of consistent evidence from prospective cohort studies that fiber-rich diets are associated with significant reductions in cardiovascular disease risk, the FNB of the Institute of Medicine established its first recommended intake levels for fiber in 2001. The adequate intake (AI) recommendations for total fiber intake are based on the findings of several large prospective cohort studies that dietary fiber intakes of 14 g/4184 kJ (1000 kcal) of energy were associated with significant reductions in the risk of coronary heart disease, as well as type 2 DM (Salmeron et al., 1997). For adults who are 50 years of age or younger, the AI for total fiber intake is 38 g/day for men and 25 g/day for women. For adults >50 years of age, the recommendation is 30 g/day for men and 21 g/day for women. The AI recommendations for males and females of all ages are presented in Table 10.8.

Eating a large amount of fiber in a short period can cause intestinal gas (flatulence), bloating, and abdominal cramps. This usually goes away once the natural bacteria in the digestive system get used to the increase in fiber in the diet. Adding fiber gradually to the diet, instead of all at one time, can help reduce gas or diarrhea.

Too much fiber may interfere with the absorption of minerals such as iron, zinc, magnesium, and calcium. However, this effect usually does not cause too much concern because high-fiber foods are typically rich in minerals.

TABLE 10.8

U.S. Institute of Medicine Adequate Intake Recommendation for Total Fiber

Life Stage	Age	Males (g/day)	Females (g/day)
Infants	0–6 months	ND	ND
Infants	7–12 months	ND	ND
Children	1–3 years	19	19
Children	4–8 years	25	25
Children	9–13 years	31	26
Adolescents	14–18 years	38	26
Adults	19–50 years	38	25
Adults	51 years and older	30	21
Pregnancy	All ages	–	28
Breastfeeding	All ages	–	29

Source: Institute of Medicine. *Dietary, Functional, and Total Fiber. Dietary Reference Intakes for Energy, Carbohydrate, Fiber, Fat, Fatty Acids, Cholesterol, Protein and Amino Acids.* Washington, DC: National Academies Press; 2002: 265–334.

Note: ND, not determined.

CANCER AND FLAVONOIDS

Although various flavonoids have been found to inhibit the development of chemically induced cancers in animal models of lung, oral, esophageal, stomach, colon, skin, prostate, and breast cancer, epidemiological studies do not provide convincing evidence that high intakes of dietary flavonoids are associated with substantial reductions in human cancer risk. Most prospective cohort studies that have assessed dietary flavonoid intake using food frequency questionnaires have not found flavonoid intake to be inversely associated with cancer risk (Higdon, 2007).

Two prospective cohort studies in Finland, where average flavonoid intakes are relatively low, found that men with the highest dietary intakes of flavonols and flavones had a significantly lower risk of developing lung cancer than those with the lowest intakes. When individual dietary flavonoids were analyzed, dietary quercetin intake, mainly from apples, was inversely associated with the risk of lung cancer, and myricetin intake was inversely associated with the risk of prostate cancer (Higdon, 2007).

There is limited evidence that low intakes of flavonoids from food are associated with increased risk of certain cancers; however, it is not clear whether these findings are related to insufficient intakes of flavonoids or other nutrients and phytochemicals in flavonoid-rich foods.

Food Sources

Although some subclasses of dietary flavonoids like flavonols are found in many different fruits and vegetables, others are not as widely distributed (see Table 10.9). Total flavonoid intakes in Western populations appear to average 150–200 mg/day.

TABLE 10.9
Subclasses of Common Dietary Flavonoids and Some Common Food Sources

Flavonoid Subclass	Dietary Flavonoids	Some Common Food Sources
Anthocyanins	Cyanidin, delphinidin, malvidin, pelargonidin, peonidin, petunidin	Red, blue, and purple berries; red and purple grapes; red wine
Flavanols		
– Monomers	Catechin, epicatechin, epigallocatechin, epicatechin gallate, epigallocatechin gallate	Teas (green and white), chocolate, grapes, berries, apples
– Polymers	Theaflavins, thearubigins, proanthocyanidis	Teas (black and oolong), chocolate, apples, berries, red grapes, red wine
Flavanones	Hesperetin, naringenin, eriodictyol	Citrus fruits and juices
Flavonols	Quercetin, kaempferol, myricetin, isorhamnetin	Yellow onions, scallions, kale, broccoli, apples, berries, teas
Flavones	Apigenin, luteolin	Parsley, thyme, celery, hot peppers
Isoflavones	Daidzein, genistein, glycitein	Soybeans, soy foods, legumes

Source: DeVries, JW, *Proc Nutr Soc*, 62, 37, 2003.

Information on the flavonoid content of some flavonoid-rich foods is presented in Table 10.10. These values should be considered approximate because several factors may affect the flavonoid content of foods, including agricultural practices, environmental factors, ripening, processing, storing, and cooking (Higdon, 2007).

Nutrition in cancer care embodies prevention of disease, treatment, cure, or supportive palliation. Caution should be exercised when considering alternative or unproven nutritional therapies during all phases of cancer treatment and supportive palliation, as these diets may prove harmful. Patient nutritional status plays an integral role in determining not only risk of developing cancer but also risk of therapy-related toxicity and medical outcomes. Whether the goal of cancer treatment is cure or palliation, early detection of nutritional problems and prompt intervention are essential.

Optimal nutritional status is an important goal in the management of individuals with cancer. Although nutrition therapy recommendations may vary throughout the continuum of care, maintenance of adequate intake is important. Therefore, a waiver from most dietary restrictions observed during religious holidays is granted for those undergoing active treatment. Individuals with cancer are encouraged to speak to their religious leaders regarding this matter before a holiday.

TABLE 10.10

Flavonoid Content of 100 g or 100 mL of Selected Foods by Flavonoid Subclass

100 g or 100 mL[a]	Anthocyanins (mg)	Flavanols (mg)	Proanthocyanidins (mg)	Flavones (mg)	Flavonols (mg)	Flavanones (mg)
Blackberry	89–211	13–19	6–47	–	0–2	–
Blueberry	67–183	1	88–261	–	2–16	–
Grapes, red	25–92	2	44–76	–	3–4	–
Strawberry	15–75	–	97–183	–	1–4	–
Red wine	1–35	1–55	24–70	0	2–30	–
Plum	2–25	1–6	106–334	0	1–2	–
Onion, red	13–25	–	–	0	4–100	–
Onion, yellow	–	0	–	0	3–120	–
Green tea	–	24–216	–	0–1	3–9	–
Black tea	–	5–158	4	0	1–7	–
Chocolate, dark	–	43–63	90–332	–	–	–
Parsley, fresh	–	–	–	24–634	8–10	0
Grapefruit juice	–	–	–	0	0	10–104

Source: DeVries, JW, *Proc Nutr Soc*, 62, 37, 2003.

[a] Per 100 g (fresh weight) or 100 mL (liquids); 100 g is equivalent to ~3.5 oz; 100 mL is equivalent to ~3.5 fl oz.

Whether patients are undergoing active therapy, recovering from cancer therapy, or in remission and striving to avoid cancer recurrence, the benefit of optimal caloric and nutrient intake is well documented.

The goals of nutrition therapy are to accomplish the following:

- Prevent or reverse nutrient deficiencies
- Preserve lean body mass
- Help patients better tolerate treatments
- Minimize nutrition-related adverse effects and complications
- Maintain strength and energy
- Protect immune function, decreasing the risk of infection
- Aid in recovery and healing
- Maximize quality of life

Patients with advanced cancer can receive nutritional support even when nutrition therapy can do little for weight gain. Such support may help accomplish the following:

- Lessen adverse effects
- Reduce risk of infection (if given enterally)
- Reduce asthenia
- Improve well-being

In individuals with advanced cancer, the goal of nutrition therapy should not be weight gain or reversal of malnutrition, but rather comfort and symptom relief.

Nutrition continues to play an integral role for individuals whose cancer has been cured or who are in remission. A healthy diet helps prevent or control comorbidities such as heart disease, diabetes, and hypertension. Following a healthful nutrition program might help prevent another malignancy from developing.

REFERENCES

Aggarwal BB, Kumar A, Aggarwal MS, Shishodial S. Curcumin derived from turmeric (*Curcuma longa*): A spice for all seasons. In: Preuss H, ed. *Phytopharmaceuticals in Cancer Chemoprevention*. Boca Raton, FL: CRC Press; 2005: 349–387.

Albanes D, Malila N, Taylor PR et al. Effects of supplemental alpha-tocopherol and beta-carotene on colorectal cancer. *Cancer Causes Control* 2000; 11(3): 197–205.

Bjelakovic G, Nikolova D, Gluud LL, Simonetti RG, Gluud C. Antioxidant supplements for prevention of mortality in healthy participants and patients with various diseases. *Cochrane Database Syst Rev* 2012; 3: CD007176.

Block G, Patterson B, Subar A. Fruit, vegetables, and cancer prevention: A review of the epidemiological evidence. *Nutr Cancer* 1992; 18(1): 1–29.

Bonithon-Kopp C, Kronborg O, Giacosa A, Rath U, Faivre J. Calcium and fibre supplementation in prevention of colorectal adenoma recurrence: A randomised intervention trial. European Cancer Prevention Organisation Study Group. *Lancet* 2000; 356(9238): 1300–1306.

Bouayed J, Bohn T. Exogenous antioxidants—Double-edged swords in cellular redox state: Health beneficial effects at physiologic doses versus deleterious effects at high doses. *Oxid Med Cell Longev* 2010; 3(4): 228–237.

Brooks JD, Metter EJ, Chan DW et al. Plasma selenium level before diagnosis and the risk of prostate cancer development. *J Urol* 2001; 166(6): 2034–2038.

Carr AC, Frei B. Toward a new recommended dietary allowance for vitamin C based on antioxidant and health effects in humans. *Am J Clin Nutr* 1999; 69(6): 1086–1107.

Choi SW, Mason JB. Folate and carcinogenesis: An integrated scheme. *J Nutr* 2000; 130(2): 129–132.

Chuang SE, Kuo ML, Hsu CH et al. Curcumin-containing diet inhibits diethylnistrosamine-induced murine hepatocarcinogenesis. *Carcinogenesis* 2000; 21(2): 331–335.

Clark LC, Combs GF, Jr., Turnbull BW et al. Effects of selenium supplementation for cancer prevention in patients with carcinoma of the skin: A randomized controlled trial. Nutritional Prevention of Cancer Study Group. *JAMA* 1996; 276(24): 1957–1963.

Clinton SK. Lycopene: Chemistry, biology, and implications for human health and disease. *Nutr Rev* 1998; 56(2 Pt 1): 35–51.

Combs GF, Jr., Gray WP. Chemopreventive agents: Selenium. *Pharmacol Ther* 1998; 79(3): 179–192.

Davis CD, Tsuji PA, Milner JA. Selenoproteins and cancer prevention. *Annu Rev Nutr* 2012; 32: 73–95.

DeVries JW. On defining dietary fibre. *Proc Nutr Soc* 2003; 62(1): 37–43.

Diplock AT, Charleux JL, Crozier-Willi G et al. Functional food science and defence against reactive oxygen species. *Br J Nutr* 1998; 80(Suppl 1): S77–S112.

EFSA Panel on Dietetic Products, Nutrition and Allergies. Scientific opinion on the substantiation of health claims related to various food(s)/food constituent(s) and protection of cells from premature aging, antioxidant activity, antioxidant content and antioxidant properties, and protection of DNA, proteins and lipids from oxidative damage pursuant to Article 13 (1) of Regulation (EC) No. 1924/20061. *EFSA J* 2010; 8(2): 1489.

Feiz HR, Mobarhan S. Does vitamin C intake slow the progression of gastric cancer in *Helicobacter pylori*–infected populations? *Nutr Rev* 2002; 60(1): 34–36.

Fenwick GR, Heaney RK, Mullin WJ. Glucosinolates and their breakdown products in food and food plants. *Crit Rev Food Sci Nutr* 1983; 18(2): 123–201.

Flood A, Velie EM, Chaterjee N et al. Fruit and vegetable intakes and the risk of colorectal cancer in Breast Cancer Detection Demonstration Project follow-up cohort. *Am J Clin Nutr* 2002; 75(5): 936–943.

Food and Nutrition Board, Institute of Medicine. *Folic acid. Dietary Reference Intakes: Thiamin, Riboflavin, Niacin, Vitamin B-6, Vitamin B-12, Pantothenic Acid, Biotin, and Choline.* Washington, DC: National Academy Press; 1998: 193–305.

Fortmann SP, Burda BU, Senger CA, Lin JS, Whitlock EP. Vitamin and mineral supplements in the primary prevention of cardiovascular disease and cancer: An updated systematic evidence review for the U.S. Preventive Services Task Force. *Ann Intern Med* 2013; 159(12): 824–834.

Fukumura H, Sato M, Kezuka K et al. Effect of ascorbic acid on reactive oxygen species production in chemotherapy and hyperthermia in prostate cancer cells. *J Physiol Sci* 2012; 62: 251–257.

Garcea G, Jones DJ, Singh R et al. Detection of curcumin and its metabolites in hepatic tissue and portal bold of patients following oral administration. *Br J Cancer* 2004; 90(5): 1011–1015.

Garcea G, Berry DP, Jones DJ et al. Consumption of the putative chemopreventive agent curcumin by cancer patients: Assessment of curcumin levels in the colorectum and their pharmacodynamic consequences. *Cancer Epidemiol Biomarkers Prev* 2005; 14(1): 120–125.

Gartner C, Stahl W, Sies H. Lycopene is more bioavailable from tomato paste than form fresh tomatoes. *Am J Clin Nutr* 1997; 66(1): 116–122.

Gaziano JM, Glynn RJ, Christen WG et al. Vitamins E and C in the prevention of prostate and total cancer in men: The Physicians' Health Study II randomized controlled trial. *JAMA* 2009; 301(1): 52–62.

Ghadirian P, Maisonneuve P, Perret C et al. A case–control study of toenail selenium and cancer of the breast, colon, and prostate. *Cancer Detect Prev* 2000; 24(4): 305–313.

Ghiselli A, Serafini M, Natella F, Scaccini C. Total antioxidant capacity as a tool to assess redox status: Critical view and experimental data. *Free Radic Biol Med* 2000; 29(11): 1106–1114.

Giovannucci E, Rimm EB, Ascherio A, Stampfer MJ, Colditz GA, Willett WC. Alcohol, low-methionine-low-folate diets, and risk of colon cancer in men. *J Natl Cancer Inst* 1995; 87(4): 265–273.

Giovannucci E, Liu Y, Platz EA, Stampfer MJ, Willett WC. Risk factors for prostate cancer incidence and progression in the Health Professionals Follow-up Study. *Int J Cancer* 2007; 121: 1571–1578.

Goodman GE, Thornquist MD, Balmes J et al. The Beta-Carotene and Retinol Efficacy Trial: Incidence of lung cancer and cardiovascular disease mortality during 6-year follow-up after stopping beta-carotene and retinol supplements. *J Natl Cancer Inst* 2004; 96(23): 1743–1750.

Gravo ML, Pinto AG, Chaves P et al. Effect of folate supplementation on DNA methylation of rectal mucosa in patients with colonic adenomas: Correlation with nutrient intake. *Clin Nutr* 1998; 17(2): 45–49.

Heaney ML, Gardner JR, Karasavvas N et al. Vitamin C antagonizes the cytotoxic effects of antineoplastic drugs. *Cancer Res* 2008; 68(9): 8031–8038.

Herbert V. Folic acid. In: Shils M, Olson JA, Shike M, Ross AC, eds. *Nutrition in Health and Disease*, 9th Ed. Baltimore, MD: Williams & Wilkins; 1999: 433–446.

Higdon J. *An Evidenced-Based Approach to Dietary Phytochemicals*. New York: Thieme; 2007.

Higdon J, Drake V. *An Evidenced-Based Approach to Vitamins and Minerals: Health Benefits and Intake Recommendations Dietary Phytochemicals*, 2nd Ed. New York: Thieme; 2011.

Huang MT, Lou YR, Ma W, Newmark HL, Reuhl KR, Conney AH. Inhibitory effects of dietary curcumin on forestomach, duodenal, and colon carcinogenesis in mice. *Cancer Res* 1994; 54(22): 5841–5847.

Hung HC, Joshipura KJ, Jiang R et al. Fruit and vegetable intake and risk of major chronic disease. *J Natl Cancer Inst* 2004; 96: 1577–1584.

Ikezaki S, Nishikawa A, Furukawa F et al. Chemopreventive effects of curcumin on glandular stomach carcinogenesis induced by N-methyl-N'-nitro-N-nitrosoguanidine and sodium chloride in rats. *Anticancer Res* 2001; 21(5): 3407–3411.

Institute of Medicine. *Dietary, Functional, and Total Fiber. Dietary Reference Intakes for Energy, Carbohydrate, Fiber, Fat, Fatty Acids, Cholesterol, Protein and Amino Acids.* Washington, DC: National Academies Press; 2002: 265–334.

International Center for Alcohol Policies. Report 5: What is a "standard drink"? Accessed June 19, 2008. Available at: http://www.icap.org/.

Karunagaran D, Rashmi R, Kumar TR. Induction of apoptosis by curcumin and its implications for cancer therapy. *Curr Cancer Drug Targets* 2005; 5(2): 117–129.

Kavanaugh CJ, Trumbo PR, Ellwood KC. The U.S. Food and Drug Administration's evidence-based review for qualified health claims: Tomatoes, lycopene, and cancer. *J Natl Cancer Inst* 2007; 99: 1074–1085.

Kawamori T, Lubet R, Steele VE et al. Chemopreventive effect of curcumin, a naturally occurring anti-inflammatory agent, during the promotion/progression stages of colon cancer. *Cancer Res* 1999; 59(3): 597–601.

Key TJ, Allen N, Appleby P et al. Fruits and vegetables and prostate cancer: No association among 1104 cases in a prospective study of 130544 men in the European Prospective Investigation into Cancer and Nutrition Prospective Investigation into Cancer and Nutrition (EPIC). *Int J Cancer* 2004; 109(1): 119–124.

Kim YI, Baik HW, Fawaz K et al. Effects of folate supplementation on two provisional molecular markers of colon cancer: A prospective, randomized trial. *Am J Gastroenterol* 2001; 96(1): 184–195.

Klein EA, Thompson IM, Tangen CM et al. Vitamin E and the risk of prostate cancer: The Selenium and Vitamin E Cancer Prevention Trial (SELECT). *JAMA* 2011; 306(14): 1549–1556.

Knekt P, Marniemi J, Teppo L, Heliovaara M, Aromaa A. Is low selenium status a risk factor for lung cancer? *Am J Epidemiol* 1998; 148(10): 975–982.

Kolonel LN, Hankin JH, Whittemore AS et al. Vegetables, fruits, legumes and prostate cancer: A multiethnic case–control study. *Cancer Epidemiol Biomarkers Prev* 2000; 9(8): 795–804.

Krishnaswamy K, Goud VK, Sesikeran B, Mukundan MA, Krishna TP. Retardation of experimental tumorigenesis and reduction in DNA adducts by turmeric and curcumin. *Nutr Cancer* 1998; 30(2): 163–166.

Kristal AR, Lampe JW. Brassica vegetables and prostate cancer risk: A review of the epidemiological evidence. *Nutr Cancer* 2002; 42(1): 1–9.

Kromhout D. Essential micronutrients in relation to carcinogenesis. *Am J Clin Nutr* 1987; 45(5 Suppl): 1361–1367.

La Vecchia C, Chatenoud L, Negri E, Franceshi S. Session: Whole cereal grains, fibre and human cancer. Wholegrain cereals and cancer in Italy. *Proc Nutr Soc* 2003; 62(1): 45–49.

Lawenda BD, Kelly KM, Ladas EJ, Sagar SM, Vickers A, Blumberg JB. Should supplemental antioxidant administration be avoided during chemotherapy and radiation therapy? *J Natl Cancer Inst* 2008; 100(11): 773–783.

Lee IM, Cook NR, Manson JE. Beta-carotene supplementation and incidence of cancer and cardiovascular disease: Women's Health Study. *J Natl Cancer Inst* 1999; 91: 2102–2106.

Lee IM, Cook NR, Gaziano JM et al. Vitamin E in the primary prevention of cardiovascular disease and cancer: The Women's Health Study: A randomized controlled trial. *JAMA* 2005; 294(1): 56–65.

Li N, Chen X, Liao J et al. Inhibition of 7,12-dimethylbenz[a]anthracene (DMBA)-induced oral carcinogenesis in hamsters by tea and curcumin. *Carcinogenesis* 2002; 23(8): 1307–1313.

Lin J, Zhang SM, Cook NR et al. Dietary intakes of fruit, vegetables and fiber, and risk of colorectal cancer in a prospective cohort of women (United States). *Cancer Causes Control* 2005; 16(3): 225–233.

Lippman SM, Klein EA, Goodman PJ et al. Effect of selenium and vitamin E on risk of prostate cancer and other cancers: The Selenium and Vitamin E Cancer Prevention Trial (SELECT). *JAMA* 2009; 301(1): 39–51.

Lonn E, Bosch J, Yusuf S et al. Effects of long-term vitamin E supplementation on cardiovascular events and cancer: A randomized controlled trial. *JAMA* 2005; 293(11): 1338–1347.

Ma J, Stampfer MJ, Giovannucci E et al. Methylenetetrahydrofolate reductase polymorphism, dietary interactions, and risk of colorectal cancer. *Cancer Res* 1997; 57(6): 1098–1102.

Mahmoud NN, Carothers AM, Grunberger D et al. Plant phenolic decrease intestinal tumors in an animal model of familial adenomatous polyposis. *Carcinogenesis* 2000; 21(5): 921–927.

Mathers JC. Pulses and carcinogenesis: Potential for the prevention of colon, breast and other cancers. *Br J Nutr* 2002; 88(Suppl 3): S273–S279.

Mattisson I, Wirfalt E, Johansson U, Gullberg B, Olsson H, Berglund G. Intakes of plant foods, fibre and fat and risk of breast cancer—A prospective study in the Malmo Diet and Cancer cohort. *Br J Cancer* 2004; 90(1): 122–127.

McCullough ML, Robertson AS, Chao A et al. A prospective study of whole grains, fruits, vegetables and colon cancer risk. *Cancer Causes Control* 2003; 14(10): 959–970.

Messina MJ. Legumes and soybeans: Overview of their nutritional profiles and health effects. *Am J Clin Nutr* 1999; 70(3 Suppl): 439S–450S.

Michaud DS, Spiegelman D, Clinton SK, Rimm EB, Willett WC, Giovannucci EL. Fruit and vegetable intake and incidence of bladder cancer in a male prospective cohort. *J Natl Cancer Inst* 1999; 91(7): 605–613.

Michaud DS, Pietinen P, Taylor PR, Virtanen M, Virtamo J, Albanes D. Intakes of fruits and vegetables, carotenoids and vitamins A, E, C in relation to the risk of bladder cancer in the ATBC cohort study. *Br J Cancer* 2002; 87(9): 960–965.

Michels KB, Edward G, Joshipura KJ et al. Prospective study of fruit and vegetable consumption and incidence of colon and rectal cancers. *J Natl Cancer Inst* 2000; 92(21): 1740–1752.

Michels KB, Holmberg L, Bergkvist L, Ljung H, Bruce A, Wolk A. Dietary antioxidant vitamins, retinol, and breast cancer incidence in a cohort of Swedish women. *Int J Cancer* 2001; 91(4): 563–567.

Mills PK, Beeson WL, Phillips RL, Fraser GE. Cohort study of diet, lifestyle, and prostate cancer in Adventist men. *Cancer* 1989; 64(3): 598–604.

National Institutes of Health. An introduction to clinical trials. 2005. Available at: http://clinical trials.gov/ct/info/whatis. Accessed July 26, 2006.

Neuhouser ML, Barnett MJ, Kristal AR et al. Dietary supplement use and prostate cancer risk in the Carotene and Retinol Efficacy Trial. *Cancer Epidemiol Biomarkers Prev* 2009; 18(8): 2202–2206.

Nomura AM, Lee J, Stemmermann GN, Combs GF, Jr. Serum selenium and subsequent risk of prostate cancer. *Cancer Epidemiol Biomarkers Prev* 2000; 9(9): 883–887.

Nomura AM, Hankin JH, Lee J, Stemmermann GN. Cohort study of tofu intake and prostate cancer; No apparent association. *Cancer Epidemiol Biomarkers Prev* 2004; 13(12): 2277–2279.

Ohigashi, H, Murakami, A. Cancer prevention with food factors: Alone and in combination. *Biofactors* 2004; 22: 49–55.

Omenn GS, Goodman GE, Thornquist MD et al. Effects of a combination of beta carotene and vitamin A on lung cancer and cardiovascular disease. *N Engl J Med* 1996; 334(18): 1150–1155.

Ovaskaimen ML, Virtamo J, Altfthan G et al. Toenail selenium as an indicator of selenium intake among middle-aged men in an area with low soil selenium. *Am J Clin Nutr* 1993; 57(5): 662–665.

Patterson RE, White E, Kristal AR, Neuhouser ML, Potter JD. Vitamin supplements and cancer risk: The epidemiologic evidence. *Cancer Causes Control* 1997; 8(5): 786–802.

Pereira MA, Grubbs CJ, Barnes LH et al. Effects of the phytochemicals, curcumin and quercentin, upon azoxymethane-induced colon cancer and 7,12-dimethylbenz[a]anthracene-induced mammary cancer in rats. *Carcinogenesis* 1996; 17(6): 1305–1311.

Perkins S, Verschoyle RD, Hill K et al. Chemopreventive efficacy and pharmacokinetics of curcumin in the min/+ mouse, a model of familial adenomatous polyposis. *Cancer Epidemiol Biomarkers Prev* 2002; 11(6): 535–540.

Rao CV, Rivenson A, Simi B, Reddy BS. Chemoprevention of colon carcinogenesis by dietary curcumin, a naturally occurring plant phenolic compound. *Cancer Res* 1995; 55(2): 259–266.

Rautalahti MT, Virtamo JR, Taylor PR et al. The effects of supplementation with alpha-tocopherol and beta-carotene on the incidence and mortality of carcinoma of the pancreas in a randomized, controlled trial. *Cancer* 1999; 86(1): 37–42.

Rayman MP, Clark LC. Selenium in cancer prevention. In: Roussel AM, ed. *Trace Elements in Man and Animals*, 10th Ed. New York: Plenum Press; 2000: 575–580.

Rohan TE, Jain MG, Howe GR, Miller AB. Dietary folate consumption and breast cancer risk. *J Natl Cancer Inst* 2000; 92(3): 266–269.

Salmeron J, Ascherio A, Rimm EB et al. Dietary fiber, glycemic load, and risk of NIDDM in men. *Diabetes Care* 1997; 20(4): 545–550.

Sato Y, Tsubono Y, Nakaya N et al. Fruit and vegetable consumption and risk of colorectal cancer in Japan: The Miyagi Cohort Study. *Public Health Nutr* 2005; 8(3): 309–314.

Sellers TA, Kushi LH, Cerhan JR et al. Dietary folate intake, alcohol, and risk of breast cancer in a prospective study of postmenopausal women. *Epidemiology* 2001; 12(4): 420–428.

Shannon J, Ray R, Wu C et al. Food and botanical groupings and risk of breast cancer: A case–control study in Shanghai, China. *Cancer Epidemiol Biomarkers Prev* 2005; 14(1): 81–90.

Sharma RA, Euden SA, Platton SL et al. Phase I clinical trial of oral curcumin: Biomarkers of systemic activity and compliance. *Clin Cancer Res* 2004; 10(20): 6847–6854.

Sharma RA, Gescher AJ, Steward WP. Curcumin: The story so far. *Eur J Cancer* 2005; 41(13): 1995–1968.

Slattery ML, Potter JD, Samowitz W, Schaffer D, Leppert M. Methylenetetrahydrofolate reductase, diet, and risk of colon cancer. *Cancer Epidemiol Biomarkers Prev* 1999; 8(6): 513–518.

Smith-Warner SA, Spiegelman D, Yaun SS et al. Intake of fruits and vegetables and risk of breast cancer: A pooled analysis of cohort studies. *JAMA* 2001; 285(6): 769–776.

Smith-Warner SA, Spiegelman D, Yaun SS et al. Fruits, vegetables and lung cancer: A pooled analysis of cohort studies. *Int J Cancer* 2003; 107(6): 1001–1011.

Steinmetz KA, Potter JD. Vegetables, fruit, and cancer prevention: A review. *J Am Diet Assoc* 1996; 96(10): 1027–1039.

Su LJ, Arab L. Nutritional status of folate and colon cancer risk: Evidence from NHANES I epidemiologic follow-up study. *Ann Epidemiol* 2001; 11(1): 65–72.

Terry P, Jain M, Miller AB, Howe GR, Rohan TE. Dietary intake of folic acid and colorectal cancer risk in a cohort of women. *Int J Cancer* 2002; 97(6): 864–867.

The Alpha-Tocopherol, Beta Carotene Cancer Prevention Study Group. The effects of vitamin E and beta carotene on the incidence of lung cancer and other cancers in male smokers. *New Engl J Med* 1994; 330: 1029–1035.

Tsubono Y, Otani T, Kobayashi M, Yamamoto S, Sobue T, Tsugane S. No association between fruit or vegetable consumption and the risk of colorectal cancer in Japan. *Br J Cancer* 2005; 92(9): 1782–1784.

U.S. Department of Agriculture, Agricultural Research Service. USDA Nutrient Database for Standard Reference, Release 17. 2004. Available at: http://www.nal.usda.gov/fnic/food comp.

U.S. Department of Agriculture, Agricultural Research Service. 2012. Oxygen Radical Absorbance Capacity (ORAC) of Selected Foods, Release 2. Available at: http://www .orac-info-portal.de/download/ORAC_R2.pdf.

U.S. Department of Agriculture, Agricultural Research Service. 2011. USDA National Nutrient Database for Standard Reference, Release 24. Available at: http://www.ars .usda.gov/ba/bhnrc/ndl.

U.S. Department of Agriculture, Agricultural Research Service. 2012. USDA National Nutrient Database for Standard Reference, Release 25. Available at: http://www.nal .usda.gov/fnic/foodcomp/search/.

U.S. Department of Agriculture and U.S. Department of Health and Human Services. *Dietary Guidelines for Americans*, 7th Ed. Washington, DC: U.S. Government Printing Office; 2010.

Valko M, Leibfritz D, Moncol J, Cronin MT, Mazur M, Telser J. Free radicals and antioxidants in normal physiological functions and human disease. *Int J Biochem Cell Biol* 2007; 39(1): 44–84.

Van Gils CH, Peeters PH, Bueno-de-Mesquita HB et al. Consumption of vegetables and fruits and risk of breast cancer. *JAMA* 2005; 293(2): 183–193.

Virtamo J, Edwards BK, Virtanen M et al. Effects of supplemental alpha-tocopherol and beta-carotene on urinary tract cancer: Incidence and mortality in a controlled trial (Finland). *Cancer Causes Control* 2000; 11(10): 933–939.

World Cancer Research Fund. *Food, Nutrition, and the Prevention of Cancer: A Global Perspective*. Washington, DC: American Institute for Cancer Research; 1997.

World Cancer Research Fund, American Institute for Cancer Research. *Food, Nutrition, Physical Activity, and the Prevention of Cancer: A Global Perspective*. Washington, DC: American Institute for Cancer Research; 2007.

Wright ME, Virtamo J, Hartman AM et al. Effects of alpha-tocopherol and beta-carotene supplementation on upper aerodigestive tract cancers in a large, randomized controlled trial. *Cancer* 2007; 109(5): 891–898.

Yoshizawa K, Willett WC, Morris SJ et al. Study of prediagnostic selenium level in toenails and the risk of advanced prostate cancer. *J Natl Cancer Inst* 1998; 90(16): 1219–1224.

Yu MW, Horng IS, Hsu KH, Chiang YC, Liaw YF, Chen CJ. Plasma selenium levels and risk of hepatocellular carcinoma among men with chronic hepatitis virus infection. *Am J Epidemiol* 1999; 150(4): 367–374.

Yu SY, Zhu YJ, Li WG. Protective role of selenium against hepatitis B virus and primary liver cancer in Quidong. *Biol Trace Elem Res* 1997; 56(1): 117–124.

Zhang S, Hunter DJ, Forman MR et al. Dietary carotenoids and vitamins A, C, and E and risk of breast cancer. *J Natl Cancer Inst* 1999a; 91(6): 547–556.

Zhang S, Hunter DJ, Hankinson SE et al. A prospective study of folate intake and the risk of breast cancer. *JAMA* 1999b; 281(17): 1632–1637.

11 Antioxidants in Neurodegeneration
Truth or Myth?

Francisco Capani, George Barreto,
Eduardo Blanco Calvo, and Christopher Horst Lillig

CONTENTS

Redox Control and Reactive Oxygen Species/Reactive Nitrogen Species 199
Thioredoxin Family Proteins in the Brain 200
Pathologies Involved in Neurodegeneration 202
    Perinatal Asphyxia 202
    Parkinson's Disease 203
    Alzheimer's Disease 204
Signaling Pathways in CNS Diseases: Role of the Thioredoxins Protein Family 205
Pharmacological Approaches 206
Conclusion 207
References 207

REDOX CONTROL AND REACTIVE OXYGEN SPECIES/REACTIVE NITROGEN SPECIES

The cell signaling theory was developed from the analysis of signal transduction from extracellular signals to intracellular effector molecules via G-protein coupled receptors by Rodbell [1] and Gilman [2]. First, an extracellular signal activates a receptor protein or protein complex. Then, this activation promotes the release of second messenger molecules. These molecules might act on transducer proteins, e.g., protein kinases, activate the production or release of third messenger molecules, or directly activate effector molecules.

The activities of the enzymes that catalyze the generation of the signals and the modifications of the effector molecules determine the transduction of the information, and the action of protein kinases and phosphatases in signal transduction pathways.

Redox signaling requires the active adjustment of the levels of redox activity of the second messengers in response to the activation of a receptor or sensor molecule [3,4]. The key compounds, i.e., the metabolites that hold the potential to induce reversible posttranslational redox modifications on proteins, are H_2O_2, $NO^{\bullet}$, and peroxynitrite/

peroxynitrous acid (ONOO⁻/ONOOH). These compounds are produced enzymatically, either as primary products of specialized enzymes, for instance $NO^\bullet$ produced by nitric oxide synthase (NOS), or as by-products of enzymes, such as superoxide $\left(O_2^{-\bullet}\right)$ produced by complex I of the inner mitochondrial membrane and a number of other enzymes. The decay of these compounds is controlled by other independent enzymes; for instance, H_2O_2 and ONOOH are reduced by glutathione peroxidases and peroxiredoxins. The levels of these redox-active second messengers are thus enzymatically regulated on both the production and the elimination side, similar to, e.g., adenylate cyclases and phosphodiesterases whose combined activities determine the level of the second messenger molecule cAMP.

The thioredoxin protein family (Trxs) is involved in this function in different ways through their thiol groups. Two protein thiols can be oxidized to a disulfide, forming a strong inter- or intramolecular bridge. A single protein thiol may also form a disulfide with GSH, termed glutathionylation, or free cysteine, termed cysteinylation or thiolation. Cysteinyl thiols may also react with hydrogen sulfide (H_2S) to form persulfides, reactive oxygen species (ROS), or reactive nitrogen species (RNS) to form sulfenic acids, or nitric oxide resulting in nitroso thiols, a process named S-nitrosylation. Not every surface-exposed, cysteinyl residue can undergo any or all of these oxidative modifications. It was repeatedly demonstrated that distinct thiol groups undergo specific modifications, such as glutathionylation, S-nitrosylation, or sulfenylation, in response to specific oxidants [5].

THIOREDOXIN FAMILY PROTEINS IN THE BRAIN

Trxs are a class of enzymes that utilize the thiol groups of cysteinyl residues for the catalysis of thiol-disulfide exchange and peroxidatic reactions. This family includes the thioredoxins (Trxs), glutaredoxins (Grxs), and peroxiredoxins (Prxs) [6–8], which are all characterized by a common structural motif known as the thioredoxin fold [9].

Trxs were first described as hydrogen donors for ribonucleotide reductase from *Escherichia coli* [10]. However, during the previous decade, these proteins were recognized as key regulators of cellular functions in the response to redox signals, for instance by the modulation of various signaling pathways, transcription factors, and the immune response [8]. Although the Trxs include more than 10 proteins, the major Trx isoforms are the cytosolic Trx1 and the mitochondrial Trx2. Trxs are thought to be tightly connected to thioredoxin reductases (TrxR). TrxR is an NADPH-dependent homodimer with one FAD cofactor per subunit and a cysteine–selenocysteine active site that reduces the disulfide in the active site of oxidized Trx [11,12]. In addition, TrxR1 can directly reduce the number of substrates, in particular lipid hydroperoxides and H_2O_2 [13–17].

Glutathione (GSH) constitutes the major intracellular redox buffer in cells [18]. GSH is synthesized in the cytosol in two steps. First, the enzyme γ-glutamylcysteine synthetase (γ-GCS) catalyzes the formation of L-γ-glutamyl-L-cysteine [19–21]. The glycine residue of the GSH tripeptide is added in the second step by glutathione synthetase. Cellular GSH exists predominantly in a reduced form; however, small amounts of the oxidized disulfide form GSSG can also be detected. GSSG is reduced by glutathione reductase (GR) at the expense of NADPH. The GSH/GSSG ratio is often taken as an indicator of the cellular redox status. Changes in this ratio have been associated with the modulation of transcription of a wide variety of genes implied in multiple cellular processes such as growth, differentiation, and cell death [22–24]. To date, four Grx isoforms have been found in mammals [24]: the cytosolic dithiol Grx1; the mainly mitochondrial Grx2 (Grx2a); testicular cells and some cancer cells express two additional cytosolic/nuclear isoforms of the protein, Grx2b and Grx2c; the cytosolic multidomain monothiol Grx3; and the mitochondrial monothiol Grx5 [8,24]. Unlike in the Trx system, electrons in the Grx system are transferred from the NADPH-dependent glutathione reductase to glutathione (GSH), which, in turn, reduces oxidized glutaredoxin [24].

Peroxiredoxins are a heterogeneous family of thiol-dependent peroxidases present in all kingdoms of life. Prxs execute enzymatic degradation of H_2O_2, organic hydroperoxides, and peroxynitrite [25]. Unlike Trxs that possess the active double-cysteine region forming an intramolecular disulfide bond when oxidized, Prxs can form intermolecular disulfide bonds. By the number of active Cys residues, mammalian peroxiredoxins fall into three groups: typical two-cysteine Prxs (Prx1–Prx4) that contain both N- and C-terminal Cys residues, atypical two-cysteine Prxs (Prx5) that contain the N-terminal conserved Cys but require an additional Cys for their peroxidase activity, and single-cysteine Prxs (Prx6) that contain only the N-terminal Cys [22,26]. Prxs are present in all subcellular compartments: Prx1, Prx2, and Prx5 are found in the cytoplasm and nuclei, Prx4 and Prx6 in the cytoplasm and secreted, and Prx3 and Prx5 in mitochondria [23,26].

The brain is more susceptible to oxidative damage than most other organs because of its high oxygen utilization, high iron content, presence of unsaturated fatty acids, and decreased activities of detoxifying enzymes such as superoxide dismutase (SOD), catalase, and GR [27–29]. Molecular oxygen is the central component in energy production in mammalians, and the drop in oxygen supply to neuronal tissue has serious consequences for cell fate and survival. Ischemia–reperfusion injury induces serious oxidative stress and, as consequence, a multitude of spatially and temporally regulated responses, ranging from changes in the gene expression pattern to biochemical alterations and, ultimately, cell death. The disturbance of redox homeostasis, low levels of GSH, and an increased production of ROS and peroxynitrite have been described for a number of central nervous system (CNS) disorders, for instance perinatal asphyxia [30–32], stroke [22], focal traumatic brain injury [33], and numerous neurodegenerative disorders including Alzheimer's disease, Parkinson's disease, multiple sclerosis, and amyotrophic lateral sclerosis [34,35]. Ischemic brain injuries, resulting either from global or focal decreases in perfusion, are among the most common and important causes of disability and death worldwide after heart infarction and cancer [36,37].

Recently, we described the cellular localization of Trxs in the CNS [38]. We have observed several remarkable differences in both abundance and regional distribution of Trx-immunopositive cells that point to a complex interplay and crosstalk between the proteins of this family. Most of the Golgi type I neurons in the different ischematic-sensitive areas showed strong staining for Trx1, Trx2, TrxR1, TrxR2, Txnip, Grx1, Grx2, Grx3, Grx5, γ-GCS, Prx1, Prx2, Prx3, Prx4, Prx5, and Prx6. In addition, one

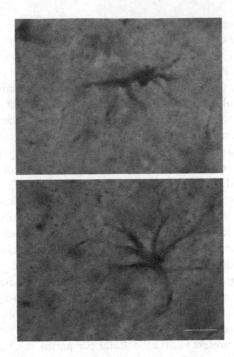

FIGURE 11.1 Hippocampal astrocytes expressing Trx2. Scale bar, 10 μm.

of the most striking localizations was in hippocampal astrocytes stained with Trx2 (Figure 11.1). These data strongly support the concept that Trxs, Grxs, and Prxs are involved in various steps during the oxidative stress response induced by CNS disease [39–52] (for more details, see the next section).

PATHOLOGIES INVOLVED IN NEURODEGENERATION

PERINATAL ASPHYXIA

Perinatal asphyxia (PA)-induced brain injury is one of the most common causes of morbidity and mortality in term and preterm neonates, accounting for 23% of neonatal deaths globally [53]. Following PA, approximately 45% of newborns die and 25% have permanent neurological deficits, including cerebral palsy, mental retardation and developmental delay, learning disabilities, and different issues in school readiness [54]. Neonatal stroke, a cerebrovascular event that occurs between 28 weeks' gestation and 1 month postnatal age, may be either hemorrhagic or hypoxia-ischemia (HI) in origin and has been associated with consequences including cerebral palsy and behavioral abnormalities [55,56].

Brain injury that occurs early during development results in significant and persistent decreases in cortical and hippocampal volumes. The type and distribution of human brain lesions differ markedly between premature and term babies, likely attributed to the stage of brain maturation and regional vulnerability, as described elsewhere [57–59]. Atrophy of both gray and white matter is also obvious in models of perinatal HI. This atrophy is attributed to both loss of ischemic infarcted tissue and impaired development of the surrounding tissue over time [59,60]. The immature brain is considerably more resistant to hypoxia presumably because of the lower density of axons and dendrites over which a membrane gradient must be maintained. Therefore, obtaining a similarly sized injury between age groups requires different durations of hypoxia–ischemia [60]. Moreover, different mechanisms of injury are activated in the immature brain versus the adult, the most obvious difference being that apoptotic mechanisms are several-fold more pronounced in immature animals [60]. It is becoming increasingly recognized that the developing brain shows marked susceptibility to both oxidative stress and neuronal apoptosis, which may underlie this age-dependent injury vulnerability [61–65].

The mechanisms that cause neurological damage after PA are divided schematically into three metabolic phases [66,67]. Hypoxia leads to primary energy failure (phase 1); then, a short time after reoxygenation, aerobic metabolism and cell functions are reestablished (phase 2). However, as a result of a cascade of cellular mechanisms [68,69], after this "latent phase" of 6–24 h, mitochondrial energy production again begins to fail. This secondary energy failure (phase 3) lasts for 24–48 h after the hypoxic event. The damage that occurs during this phase is considerable [70]. In addition, the reoxygenation part of the hypoxia is necessary but also induces the most damage after AP: during the reoxygenation period, extracellular glutamate levels are increased, enhancing the activation of Na^+/ATPase, increasing further ATP consumption. Extracellular glutamate levels override the buffer capacity of astrocytes, resulting in sustained overactivation of glutamate receptors, mainly of the N-methyl-D-aspartate (NMDA) increasing Ca^{2+} conductance. All these changes activate molecular and cell cascades, prolonging the energy deficit and oxidative stress associated with further cell damage and apoptotis or necrosis.

Oxidative stress is inherent to reoxygenation, resulting in overactivation, but also inactivation of a number of enzymes, mainly those modulating the activity of mitochondria [29,31]. In the clinical situation, resuscitation may even imply hyperoxemia, leading to further production of free radicals and oxidative stress, worsening brain injury [30,31,71–73].

PARKINSON'S DISEASE

Parkinson's disease (PD) manifests itself in most patients with prominent movement abnormalities, including a 4–6 Hz tremor at rest, muscular rigidity, slowness of movement (bradykinesia), and a failure of movement initiation (akinesia). Several environmental factors may have an impact on the occurrence of the disease. Living in rural areas, drinking well water, pesticide exposure, and head trauma are associated with an increased risk of developing PD, while caffeine consumption, taking nonsteroidal anti-inflammatory medications, and smoking appear to protect against it.

The prominent motor abnormalities in PD appear to arise in large part from degeneration of neurons in the substantia nigra (SNc), with resulting loss of dopamine in the basal ganglia. Degenerating dopaminergic cells leave characteristic eosinophilic inclusions in their wake, the so-called Lewy neurites and Lewy bodies [74].

Most cases of PD are "sporadic" and appear to arise from a combination of genetic predisposition and environmental or toxic factors. Purely genetic forms of the disease probably account for less than 10% of cases; however, the risk of family members of an affected patient to develop PD is significantly increased even in sporadic PD. Cells in the SNc are among the most vulnerable cells in the brain due to a relative deficiency in neuroprotective factors, such as the antioxidant glutathione, and because they are exposed to a high level of oxidative stress due to the presence of dopaminergic metabolism and other factors.

This environment may induce these neurons particularly vulnerable to nonspecific genetic or environmental insults that, by themselves, would not be sufficient to induce cell death in other cells. Interestingly, many of the factors known to be involved in neuronal damage in PD appear to interfere with the cell's ability to eliminate damaged or mutated proteins through the ubiquitin proteasome system [74]. One example of a genetically determined form of parkinsonism, which results directly in degeneration of dopaminergic neurons, are mutations of the gene coding for α-synuclein [75]. Mutated α-synuclein tends to aggregate as the result of a conformational change of the molecule from its usual unfolded, soluble form into a β-pleated sheath. Aggregated α-synuclein is a prominent component of Lewy bodies.

A number of genetic mutations have been associated with autosomal recessive juvenile Parkinson's disease. The most frequent of these is the gene *PARK2*, coding for parkin, which accounts for about half of patients with juvenile onset, below the age of 40 years. Parkin is an E3 ubiquitin ligase that is necessary for ubiquitination of proteins for their subsequent degradation in proteasomes. Loss of function of the mutated enzyme may result in failure to direct its substrates to the proteasome system for degradation [76]. However, the mechanism involved in Parkinson disease is not well known.

ALZHEIMER'S DISEASE

Alzheimer's disease (AD) is the most common form of dementia among older adults, affecting more than 4 million people in the United States and almost 30 million worldwide [77]. AD is the most common form of dementia and characterized by deposition of amyloid-β (Aβ) plaques, neurofibrillary tangles, and progressive neurodegeneration. AD manifests as progressive memory loss and cognitive impairments [77,78]. This syndrome results from abnormalities associated with dysfunction and death of the neurons involved in memory and cognition [78]. Genetic evidence indicates that the inheritance of mutations in several genes causes autosomal dominant familial AD (fAD), while the presence of certain alleles of *ApoE4* are significant risk factors for putative sporadic disease [79,80].

Multiple lines of evidence have implicated oxidative stress and free radical damage to the pathogenesis and possible etiology of AD. Such damage found in AD includes advanced glycation end products [81–83], nitration [82], lipid peroxidation adduction products [78], and carbonyl-modified neurofilament protein and free carbonyls [84]. The cytopathological significance of oxidative damage is seen by the upregulation of antioxidant enzymes. Heme oxygenase-1 (HO-1) is among the most sensitive and selective indicators of the cellular oxidative stress response [85,86].

However, the most crucial aspects of the cellular oxidative damage in AD pathogenesis appear to be the cytoskeletal modifications in neurons susceptible to AD, which in turn play a key role in the irreversible cellular dysfunction that ultimately leads to neuronal death [87]. The neuropathological hallmarks of AD are senile plaques and neurofibrillary tangles [88,89]. Evidence of an increased oxidation of macromolecules (lipids, carbohydrates, proteins, and DNA) and oxidative stress products has been found in senile plaques and neurofibrillary tangles [90]. Biomarkers of these forms of oxidation have been observed not only in AD brains but also in peripheral tissues (e.g., blood cells) and biological fluids (e.g., urine) of individuals affected by AD [91–95].

SIGNALING PATHWAYS IN CNS DISEASES: ROLE OF THE THIOREDOXINS PROTEIN FAMILY

Oxidative stress and a misbalance in the production or free radicals have been implicated in different diseases of the CNS. Since Trxs are key proteins related to the regulation of redox signaling, it is logical to think that they might be involved in the pathogenesis of CNS disorders. Regarding thioredoxins (Trx1), using amyloid-β treatment in an AD model led to oxidation of Trx1 in the neuroblastoma cell line SH-SY5Y [96]. Overexpression of Trx1 protected SH-SY5Y cells against amyloid-β-induced cell death [96]. Trx1 expression was suppressed in a rat pheochromocytoma cell line (PC12) after treatment with 1-methyl-4-phenylpyridinium (MPP+), an active metabolite of 1-methyl-4-phenyl-1,2,3,6-tetrahydropyridine (MPTP) that causes parkinsonism [97]. Trx1 is also induced after cerebral ischemia induced by middle cerebral artery occlusion [98], and mice overexpressing Trx1 showed attenuation of apoptosis and thereby neuroprotection after both permanent and transient focal ischemia [99].

Although proper mitochondrial function is crucial for the progression of most neurological diseases, almost nothing is known about the role of the mitochondrial Trx2, except for the finding that Trx2 levels were increased in the hippocampus of gerbils after ischemia–reperfusion [100]. Treatment of rat primary hippocampal neurons with TrxR1 attenuated amyloid-β-mediated toxicity. In AD patients, TrxR1 activity was generally enhanced compared with controls [101], whereas TrxR1 levels in cerebrospinal fluid and blood of multiple sclerosis patients were decreased [102].

In relation to glutaredoxins, overexpression of Grx1 protected SH-SY5Y cells against amyloid-β-induced cell death [96]. Several proteins have been described to be involved in PD development and progression. The expression of one of these proteins, DJ-1 [98], correlates with the expression of Grx1 [103,104]. In a mouse model for PD based on MPTP toxicity, loss of dopaminergic neurons was associated with inactivation of mitochondrial complex I, a hallmark of the disease. Recovery of complex I activity correlated with an increase of Grxs activity following MPTP treatment. Whereas knockout of both Grx1 and Grx2 inhibited this recovery [105], overexpression of Grx2 diminished MPTP-induced neuronal apoptosis via decreased complex I activity [106]. After induction of focal ischemia in rat brains, Grx1 levels decreased parallel to the rate of neuronal damage. In AD brain tissue, Grx1 was upregulated in healthy neurons of the hippocampus and the frontal cortex but downregulated in degenerating neurons [96]. Deglutathionylation/glutathionylation, specifically catalyzed by Grxs, is associated with several aspects of neurodegeneration, like apoptosis, mitochondrial function, and plaque formation, summarized for instance in Ref. [107].

Several other studies demonstrated the important role of GSH in pathologies of the CNS. Amyloid-β treatment of SH-SY5Y cells decreased the total cellular GSH amount [96]. In the substantia nigra of PD patients, total GSH levels were not only decreased, but GSH was also virtually absent. This loss of GSH is one of the first signs of the disease. Knockdown of GSH synthesis in PC12 cells, rat dopaminergic N27 cells, as well as in mice by catecholaminergic neuron-specific downregulation of γ-glutamyl cysteine ligase, the rate-limiting enzyme in the *de novo* glutathione synthesis, resulted in inhibition of complex I activity [108,109]. These data highlight the importance of the GSH/Grx system in maintenance of mitochondrial function in the early onset of PD.

Finally, some functions have been attributed to Prxs in CNS disease. In amyloid-β-resistant clones of the PC12 cell line, Prx1, Prx2, and Prx6 expression was significantly increased. PC12 cells and primary neurons overexpressing Prx1 exhibited attenuated amyloid-β and MPP+/MPTP toxicity [110]. Treatment with 6-hydroxy-dopamine (6-OHDA) led to an oxidation of Prx1. Increased levels of Prx1 and Prx2 protected dopaminergic cells *in vitro* and *in vivo* against 6-OHDA-induced apoptosis, whereas silencing of Prx1 sensitized the cells [111]. In addition, elevated Prx2 levels protected against amyloid-β toxicity in a transgenic mouse model for AD [112]. In whole brain samples, the expression levels of Prx1 and Prx2 were elevated in AD patients [113]. Two other studies, however, could not confirm a higher Prx1 expression in AD brains [114]. Prx2 levels were also increased in the hippocampus and the frontal cortex of AD patients [114] and in the substantia nigra of PD patients [115]. Prx3 expression was decreased in the brains of AD patients [116]. In addition, Prx6 was upregulated in astrocytes of AD patients [117]. In PD patients, peroxidase activity of Prx2 was inhibited by *S*-nitrosylation [118,119] and phosphorylation [114]. The redox states of Prx2 and Prx6 were more oxidized in the brains and serum of AD patients [120]. In circulating endothelial progenitor cells of ischemia stroke patients, Prx1 was 10-fold more highly expressed than in healthy controls [121]. Prx2 in rat brains was downregulated after cerebral ischemia [122] and protected against stroke-related insults, such as ischemia and glutamate treatment *in vitro* and *in vivo* [99]. Prx3 was increased in the hippocampus of gerbils after cerebral ischemia–reperfusion and protected against ischemic damage [123,124].

PHARMACOLOGICAL APPROACHES

A body of studies have been published about antioxidant properties; however, they have not had a positive effect on clinical studies [117]. Since Trx family proteins show specific alterations in various pathological conditions, including changes in protein expression, enzymatic activity, tissue distribution, and intra- and extracellular localization, they have been used as therapeutic tools in different experimental models. For instance, ebselen, reviewed in Ref. [119], a chemical mimic of glutathione peroxidase that was shown to reduce hydrogen peroxide levels and oxidize Trx

[120], was analyzed as potential drug, e.g., for cerebral ischemia [121] and stroke [122]. Two drugs, nipradilol and timolol, used in glaucoma therapy increase the protein levels of Prx2 and thereby protect cells of the trabecular meshwork, the tissue surrounding the base of the cornea, against hydrogen peroxide–induced apoptosis [123]. Another potential target in the clinic is Prx6. Overexpression of the peroxidase could be used to prevent the progression of hypoxia-dependent disorders, such as glaucoma [124]. These studies suggest Trxs as a promising tool for a new therapeutic approach.

CONCLUSION

The importance of redox signaling is increasingly recognized despite the highly transient nature of the redox modifications that makes them very difficult to investigate deeply. The various redox modifications are highly target specific and site specific, and the Trx protein family systems are key players in redox signal transduction both as transducers and regulators of second messenger levels.

Thus far, neuroprotective treatment may limit the secondary neuron damage. New knowledge about cellular repair mechanisms can also pave the way for types of treatment that not merely limit damage but can also repair defects. Therefore, redox signaling studies will be able to answer several questions about the functions of oxidative stress contributing to the development of new clinical applications.

REFERENCES

1. Rodbell, M. 1995. Nobel Lecture. Signal transduction: Evolution of an idea. *Biosci. Rep.* 15: 117–133.
2. Gilman, A.G. 1995. Nobel Lecture. G proteins and regulation of adenylyl cyclase. *Biosci. Rep.* 15: 65–97.
3. Jomova, K., Valko, M. 2011. Advances in metal-induced oxidative stress and human disease. *Toxicology* 283: 65–87.
4. Ullrich, V., Kissner, R. 2006. Redox signaling: Bioinorganic chemistry at its best. *J. Inorg. Biochem.* 100: 2079–2086.
5. Giustarini, D., Milzani, A., Aldini, G., Carini, M., Rossi, R., Dalle-Donne, I. 2005. *S*-Nitrosation versus *S*-glutathionylation of protein sulfhydryl groups by *S*-nitrosoglutathione. *Antioxid. Redox Signal.* 7: 930–939.
6. Holmgren, A. 1989. Thioredoxin and glutaredoxin systems. *J. Biol. Chem.* 264: 13963–13966.
7. Wells, W.W., Yang, Y., Deits, T.L., Gan, Z.R. 1993. Thioltransferases. *Adv. Enzymol. Relat. Areas Mol. Biol.* 66: 149–201.
8. Lillig, C.H., Holmgren, A. 2007. Thioredoxin and related molecules—From biology to health and disease. *Antioxid. Redox Signal.* 9: 25–47.
9. Martin, J.L. 1995. *S*-thioredoxin—A fold for all reasons. *Structure* 3: 245–250.
10. Laurent, T.C., Moore, E.C., Reichard, P. 1964. Enzymatic synthesis of deoxyribonucleotides. IV. Isolation and characterization of thioredoxin, the hydrogen donor from *Escherichia coli* B. *J. Biol. Chem.* 239: 3436–3444.
11. Arner, E.S., Holmgren, A. 2000. Physiological functions of thioredoxin and thioredoxin reductase. *Eur. J. Biochem.* 267: 6102–6109.
12. Arner, E.S. 2009. Focus on mammalian thioredoxin reductases—Important selenoproteins with versatile functions. *Biochim. Biophys. Acta* 1790: 495–526.

13. Zhong, L., Holmgren, A. 2000. Essential role of selenium in the catalytic activities of mammalian thioredoxin reductase revealed by characterization of recombinant enzymes with selenocysteine mutations. *J. Biol. Chem.* 275: 18121–18128.
14. Bjornstedt, M., Hamberg, M., Kumar, S., Xue, J., Holmgren, A. 1995. Human thioredoxin reductase directly reduces lipid hydroperoxides by NADPH and selenocystine strongly stimulates the reaction via catalytically generated selenols. *J. Biol. Chem.* 270: 11761–11764.
15. May, J.M., Mendiratta, S., Hill, K.E., Burk, R.F. 1997. Reduction of dehydroascorbate to ascorbate by the selenoenzyme thioredoxin reductase. *J. Biol. Chem.* 272: 22607–22610.
16. Watabe, S., Makino, Y., Ogawa, K., Hidro, T., Yamamoto, Y., Takahashi, S.Y. 1994. Mitochondrial thioredoxin reductase in bovine adrenal cortex its purification, properties, nucleotide/amino acid sequences, and identification of selenocysteine. *Eur. J. Biochem.* 264: 74–84.
17. Nishiyama, A., Matsui, M., Iwata, S. et al. 1999. Identification of thioredoxin-binding protein-2/vitamin D(3) up-regulated protein 1 as a negative regulator of thioredoxin function and expression. *J. Biol. Chem.* 274: 21645–21650.
18. Filomeni, G., Rotilio, G., Ciriolo, M.R. 2002. Cell signaling and the glutathione redox system. *Biochem. Pharmacol.* 64: 1057–1064.
19. Pacheco, C.C., Passos, J.F., Castro, A.R., Moradas-Ferreira, P., De Marco, P. 2008. Role of respiration and glutathione in cadmium-induced oxidative stress in *Escherichia coli* K-12. *Arch. Microbiol.* 189: 271–278.
20. Meister, A., Anderson, M.E. 1993. Glutathione. *Annu. Rev. Biochem.* 52: 711–760.
21. Van Elzen, R., Moens, L., Dewilde, S. 2008. Expression profiling of the cerebral ischemic and hypoxic response. *Expert Rev. Proteomics* 5: 263–282.
22. Hoffmann, B., Hecht, H.J., Flohe, L. 2002. Peroxiredoxins. *Biol. Chem.* 383: 347–364.
23. Wood, Z.A., Schroder, E., Robin Harris, J., Poole, L.B. 2003. Structure, mechanism and regulation of peroxiredoxins. *Trends Biochem. Sci.* 28: 32–40.
24. Lillig, C.H., Berndt, C., Holmgren, A. 2008. Glutaredoxin systems. *Biochim. Biophys. Acta* 1780: 1304–1317.
25. Rubartelli, A., Bajetto, A., Allavena, G., Wollman, E., Sitia, R. 1992. Secretion of thioredoxin by normal and neoplastic cells through a leaderless secretory pathway. *J. Biol. Chem.* 267: 24161–24164.
26. Rhee, S.G., Kang, S.W., Chang, T.G., Jeong, W., Kim, K. 2001. Peroxiredoxin, a novel family of peroxidases. *IUBMB Life* 52: 35–41.
27. Bharath, S., Hsu, M., Kaur, D., Rajagopalan, S., Andersen, J.K. 2002. Glutathione, iron and Parkinson's disease. *Biochem. Pharmacol.* 64: 1037–1048.
28. Dringen, R. 2000. Glutathione metabolism and oxidative stress in neurodegeneration. *Eur. J. Biochem.* 267: 4903.
29. Rodriguez, V.M., Del Razo, L.M., Limon-Pacheco, J.H. et al. 2005. Glutathione reductase inhibition and methylated arsenic distribution in Cd1 mice brain and liver. *Toxicol. Sci.* 84: 157–166.
30. Capani, F., Aguirre, F., Piehl, L. et al. 2001. Changes in reactive oxygen species (ROS) production in rat brain during global perinatal asphyxia: An ESR study. *Brain Res.* 914: 204–207.
31. Capani, F., Loidl, C.F., Piehl, L.L., Facorro, G., De Paoli, T., Hager, A. 2003. Long-term production of reactive oxygen species during perinatal asphyxia in the rat central nervous system: Effects of hypothermia. *Int. J. Neurosci.* 113: 641–654.
32. Eliasson, M.J., Huang, Z., Ferrante, R.J. et al. 1999. Neuronal nitric oxide synthase activation and peroxynitrite formation in ischemic stroke linked to neural damage. *J. Neurosci.* 19: 5910–5918.

33. Singh, I.N., Sullivan, P.G., Deng, Y., Mbye, L.H., Hall, E.D. 2006. Time course of post-traumatic mitochondrial oxidative damage and dysfunction in a mouse model of focal traumatic brain injury: Implications for neuroprotective therapy. *J. Cereb. Blood Flow Metab.* 26: 1407–1418.

34. Torreilles, F., Salman-Tabcheh, S., Guerin, M., Torreilles, J. 1999. Neurodegenerative disorders: The role of peroxynitrite. *Brain Res. Brain Res. Rev.* 30: 153–163.

35. Bains, J.S., Shaw, C.A. 1997. Neurodegenerative disorders in humans: The role of glutathione in oxidative stress-mediated neuronal death. *Brain Res. Brain Res. Rev.* 25: 335–358.

36. Dirnagl, U., Becker, K., Meisel, A. 2009. Preconditioning and tolerance against cerebral ischemia: From experimental strategies to clinical use. *Lancet Neurol.* 8: 398–412.

37. Martensson, J., Meister, A. 1991. Glutathione deficiency decreases tissue ascorbate levels in newborn rats: Ascorbate spares glutathione and protects. *Proc. Natl. Acad. Sci. U. S. A.* 88: 4656–4660.

38. Aón-Bertolino, M.L., Romero, J.L., Galeano, P. et al. 2011. Thioredoxin and glutaredoxin system proteins—Immunolocalization in the rat central nervous system. *Biochim. Biophys. Acta* 1810: 93–110.

39. Hansson, H.A., Rozell, B., Stemme, S., Engstrom, Y., Thelander, L., Holmgren, A. 1986. Different cellular distribution of thioredoxin and subunit M1 of ribonucleotide reductase in rat tissues. *Exp. Cell Res.* 163: 363–369.

40. Rybnikova, E., Damdimopoulos, A.E., Gustafsson, J.A., Spyrou, G., Pelto-Huikko, M. 2000. Expression of novel antioxidant thioredoxin-2 in the rat brain. *Eur. J. Neurosci.* 12: 1669–1678.

41. Leifer, D., Kowall, N.W. 1993. Immunohistochemical patterns of selective cellular vulnerability in human cerebral ischemia. *J. Neurol. Sci.* 119: 217–228.

42. Ordy, J.M., Wengenack, T.M., Bialobok, P. et al. 1993. Selective vulnerability and early progression of hippocampal CA1 pyramidal cell degeneration and GFAP-positive astrocyte reactivity in the rat four-vessel occlusion model of transient global ischemia. *Exp. Neurol.* 119: 128–139.

43. Neumann-Haefelin, T., Wiessner, C., Vogel, P., Back, T., Hossmann, K.A. 1994. Differential expression of the immediate early genes c-fos, c-jun, junB, and NGFI-B in the rat brain following transient forebrain ischemia. *J. Cereb. Blood Flow Metab.* 14: 206–216.

44. Rozell, B., Hansson, H.A., Luthman, M., Holmgren, A. 1985. Immunohistochemical localization of thioredoxin and thioredoxin reductase in adult rats. *Eur. J. Cell Biol.* 38: 79–86.

45. Takagi, Y., Tokime, T., Nozaki, K., Gon, Y., Kikuchi, H., Yodoi, J. 1998. Redox control of neuronal damage during brain ischemia after middle cerebral artery occlusion in the rat: Immunohistochemical and hybridization studies of thioredoxin. *J. Cereb. Blood Flow Metab.* 18: 206–214.

46. Takagi, Y., Horikawa, F., Nozaki, K., Sugino, T., Hashimoto, N., Yodoi, J. 1998. Expression and distribution of redox regulatory protein, thioredoxin during transient focal brain ischemia in the rat. *Neurosci Lett.* 251: 25–28.

47. Takagi, Y., Nakamura, T., Nishiyama, A. et al. 1999. Localization of glutaredoxin (thioltransferase) in the rat brain and possible functional implications during focal ischemia. *Biochem. Biophys. Res. Commun.* 10: 390–394.

48. Wang, X.W., Tan, B.Z., Sun, M., Ho, B., Ding, J.L. 2008. Thioredoxin-like 6 protects retinal cell line from photooxidative damage by upregulating NF-kappaB activity. *Free Radic. Biol. Med.* 45: 336–344.

49. Lillig, C.H., Lonn, M.E., Enoksson, M., Fernandes, A.P., Holmgren, A. 2004. Short interfering RNA-mediated silencing of glutaredoxin 2 increases the sensitivity of HeLa cells toward doxorubicin and phenylarsine oxide. *Proc. Natl. Acad. Sci. U. S. A.* 101: 13227–13232.

50. Lillig, C.H., Lonn, M.E., Enoksson, M., Fernandes, A.P., Holmgren, A. 2004. Short interfering RNA-mediated silencing of glutaredoxin 2 increases the sensitivity of HeLa cells toward doxorubicin and phenylarsine oxide. *Proc. Natl. Acad. Sci. U. S. A.* 101: 13227–13232.

51. Nakaso, K., Kitayama, M., Mizuta, E. et al. 2000. Co-induction of heme oxygenase-1 and peroxiredoxin I in astrocytes and microglia around hemorrhagic region in the rat brain. *Neurosci. Lett.* 293: 49–52.

52. Lawn, J.E., Cousens, S., Zupan, J., Lancet Neonatal Survival Steering Team. 2005. 4 million neonatal deaths: When? Where? Why? *Lancet* 365: 891–900.

53. Amiel-Tison, C., Ellison, P. 1986. Birth asphyxia in the full-term newborn: Early assessment and outcome. *Dev. Med. Child Neurol.* 28: 671–682.

54. Lee, J., Croen, L.A., Lindan, C. et al. 2005. Predictors of outcome in perinatal arterial stroke: A population-based study. *Ann. Neurol.* 58: 303–308.

55. Lynch, J.K. 2009. Epidemiology and classification of perinatal stroke. *Semin. Fetal Neonatal Med.* 14: 245–249.

56. Miller, S.P., Ferriero, D.M. 2009. From selective vulnerability to connectivity: Insights from newborn brain imaging. *Trends Neurosci.* 32: 496–505.

57. Verger, K., Junque, C., Levin, H.S. et al. 2001. Correlation of atrophy measures on MRI with neuropsychological sequelae in children and adolescents with traumatic brain injury. *Brain Injury* 15: 211–221.

58. Yager, J.Y., Thornhill, J.A. 1997. The effect of age on susceptibility to hypoxic ischemic brain damage. *Neurosci. Biobehav. Rev.* 21: 167–174.

59. Li, H., Li, Q., Du, X. et al. 2011. Lithium-mediated long-term neuroprotection in neonatal rat hypoxia–ischemia is associated with anti-inflammatory effects and enhanced proliferation and survival of neural stem/progenitor cells. *J. Cereb. Blood Flow Metab.* 31: 2106–2115.

60. Li, Q., Li, H., Roughton, K. et al. 2010. Lithium reduces apoptosis and autophagy after neonatal hypoxia–ischemia. *Cell Death Dis.* 1: e56. doi: 10.1038/cddis.2010.33.

61. Zhu, C., Wang, X., Xu, F. et al. 2005. The influence of age on apoptotic and other mechanisms of cell death after cerebral hypoxia–ischemia. *Cell Death Differ.* 12: 162–176.

62. Bayir, H., Kochanek, P.M., Kagan, V.E. 2006. Oxidative stress in immature brain after traumatic brain injury. *Dev. Neurosci.* 28: 420–431.

63. Blomgren, K., Leist, M., Groc, L. 2007. Pathological apoptosis in the developing brain. *Apoptosis* 12: 993–1010.

64. Blomgren, K., Zhu, C., Hallin, U., Hagberg, H. 2003. Mitochondria and ischemic reperfusion damage in the adult and in the developing brain. *Biochem. Biophys. Res. Commun.* 304: 551–559.

65. Ikonomidou, C., Kaindl, A.M. 2011. Neuronal death and oxidative stress in the developing brain. *Antioxid. Redox Signal.* 14: 1535–1550.

66. Potts, M., Koh, S.-E., Whetstone, W. et al. 2006. Traumatic injury to the immature brain: Inflammation, oxidative injury, and iron-mediated damage as potential therapeutic targets. *Neuroreport* 3: 143–153.

67. Gunn, A.J., Gunn, T.R., de Haan, H.H., Williams, C.E., Gluckman, P.D. 1997. Dramatic neuronal rescue with prolonged selective head cooling after ischemia in fetal lambs. *J. Clin. Invest.* 99: 248–256.

68. Roelfsema, V., Bennet, L., George, S. et al. 2004. Window of opportunity of cerebral hypothermia for postischemic white matter injury in the near-term fetal sheep. *J. Cereb. Blood Flow Metab.* 24: 877–886.

69. Hobbs, C., Thoresen, M., Tucker, A., Aquilina, K., Chakkarapani, E., Dingley, J. 2008. Xenon and hypothermia combine additively, offering long-term functional and histopathologic neuroprotection after neonatal hypoxia/ischemia. *Stroke* 39: 1307–1313.

70. Kittaka, M., Giannotta, S.L., Zelman, V. et al. 1997. Attenuation of brain injury and reduction of neuron-specific enolase by nicardipine in systemic circulation following focal ischemia and reperfusion in a rat model. *J. Neurosurg.* 87: 731–737.
71. Vannucci, R.C., Towfighi, J., Vannucci, S.J. 2004. Secondary energy failure after cerebral hypoxia–ischemia in the immature rat. *J. Cereb. Blood Flow Metab.* 24: 1090–1097.
72. Sejersted, Y., Hildrestrand, G.A., Kunke, D. et al. 2011. Endonuclease VIII-like 3 (Neil3) DNA glycosylase promotes neurogenesis induced by hypoxia–ischemia. *Proc. Natl. Acad. Sci. U. S. A.* 108: 18802–18807.
73. Kapadia, V.S., Chalak, L.F., DuPont, T.L., Rollins, N.K., Brion, L.P., Wyckoff, M.H. 2013. Perinatal asphyxia with hyperoxemia within the first hour of life is associated with moderate to severe hypoxic–ischemic encephalopathy. *J. Pediatr.* 163: 949–954. doi: 10.1016/j.jpeds.2013.04.043.
74. Gitto, E., Reiter, R.J., Karbownik, M. et al. 2002. Causes of oxidative stress in the pre- and perinatal period. *Biol. Neonate* 81: 146–157. doi: 10.1159/000051527.
75. McNaught, K.S., Olanow, C.W., Halliwell, B., Isacson, O., Jenner, P. 2001. Failure of the ubiquitin–proteasome system in Parkinson's disease. *Nat. Rev. Neurosci.* 2: 589–594.
76. Polymeropoulos, M.H., Lavedan, C., Leroy, E. et al. 1997. Mutation in the alpha-synuclein gene identified in families with Parkinson's disease. *Science* 276: 2045–2047.
77. Healy, D.G., Abou-Sleiman, P.M., Wood, N.W. 2004. PINK, PANK, or PARK? A clinicians' guide to familial parkinsonism. *Lancet Neurol.* 3: 652–662.
78. Brookmeyer, R., Gray, S., Kawas, C. 1998. Projections of Alzheimer's disease in the United States and the public health impact of delaying disease onset. *Am. J. Public Health* 88: 1337–1342.
79. Pohanka, M. 2013. Alzheimer's disease and oxidative stress: A link to etiology? A review. *Curr. Med. Chem.* 21: 356–364.
80. Sisodia, S.S., George-Hyslop, P.H. 2002. Γ-Secretase, Notch, Aβ and Alzheimer's disease: Where do the presenilins fit in? *Nat. Rev. Neurosci.* 3: 281–290.
81. Tanzi, R.E., Bertram, L. 2001. New frontiers in Alzheimer's disease genetics. *Neuron* 32: 181–184.
82. Smith, M.A., Taneda, S., Richey, P.L. et al. 1994. Advanced Maillard reaction end products are associated with Alzheimer disease pathology. *Proc. Natl. Acad. Sci. U. S. A.* 91(12): 5710–5714.
83. Smith, M.A., Richey Harris, P.L., Sayre, L.M., Beckman, J.S., Perry, G. 1997. Widespread peroxynitrite-mediated damage in Alzheimer's disease. *J. Neurosci.* 17(8): 2653–2657.
84. Montine, T.J., Amarnath, V., Martin, M.E., Strittmatter, W.J., Graham, D.G. 1996. E-4-hydroxy-2-nonenal is cytotoxic and cross-links cytoskeletal proteins in P19 neuroglial cultures. *Am. J. Pathol.* 148(1): 89–93.
85. Sayre, L.M., Zelasko, D.A., Harris, P.L., Perry, G., Salomon, R.G., Smith, M.A. 1997. 4-Hydroxynonenal-derived advanced lipid peroxidation end products are increased in Alzheimer's disease. *J. Neurochem.* 68(5): 2092–2097.
86. Smith, M.A., Kutty, R.K., Richey, P.L. et al. 1994. Heme oxygenase-1 is associated with the neurofibrillary pathology of Alzheimer's disease. *Am. J. Pathol.* 145(1): 42–47.
87. Premkumar, D.R., Smith, M.A., Richey, P.L. et al. 1995. Induction of heme oxygenase-1 mRNA and protein in neocortex and cerebral vessels in Alzheimer's disease. *J. Neurochem.* 65(3): 1399–1402.
88. Smith, M.A., Sayre, L.M., Monnier, V.M., Perry, G. 1995. Radical AGEing in Alzheimer's disease. *Trends Neurosci.* 8(4): 172–176.
89. Gou, J.P., Eyer, J., Leterrier, J.F. 1995. Progressive hyperphosphorylation of neurofilament heavy subunits with aging: Possible involvement in the mechanism of neurofilament accumulation. *Biochem. Biophys. Res. Commun.* 215: 368–376.

90. Tuppo, E., Forman, L., Spur, B., Chan-Ting, R.E., Chopra, A., Cavalieri, T.A. 2001. Sign of lipid peroxidation as measured in the urine of patients with probable Alzheimer's disease. *Brain Res. Bull.* 565: 568.

91. Markesbery, W., Carney, J. 1999. Oxidative alterations in Alzheimer's disease. *Brain Pathol.* 133: 146.

92. Migliore, L., Coppedè, F. 2009. Environmental-induced oxidative stress in neurodegenerative disorders and aging. *Mutat. Res.* 73: 84.

93. Behl, C. 2005. Oxidative stress in Alzheimer's disease: Implications for prevention and therapy, in *Subcellular Biochemistry*, 38th edition, vol. 38, J. Harris and F. Fahrenholz, Eds., pp. 65–79, Springer, New York.

94. Mancuso, M., Coppede, F., Migliore, L., Siciliano, G., Murri, L. 2006. Mitochondrial dysfunction, oxidative stress and neurodegeneration. *J. Alzheimers Dis.* 59: 73.

95. Lee, H.G., Zhu, X., Nunomura, A., Perry, G., Smith, M.A. 2006. Amyloid β: The alternate hypothesis. *Curr. Alzheimer Res.* 3: 75–80.

96. Kontush, A., Berndt, C., Weber, W. et al. 2001. Amyloid-β is an antioxidant for lipoproteins in cerebrospinal fluid and plasma. *Free Radic. Biol. Med.* 119: 128–131.

97. Akterin, S., Cowburn, R.F., Miranda-Vizuete, A. et al. 2006. Involvement of glutaredoxin-1 and thioredoxin-1 in beta-amyloid toxicity and Alzheimer's disease. *Cell Death Differ.* 13: 1454–1465.

98. Bai, J., Nakamura, H., Hattori, I., Tanito, M., Yodoi, J. 2002. Thioredoxin suppresses 1-methyl-4-phenylpyridinium-induced neurotoxicity in rat PC12 cells. *Neurosci. Lett.* 321: 81–84.

99. Koh, P.-O. 2010. Proteomic analysis of focal cerebral ischemic injury in male rats. *J. Vet. Med. Sci.* 72: 181–185.

100. Takagi, Y., Mitsui, A., Nishiyama, A. et al. 1999. Overexpression of thioredoxin in transgenic mice attenuates focal ischemic brain damage [Online]. *Proc. Natl. Acad. Sci. U. S. A.* 96: 4131–4136.

101. Hwang, I.K., Yoo, K.-Y., Kim, D.W. et al. 2010. Changes in the expression of mitochondrial peroxiredoxin and thioredoxin in neurons and glia and their protective effects in experimental cerebral ischemic damage. *Free Radic. Biol. Med.* 48: 1242–1251.

102. Lovell, M.A., Xie, C., Gabbita, S.P., Markesbery, W.R. 2000. Decreased thioredoxin and increased thioredoxin reductase levels in Alzheimer's disease brain. *Free Radic. Biol. Med.* 28: 418–427.

103. da Costa, C.A. 2007. DJ-1: A newcomer in Parkinson's disease pathology. *Curr. Mol. Med.* 7: 650–657.

104. Saeed, U., Ray, A., Valli, R.K., Kumar, A.M.R., Ravindranath, V. 2010. DJ-1 loss by glutaredoxin but not glutathione depletion triggers Daxx translocation and cell death. *Antioxid. Redox Signal.* 13: 127–144.

105. Kenchappa, R.S., Ravindranath, V. 2003. Glutaredoxin is essential for maintenance of brain mitochondrial complex I: Studies with MPTP. *FASEB J.* 17: 717–719.

106. Sabens Liedhegner, E.A., Gao, X.-H., Mieyal, J.J. 2012. Mechanisms of altered redox regulation in neurodegenerative diseases—Focus on *S*-glutathionylation. *Antioxid. Redox Signal.* 16: 543–566.

107. Perry, T.L., Yong, V.W. 1986. Idiopathic Parkinson's disease, progressive supranuclear palsy and glutathione metabolism in the substantia nigra of patients. *Neurosci. Lett.* 67: 269–274.

108. Jha, N., Jurma, O., Lalli, G. et al. 2000. Glutathione depletion in PC12 results in selective inhibition of mitochondrial complex I activity. Implications for Parkinson's disease. *J. Biol. Chem.* 275: 26096–26101.

109. Hu, X., Weng, Z., Chu, C.T. et al. 2011. Peroxiredoxin-2 protects against 6-hydroxydopamine-induced dopaminergic neurodegeneration via attenuation of the apoptosis signal-regulating kinase (ASK1) signaling cascade. *J. Neurosci.* 31: 247–261.

110. Sultana, R., Boyd-Kimball, D., Cai, J. et al. 2007. Proteomics analysis of the Alzheimer's disease hippocampal proteome. *J. Alzheimers Dis.* 11: 153–164.

111. Basso, M., Giraudo, S., Corpillo, D., Bergamasco, B., Lopiano, L., Fasano, M. 2004. Proteome analysis of human substantia nigra in Parkinson's disease. *Proteomics* 4: 3943–3952.

112. Power, J.H.T., Asad, S., Chataway, T.K. et al. 2008. Peroxiredoxin 6 in human brain: Molecular forms, cellular distribution and association with Alzheimer's disease pathology. *Acta Neuropathol.* 115: 611–622.

113. Fang, J., Nakamura, T., Cho, D.-H., Gu, Z., Lipton, S.A. 2007. *S*-nitrosylation of peroxiredoxin 2 promotes oxidative stress-induced neuronal cell death in Parkinson's disease. *Proc. Natl. Acad. Sci. U. S. A.* 104: 18742–18747.

114. Qu, D., Rashidian, J., Mount, M.P. et al. 2007. Role of Cdk5-mediated phosphorylation of Prx2 in MPTP toxicity and Parkinson's disease. *Neuron* 55: 37–52.

115. Brea, D., Rodriguez-Gonzalez, R., Sobrino, T., Rodriguez-Yanez, M., Blanco, M., Castillo, J. 2011. Proteomic analysis shows differential protein expression in endothelial progenitor cells between healthy subjects and ischemic stroke patients. *Neurol. Res.* 33: 1057–1063.

116. Rashidian, J., Rousseaux, M.W., Venderova, K. et al. 2009. Essential role of cytoplasmic cdk5 and Prx2 in multiple ischemic injury models, in vivo. *J. Neurosci.* 29: 12497–12505.

117. Hwang, I.K., Yoo, K.-Y., Kim, D.W. et al. 2010. Changes in the expression of mitochondrial peroxiredoxin and thioredoxin in neurons and glia and their protective effects in experimental cerebral ischemic damage. *Free Radic. Biol. Med.* 48: 1242–1251.

118. Li, J., Wuliji, O., Li, W., Jiang, Z.G., Ghanbari, H.A. 2013. Oxidative stress and neurodegenerative disorders. *Int. J. Mol. Sci.* 16: 24438–24475. doi: 10.3390/ijms141224438.

119. Fang, J., Zhong, L., Zhao, R., Holmgren, A. 2005. Ebselen: A thioredoxin reductase-dependent catalyst for alpha-tocopherol quinone reduction. *Toxicol. Appl. Pharmacol.* 207: 103–109.

120. Zhao, R., Holmgren, A. 2002. A novel antioxidant mechanism of ebselen involving ebselen diselenide, a substrate of mammalian thioredoxin and thioredoxin reductase. *J. Biol. Chem.* 277: 39456–39462.

121. Parnham, M., Sies, H. 2000. Ebselen: Prospective therapy for cerebral ischaemia. *Expert Opin. Investig. Drugs* 9: 607–619.

122. Yamaguchi, T., Sano, K., Takakura, K. et al. 1998. Ebselen in acute ischemic stroke: A placebo-controlled, double-blind clinical trial. Ebselen Study Group. *Stroke* 29: 12–17.

123. Miyamoto, N., Izumi, H., Miyamoto, R. et al. 2009. Nipradilol and timolol induce Foxo3a and peroxiredoxin 2 expression and protect trabecular meshwork cells from oxidative stress. *Invest. Ophthalmol. Vis. Sci.* 50: 2777–2784.

124. Tulsawani, R., Kelly, L.S., Fatma, N. et al. 2010. Neuroprotective effect of peroxiredoxin 6 against hypoxia-induced retinal ganglion cell damage. *BMC Neurosci.* 11: 125. doi: 10.1186/1471-2202-11-125.

12 Gastrointestinal Disorders

Michael Georgoulis, Ioanna Kechribari, and Meropi D. Kontogianni

CONTENTS

Preface...215
Celiac Disease...216
    Introduction...216
    Oxidative Stress and Celiac Disease..217
    Antioxidants and Celiac Disease Risk...217
    Antioxidants and Treatment of Celiac Disease...219
    Conclusions...220
Inflammatory Bowel Diseases 221
    Introduction...221
    Oxidative Stress and IBDs 222
    Antioxidants and IBD Risk..223
        Dietary Antioxidant Intake and IBD Risk..223
        Blood Antioxidant Levels and IBD Risk..224
    Antioxidants and Treatment of IBDs 225
    Conclusions...228
References..229

PREFACE

Oxidative stress, defined as a persistent imbalance between the formation of pro-oxidant molecules and antioxidant defenses, in favor of the former, has recently emerged as a key factor contributing to the development and progression of inflammation-based gastrointestinal diseases. Considerable evidence from both human and animal studies support that the consequences of oxidative stress, including the peroxidation of cellular constituents, disruption of intracellular signaling pathways, and perpetuation of the inflammatory response, induce intestinal damage and contribute to intestinal pathology. There is also a limited number of reports testing the use of antioxidants as a part of the management of various gastrointestinal disorders; however, their preliminary data cannot support a definite therapeutic advantage thus far. The present chapter provides an overview of the role of oxidative stress in the pathogenesis of inflammation-based gastrointestinal tract diseases, namely celiac disease and inflammatory bowel diseases, as well as the potential role of antioxidants in their prevention and treatment.

CELIAC DISEASE

INTRODUCTION

Celiac disease, also defined as gluten-sensitive enteropathy, is a multiorgan, chronic inflammatory disorder induced by permanent intolerance to gluten, a protein found in cereal grains, namely wheat, barley, and rye (Troncone et al. 2008b; Hall et al. 2009; Ferretti et al. 2012). Alcohol extraction of gluten produces a soluble fraction, the prolamins (gliadin in wheat, secalin in rye, and hordein in barley), and an insoluble fraction, the glutenins, which are both toxic for patients with celiac disease and consist the environmental stimuli responsible for the development of the intestinal damage (Ciclitira et al. 1984). The disease is characterized by histopathological damage mainly located in the proximal small intestine, including villus atrophy, crypt hyperplasia, flattened mucosa, and increased epithelial lymphocytic infiltration (Stojiljkovic et al. 2009; Ferretti et al. 2012). It affects approximately 0.5–1% of the worldwide population; however, more than half of the patients remain undetected.

Although celiac disease can have its onset at any age, it is usually first diagnosed in adulthood (Troncone et al. 2008b; Hall et al. 2009). Typical clinical manifestations of celiac disease include chronic diarrhea, weight loss, abdominal distension, lassitude, and malaise. However, a significant proportion of patients experience other extradigestive symptoms, such as anemia, skin lesions, isolated hypertransaminasemia, osteopenia, infertility, dermatitis herpetiformis, ataxia, or polyneuropathia. It is important that there are also patients with no or atypical symptoms (silent celiac disease), resulting in underdiagnosis of the disease (Troncone et al. 2008a,b).

Celiac disease is associated with serious consequences on health, such as malabsorption of nutrients, osteoporosis, gastrointestinal malignancies, and the onset of other autoimmune diseases, such as diabetes mellitus, making it a serious public health problem, which needs to be treated. The cornerstone of the disease treatment is the lifelong adherence to a gluten-free diet (GFD), which has been associated with clinical and histological recovery, a better quality of life, and the prevention of disease complications (Troncone et al. 2008a; Hall et al. 2009).

Although the exact mechanisms by which gluten and its fractions (prolamins and glutenins) cause intestinal damage remain unclear, it seems that an interaction of genetic, environmental, and immunological factors occurs. Celiac disease has a genetic basis, indicated by a concordance in monozygotic twins and an increased prevalence in first-degree relatives. The determinants of genetic heritability are the human leukocyte antigen (HLA) class II *DQA* and *DQB* genes located in the major histocompatibility complex on chromosome 6. The combination of *HLA-DQA1*0501* and *DQB1*0201* alleles encode the HLA-DQA2 class II protein, which is responsible for prolamins' presentation to positive T-cell receptors of CD4 lymphocytes. However, these alleles are critical but not sufficient for celiac disease development (Ferretti et al. 2012). The proposed theory is that gluten and its fractions, as well as other environmental factors, trigger the inflammatory injury and the development of intestinal damage, by activating various pathological immune responses in genetically susceptible individuals (Troncone et al. 2008b).

OXIDATIVE STRESS AND CELIAC DISEASE

Evidence acquired during the last decade suggests that most of the cytotoxic, inflammatory, and immunogenic effects of gluten peptides on the intestinal epithelium are mediated by increased oxidative stress. Some gluten peptides have the ability to penetrate cells in celiac disease patients. Then, they accumulate in lysosomes and trigger the activation of some signal transduction pathways, leading to an overproduction of free radicals (reactive oxygen species [ROS] and reactive nitrogen species [RNS]). In turn, free radicals disturb the pro-oxidant/antioxidant balance in the intestinal mucosa, by increasing levels of lipid peroxidation products and oxidized (GSSG)/reduced (GSH) glutathione ratio (oxidative stress markers), and decreasing protein-bound sulfhydryl groups (which are involved in the cell regulation of ROS levels together with antioxidants). The altered oxidative balance leads to the activation of pro-inflammatory transcription protein complex of the nuclear factor-kappa B (NF-κB), which results in the transcription of pro-inflammatory cytokines like tumor necrosis factor-α (TNF-α), interleukin-8 (IL-8), and interferon-γ (IFN-γ), and enzymes such as cyclooxygenase 2 (COX-2) and inducible nitric oxide synthase (iNOS). Consequently, prostaglandins and nitric oxide (NO) metabolites are produced, which further contribute to oxidative stress, perpetuating a vicious cycle as illustrated in Figure 12.1. The increased oxidative stress also downregulates the production of peroxisome proliferator-activated receptor gamma, mediated by tissue transglutaminase, leading equally to NF-κB activation. As a result, the epithelial barrier dysfunction and the intestinal permeability increase and gluten peptides pass through the enterocytes, activating various immune responses, which further lead to cell damage and villous atrophy in celiac disease patients (Ferretti et al. 2012).

Data from several studies assessing the oxidative or antioxidant status of patients with celiac disease also support the involvement of oxidative stress in the disease pathogenesis and have been recently reviewed (Ferretti et al. 2012). As reported in this review, it seems that celiac disease patients demonstrate increased markers of oxidative stress and damage (e.g., increased iNOS expression in intestine and NO metabolite levels in plasma) and decreased levels of antioxidant enzymes (e.g., decreased glutathione peroxidase activity in the intestine and in blood, respectively) and nuclear factors in intestinal cells and biological fluids, compared with healthy controls (Ferretti et al. 2012).

ANTIOXIDANTS AND CELIAC DISEASE RISK

Celiac disease patients' dietary habits, in terms of macro- and micronutrient intake, have been thus far explored in many studies, with most of the data suggesting that both newly diagnosed and long-term patients are characterized by inadequate dietary vitamin and mineral intake. Reasons for the observed nutritional inadequacies include habitual poor food choices in addition to inherent deficiencies in the GFD, as well as the lack of a proper dietary counseling (Shepherd and Gibson 2013; Wierdsma et al. 2013). However, studies exploring the relationship between dietary antioxidants intake and the risk of celiac disease are currently unavailable. On the other hand, few cross-sectional studies have assessed the antioxidant body content

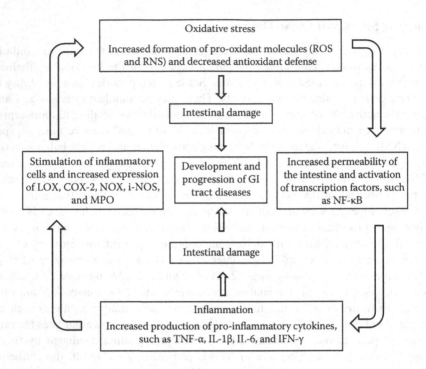

FIGURE 12.1 Schematic illustration of the interaction between oxidative stress and inflammation in the pathophysiology of inflammatory-based gastrointestinal (GI) tract diseases. As depicted, oxidative stress contributes to intestinal inflammation by (i) increasing intestinal permeability and the exposure of intestinal cells to harmful stimuli (gluten in the case of celiac disease or intestinal pathogens in the case of inflammatory bowel diseases), and (ii) stimulating signaling pathways, especially the redox-sensitive transcription factor nuclear factor kappa B (NF-κB), which in turn promotes the production of inflammatory cytokines, such as tumor necrosis factor-α (TNF-α), interleukin-1β (IL-1β), interleukin-6 (IL-6), and interferon-γ (IFN-γ). On the other hand, inflammation augments oxidative stress by stimulating the expression of inflammatory cells' reactive oxygen and nitrogen species (ROS and RNS) generating systems, such as lipoxygenase (LOX), cycloxygenase-2 (COX-2), NAD(P)H oxidases (NOXs), inducible-nitric oxide synthase (i-NOS), and myeloperoxidase (MPO).

of patients with celiac disease and reported decreased levels of antioxidant vitamin E (α-tocopherol) in both patients' circulating cells and plasma (Stojiljkovic et al. 2007; Szaflarska-Poplawska et al. 2010), as well as low serum selenium levels (Yuce et al. 2004). Nevertheless, the above-mentioned decreased levels of antioxidants are probably the result of intestinal malabsorption, rather than inadequate dietary intake. Given the fact that cross-sectional studies do not provide a good basis for establishing causality, the conduction of prospective studies in genetically predisposed individuals is clearly needed, to assess the relationship between dietary antioxidant intake and the risk of celiac disease development.

Despite the lack of strong evidence regarding the role of specific antioxidants in celiac disease risk, it is worth mentioning that current theories support the important role of selenium in celiac disease development and severity for two main reasons.

First, selenium is a part of glutathione peroxidase, one of the strongest antioxidant enzymes in the human body, which is involved in the protection of intestinal cells against oxidative damage. Second, selenium deficiency seems to be associated with the development of autoimmune thyroid diseases (AITDs), a common extraintestinal complication of celiac disease, since selenoproteins are necessary for the biosynthesis and activity of thyroid hormones and the maintenance of normal thyroid gland function. Given the aforementioned, selenium malabsorption in celiac disease has recently emerged as a key factor directly leading to both thyroid and intestinal damage. Under this scope, the correction of selenium deficiency, possibly via selenium supplementation, should be considered in patients with celiac disease in parallel with the adoption of GFD, to prevent both further oxidative stress–induced intestinal damage and the development of AITDs (Stazi and Trinti 2010).

ANTIOXIDANTS AND TREATMENT OF CELIAC DISEASE

There is much evidence that dietary antioxidants, such as plant polyphenols, carotenoids, and vitamins have the potential to modulate predisposition to intestinal chronic inflammatory diseases. They act through a plethora of mechanisms, including the decrease of inflammatory mediator production through effects on cell signaling and gene expression, the reduction of damaging oxidants production, and the promotion of gut barrier function and anti-inflammatory responses (Calder et al. 2009).

Data investigating the role of antioxidants in celiac disease treatment are scarce. Perhaps one reason explaining this fact is that during the past decades, scientific interest has focused on the effectiveness of GFD, which remains the cornerstone of disease treatment (Hall et al. 2009). Thus far, there is no human clinical trial available investigating the effect of antioxidant intake on celiac disease treatment. There is, however, only one study in a mouse model of celiac disease with unexpected results, concerning the role of retinoic acid (metabolite of vitamin A) in gliadin tolerance and inflammation. According to this study, retinoic acid promoted rather than prevented inflammatory cellular responses in a stressed intestinal environment and worked together with interleukin-15 (IL-15) to drive pro-inflammatory responses against gliadin (De Paolo et al. 2011).

Most of the data regarding the potential role of antioxidants in celiac disease management come from *in vitro* studies. Previously, one study reported that synthetic (pyrrolidine dithiocarbammate) and natural (genistein and tyrphostin) antioxidants inhibited the *iNOS* gene expression in a mouse monocyte/macrophage RAW 264.7 cell line, which were stimulated by gliadin and IFN-γ (De Stefano et al. 2006). iNOS production significantly increased in the stimulated cells; however, in the presence of the above-mentioned antioxidants, this response was attenuated. One year later, members of the same research team found that lycopene (carotenoid), quercetin (flavonoid), and tyrosol (polyphenol) decreased *iNOS* and *COX-2* gene expression induced by gliadin and IFN-γ in RAW 246.7 macrophages (De Stefano et al. 2007). These results suggest that antioxidants may control the genes encoding pro-inflammatory cytokines that are involved in celiac disease pathogenesis. In another recent *in vitro* study, the addition of vitamin C (ascorbate) to a culture of gliadin-challenged, duodenal biopsy extracts from treated celiac disease patients (for a minimum of 6 months on GFD) blocked the secretion of nitrites and pro-inflammatory cytokines (IFN-α, IFN-γ, TNF-α, and IL-6), and inhibited the expression of IL-15 triggered by gliadin, compared with samples from a non-ascorbate-supplemented culture (Bernardo et al. 2012). The authors suggested in their conclusions that vitamin C supplementation might be beneficial for patients with celiac disease and can be considered as a future treatment option. The conclusions of one recent review are also promising, suggesting that flavonoids such as epigallocatechin gallate, genistein, myricetin, and quercetin have a protective effect on intestinal intracellular tight junction (Tj) barrier function. The Tjs play an important role in the transport of gluten through enterocytes and in the function of the intestinal barrier. Oxidative stress and pro-inflammatory cytokines causes dysfunction of Tjs in celiac disease patients, and the aforementioned flavonoids have been suggested to protect their function (Suzuki and Hara 2011).

Conclusions

To sum up, oxidative stress seems to be involved in celiac disease pathogenesis and celiac patients are characterized by a low antioxidant status. According to the aforementioned studies, dietary antioxidants (antioxidant vitamins and phytochemicals) may have a role in the nutritional treatment of celiac disease, by exerting protective effects against toxic gluten fractions on intestinal cells (Figure 12.2). However, the benefits of antioxidants observed in cell cultures must also be confirmed in animal and human studies, to clarify the conclusions that remain ambiguous until now. Further research should also focus on the optimal dosage of antioxidant intake and on the possible differences between dietary sources of antioxidants and supplements. Until then, GFD remains the only step of treatment after the diagnosis of the disease.

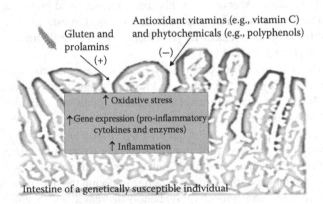

FIGURE 12.2 Potential beneficial effect of dietary antioxidant vitamins and phytochemicals on celiac disease patients. Dietary antioxidants may attenuate the toxic effects of gluten fractions on the intestinal cells.

INFLAMMATORY BOWEL DISEASES

INTRODUCTION

Inflammatory bowel diseases (IBDs) represent a group of chronic idiopathic intestinal diseases, with Crohn's disease (CD) and ulcerative colitis (UC) being the two major phenotypes. Although both pathological conditions are characterized by intestinal inflammation, the site, nature, and extent of intestinal involvement differ significantly among them. CD usually involves the terminal ileum and the colon; however, it can practically affect any part of the gastrointestinal tract from the mouth to the anus in a segmental way (skip lesions), while inflammation is transmural. By contrast, UC always affects the rectum and can spread proximally up to the cecum in an uninterrupted retrograde pattern (continuous areas of inflammation and ulceration with no segments of normal tissue), while inflammation is typically confined to the mucosa (Assadsangabi and Lobo 2013). According to epidemiological data, the highest prevalence of IBD is reported in westernized nations (Europe and North America) and their incidence appears to be gradually increasing in different regions worldwide, indicating their emergence as global diseases imposing great health and economic burdens (Molodecky et al. 2012).

IBDs can occur anytime in life; however, they usually have an onset in early adulthood and a lifelong impact characterized by periods of remission and periods of active disease. The onset and active phases of IBD usually involve symptoms of abdominal and/or rectal pain and diarrhea (with blood or mucus in UC), frequently accompanied by other manifestations such as anorexia, weight loss, nausea and vomiting, arthralgia, and fever. Patients with IBD are at a high risk of developing intestinal cancer (mostly colorectal cancer in UC), while both CD and UC are also associated with several extraintestinal manifestations, including cutaneous lesions, ophthalmologic and joint disorders, biliary and liver complications, osteoporosis, and anemia. The primary end points of active IBD therapy include induction and maintenance of remission, as well as management of IBD-related complications. Currently, therapeutic options include salicylates, corticosteroids, immunosuppressants, immunomodulators, and biologic agents; however, if these treatments fail, the surgical removal of the highly affected intestinal parts remains the only available therapeutic choice (Engel and Neurath 2010).

It has been proposed that IBD occurs due to inappropriate inflammatory and immune response to luminal pathogens and the resulting host–microbe interactions in genetically susceptible individuals; however, the exact pathogenetic mechanisms responsible for their development remain partly elucidated. In brief, data thus far suggest that genetic factors, gut microbiota disorders, defects in the intestinal barrier function that lead to increased intestinal permeability and increased exposure to pathogens, dysregulated innate and adaptive immune system response resulting in an increased secretion of pro-inflammatory cytokines, and the presence of various types of potentially cytotoxic autoantibodies represent the most important determinants of IBD pathogenesis (Fries and Comunale 2011; Zhang and Li 2014). Among the mediators of the dysfunctional immunoregulation of the gut, oxidative stress is considered as a potential etiological and/or triggering factor for IBD.

OXIDATIVE STRESS AND IBDs

Current theories on IBD pathogenesis suggest that interactions among various genetic, environmental, and immune factors lead to an uncontrolled, dysregulated immune response in the intestinal mucosa. Underlying mechanisms are not entirely clear; however, substantial evidence suggests that chronic intestinal inflammation is associated with enhanced production of ROS and RNS, which in turn contributes to the initiation and perpetuation of the abnormal immune response (Zhu and Li 2012).

There is much direct evidence that a state of increased oxidative stress is present in human and experimental IBD. Several studies have demonstrated that compared with controls, both CD and UC patients and animals with experimental IBD exhibit increased formation of ROS/RNS and excessive levels of oxidized molecules (lipid and DNA oxidation markers), both in blood and in the gastrointestinal tract (Thomson et al. 1998; Rezaie et al. 2007). The intestinal epithelium contains multiple antioxidant systems, such as antioxidant enzymes (i.e., superoxide dismutase, catalase, glutathione peroxidase, myeloperoxidase, and glutathione reductase) and low molecular-weight antioxidant molecules (i.e., reduced glutathione and metallothionein), all of which are involved in protecting the intestinal cells against oxidative stress. In line with the augmented formation of oxidized molecules, both human and *in vivo* studies have reported an imbalance (either increase or decrease) in blood and intestinal mucosa concentrations of the aforementioned antioxidants in IBD (Thomson et al. 1998; Rezaie et al. 2007). This suggests either an induction of their synthesis in response to the oxidative molecules produced during the inflammatory response or their depletion due to severe persistent oxidative stress.

Oxidative stress is considered to contribute both to the development and the progression of IBD. It has been proposed that the augmented formation of ROS/RNS may occur at the very early stage of the disease process or even before the disease onset, suggesting a possible causative role of oxidative stress in the genesis of IBD. This notion is largely supported by several *in vivo* studies, recently reviewed by Zhu and Li (2012), showing that the direct inoculation of ROS/RNS to the intestine of experimental animals leads to intestinal inflammation and the development of colitis. Moreover, the chemical or genetic depletion of endogenous antioxidants (e.g., glutathione or glutathione peroxidase) has been shown to lead to spontaneous development of experimental colitis, while both the administration of exogenous antioxidants and the chemical or genetic amplification of endogenous antioxidants, such as superoxide dismutase, have been proven to attenuate the progression of chemically induced colitis in mice (Zhu and Li 2012). Regarding IBD progression, overproduction of ROS/RNS via various sources, especially the activated neutrophils and macrophages, can cause direct damage to intestinal cells via interacting with cellular constituents, including lipids. The subsequent formation of lipid peroxidation products, such as reactive aldehydes, has been shown to induce the infiltration and activation of inflammatory cells, leading to additional mucosal injury and the perpetuation of the inflammatory response (Kumagai et al. 2004; Trevisani et al. 2007).

It is still unclear whether oxidative stress precedes or follows intestinal inflammation. ROS/RNS can disintegrate the intestinal epithelium and increase intestinal permeability, leading to an increased exposure to intestinal pathogens and induction of the inflammatory response. Moreover, oxidative stress can lead to the activation of NF-κB, a pro-inflammatory redox-sensitive transcription factor that is known to result in a further overexpression of pro-inflammatory cytokines, hence contributing to the perpetuation of intestinal inflammation in IBD. On the other hand, inflammation can result in oxidative stress by stimulating ROS/RNS-generating systems. The increased activity of infiltrating immune cells in IBD patients is known to result in an increased production of pro-inflammatory cytokines, such as TNF-α, IL-1β, and IFN-γ, which in turn lead to an increased formation of ROS/RNS by phagocytic cells accumulating within the gastrointestinal tract, during times of active inflammation (Abraham and Cho 2009; Jena et al. 2012). It is therefore obvious that oxidative stress and intestinal inflammation consist of two closely related mechanistic aspects, both implicated in the development and the progression of IBD, as shown in Figure 12.1.

ANTIOXIDANTS AND IBD RISK

As previously described, oxidative stress plays an important role in IBD pathogenesis. Several studies have thus far attempted to investigate any potential relationship between dietary antioxidant intake or blood circulating antioxidant levels and IBD risk, which are presented and discussed in detail below.

Dietary Antioxidant Intake and IBD Risk

Although genetic and immune factors are the most important determinants of IBD development, nutrition has also been proposed as a potential environmental factor affecting IBD risk. For instance, it has been hypothesized that dietary components could influence the risk of intestinal inflammation through several mechanisms, including a direct contact with the colonic mucosa, changes in the chemical composition of mucosal cell membranes, or even an effect on the balance of intestinal flora. Indeed, several studies have thus far explored potential associations between long-term dietary habits, in terms of nutrients and foods or food groups, and IBD risk. According to a recent review of prospective cohorts, mainly including middle-aged Europeans, a diet high in protein from meat and fish has been consistently found to increase the risk of both CD and UC development, while an increased intake of linoleic acid and a decreased intake of omega-3 polyunsaturated fatty acids seem to be associated with increased UC risk (Andersen et al. 2012). Retrospective case–control studies also demonstrate a positive association between the dietary intake of total polyunsaturated fatty acids and omega-6 fatty acids, as well as the consumption of meat and the likelihood of both CD and UC, while they also provide limited data on food groups rich in antioxidants; in specific, a high consumption of fruits has been associated with a lower likelihood of CD, while a high consumption of vegetables has been associated with a lower likelihood of UC (Hou et al. 2011).

Regarding dietary antioxidants, given the involvement of oxidative stress in IBD pathogenesis, one could speculate that an increased dietary antioxidant intake could protect against the development of IBD; however, such evidence is currently limited. Thus far, only one prospective study provided results regarding the potential associations between specific dietary antioxidants and UC risk (Hart et al. 2008). In this nested case–control study within a European prospective investigation, 260,686 men and women aged 20–80 years residing in the United Kingdom, Sweden, Denmark, Germany, and Italy, selected from the European Prospective Investigation into Cancer and Nutrition (EPIC) Study cohort, provided information on their dietary habits through country-specific food-frequency questionnaires and were followed for the development of UC. According to the study's results, no significant association between dietary vitamin C, vitamin E, carotene, and retinol intake and UC risk was observed. Prospective studies testing associations between dietary antioxidants and CD risk are currently unavailable. Evidence regarding the potential role of dietary antioxidants in IBD development is also available through some case–control studies, comparing the dietary habits of either newly diagnosed or long-term IBD patients with those of healthy individuals (Reif et al. 1997; Geerling et al. 1998, 2000a; Sakamoto et al. 2005; Filippi et al. 2006; Rosman-Urbach et al. 2006; Kawakami et al. 2007; Sousa Guerreiro et al. 2007). Most of the data support that both CD and UC patients tend to report lower vitamin C intake, compared with controls, while data on other dietary antioxidants, such as vitamin A or vitamin E, are largely conflicting. Moreover, in most studies, patients with CD exhibit a higher frequency of inadequate dietary antioxidant intake (defined as a dietary intake below the country-specific recommended intake) compared with healthy individuals.

Prospective studies undoubtedly provide the most reliable data regarding disease risk. Given the lack of such studies evaluating the association between dietary antioxidants and IBD risk, a definite conclusion cannot be drawn. On the other hand, case–control studies can provide valuable information regarding the role of dietary antioxidants in IBD development, given that the interval between the diagnosis and participants' recruitment into the study is short, so that the prediagnosis diet is accurately reported. However, it should be mentioned that they also present many methodological limitations, mainly due to being largely susceptible to recall bias, while their retrospective design does not allow the reporting of causal associations between dietary antioxidant intake and IBD risk, as does a prospective design. Particularly, case–control studies on long-term IBD patients are of little value, since patients' dietary habits are most probably already influenced by the disease itself. It has been reported that patients with IBD in remission modify their dietary habits to prevent a possible disease relapse; food groups usually avoided or completely excluded include fruits, vegetables, legumes, pulses, and whole grains (Zallot et al. 2013), which are among the most important dietary sources of antioxidants. In addition, IBD patients are usually advised to follow a low-fat diet to prevent symptoms of diarrhea resulting from fat malabsorption due to intestinal inflammation (Brown et al. 2011). This possibly contributes to a decreased intake of the fat-soluble antioxidants vitamins A and E. Given the aforementioned, the low antioxidant intake of IBD patients observed in case–control studies could actually reflect disease-associated dietary modifications rather than dietary habits contributing to IBD development.

Blood Antioxidant Levels and IBD Risk

Evidence regarding the association between antioxidants and IBD is also available through studies exploring the blood antioxidant status of patients with CD and UC in comparison with healthy subjects (Ringstad et al. 1993; Ramakrishna et al. 1997; Bousvaros et al. 1998; D'Odorico et al. 2001; Koutroubakis et al. 2004; Rezaie et al. 2007). Briefly, patients with IBD tend to exhibit lower total plasma antioxidant capacity and lower plasma vitamin C, vitamin A, and vitamin E levels compared with healthy individuals; however, not all studies confirm these differences between patients and controls. Interestingly, some studies have also reported lower serum selenium levels both in adults and children with IBD compared with healthy controls, as well as an inverse association between serum selenium levels and disease extent. Given that patients with IBD have an increased risk of intestinal cancer and that selenium may inhibit intestinal carcinogenesis through multiple mechanisms (e.g., by protecting cellular membranes against oxidative damage, by reducing the mutagenicity of cancer-causing chemicals, or by affecting carcinogen metabolism) (Meplan and Hesketh 2012), reduced selenium levels may be of special importance in patients with IBD.

Although it is clear that IBD patients present an imbalance in blood antioxidant levels, this observation could be a result of the established disease rather than a preceding phenomenon. For instance, low blood antioxidant levels could reflect a poor dietary antioxidant intake, caused by IBD patients' strict dietary modifications to prevent and/or manage gastrointestinal symptoms or prevent disease relapse as previously mentioned. Most important, decreased blood levels of antioxidants could be the result of IBD patients' general state of malnutrition. It is estimated that malnutrition occurs in up to 85% of patients with CD and up to 60% of patients with UC both in active phases of the disease and in periods of remission. Nutritional deficiencies are prevalent, particularly in relation to anemia and osteoporosis, but also vitamin and mineral deficiencies, and result from extensive intestinal inflammation leading to nutrient malabsorption, poor appetite leading to low energy intake and consequent weight loss, gastrointestinal symptoms including nausea, vomiting and diarrhea, intestinal surgery complications, or medication-related adverse effects (Lomer 2011).

ANTIOXIDANTS AND TREATMENT OF IBDS

Given the strong involvement of oxidative stress in IBD pathogenesis and progression, antioxidant supplementation has been proposed as a potential alternative therapeutic option combined with established pharmacological treatment for IBD patients. In fact, the oldest and most commonly used drug for the treatment of patients with IBD, mesalazine, also known as 5-aminosalicylic acid, has shown ROS scavenging capabilities, as well as a synergistic interaction with other antioxidants, such as α-tocopherol (Rezaie et al. 2007).

Thus far, only few interventional studies have been conducted to examine the efficacy of specific antioxidants in patients with IBD, which are briefly presented in Table 12.1. The main antioxidants studied are vitamins C and E, β-carotene, and selenium (Geerling et al. 2000b; Aghdassi et al. 2003; Trebble et al. 2004, 2005; Seidner et al. 2005; Mirbagheri et al. 2008; Wiese et al. 2011), while two other studies investigated the role of curcumin in IBD treatment (Holt et al. 2005; Hanai et al. 2006). Curcumin (plant name *Curcuma longa*) is the principal natural polyphenolic compound found in the Indian spice, turmeric, and seems to exert strong anti-inflammatory and antioxidant properties (Holt et al. 2005). Thus far, the studies' results are quite

TABLE 12.1

Human Studies Assessing the Efficacy of Specific Antioxidants in IBD Treatment

Reference	Study Sample and Methods	Results
Geerling et al. 2000b	RCT: 25 CD patients in remission were supplemented either with antioxidants (12.4 µg selenium, 150 µg β-carotene, 4 mg vitamin E, and 20 mg vitamin C), or antioxidants plus n-3 fatty acids or placebo daily for 3 months.	Total antioxidant capacity and superoxide dismutase activity significantly increased, whereas the activity of glutathione peroxidase decreased. No change was observed between the groups considering lipid peroxidation or disease activity.
Seidner et al. 2005	RCT: 121 patients with mild or moderate UC were given either an oral supplement enriched with fish oil, fructooligosaccharides, gum arabic, and antioxidants (72 IU vitamin E, 156 mg vitamin C and 30 µg selenium) ($n = 59$), or a carbohydrate-based placebo formula ($n = 62$) for 6 months. Clinical and histologic responses were assessed at 3 and 6 months or at the final visit.	Both groups showed histological improvements and similar reduction in the degree of disease activity, which was significantly different from the baseline. UC patients given the oral supplement required significantly reduced doses of corticosteroids to control clinical symptoms, compared with the control group. However, no marker of OS was measured in this study.
Wiese et al. 2011	Pilot study: 28 patients with active CD on stable medication were asked to consume 16 oz of IBD Nutrition Formula containing fish oil, a fermentable prebiotic/fiber system, and increased levels of antioxidant vitamins and minerals (1185 µg β-carotene, 1320 IU vitamin A, 72 IU vitamin E, 156 mg vitamin C, and 22 µg selenium) daily for 4 months.	Plasma phospholipid levels of arachidonic acid decreased, while eicosapentaenoic acid and docosahexaenoic acid levels increased. Vitamin D (25-OH) levels improved in all patients. There was a significant decrease in disease activity and a significant improvement in quality of life in patients with final EPA >2%.
Aghdassi et al. 2003	RCT: 57 stable but oxidatively stressed CD patients were supplemented either with antioxidants (800 IU vitamin E and 1000 mg vitamin C) or placebo daily for 4 weeks.	Plasma vitamin C and E increased while all indices of oxidative stress (breath pentane and ethane output, plasma lipid peroxides, and F2-isoprostane) decreased. Disease activity remained stable.

(Continued)

TABLE 12.1 (CONTINUED)

Human Studies Assessing the Efficacy of Specific Antioxidants in IBD Treatment

Reference	Study Sample and Methods	Results
Mirbagheri et al. 2008	Case series study: 15 patients with mild and moderately active UC received D-α-tocopherol enema (8000 U) plus medication daily for 12 weeks.	Rectal D-α-tocopherol administration significantly reduced disease activity and was related with less need for corticosteroids.
Trebble et al. 2004, 2005	RCT: 62 CD patients were supplemented either with fish oil (EPA and DHA) and antioxidants (150 μg β-carotene, 200 μg selenium, 30 mg vitamin E, and 90 mg vitamin C) ($n = 31$) or with placebo ($n = 31$) daily for 24 weeks.	Supplementation was associated with reduced plasma, interferon-γ, and prostaglandin E_2. No differences were detected in disease activity or indices of bone turnover.
Hanai et al. 2006	RCT: 88 patients with quiescent UC were supplemented either with curcumin (2 g/day: 1 g after breakfast and 1 g after the evening meal) plus medication ($n = 44$) or with placebo plus medication ($n = 44$) for 6 months.	Curcumin supplementation resulted in greater improvements in disease severity and greater reduction in relapse rates, compared with the placebo group.
Holt et al. 2005	Pilot study: 5 patients with UC were treated with 550 mg curcumin twice daily for 1 month and then 550 mg three times daily for another month. In addition, 5 patients with CD were treated with 360 mg curcumin for 1 month and then 360 mg four times daily for 2 months.	All 5 UC patients improved, 4 of 5 reduced concomitant medications, while in 4 CD patients disease activity (symptomatic improvements of fewer bowel movements, less diarrhea, less abdominal pain and cramping) was reduced, as well as sedimentation rates.

Note: CD, Crohn's disease; g, gram; IBD, inflammatory bowel diseases; (I)U, (international)units; mg, milligram; RCT, randomized controlled trial; UC, ulcerative colitis; μg, microgram.

promising, suggesting that antioxidants may be a therapeutic option in IBD treatment. However, they also present various limitations, such as the low dose of administered antioxidants, small sample size, short duration, and no or short follow-up period. In addition, in five of the above-mentioned studies (Geerling et al. 2000b; Trebble et al. 2004; Seidner et al. 2005; Trebble 2005; Wiese et al. 2011), the supplement given to IBD patients, apart from antioxidants, also contained other dietary components such as fish oil, vitamins, and minerals; hence, the effect of antioxidants per se on IBD activity and severity is largely unclear.

Despite the lack of interventional studies in humans with IBD, most of the data assessing the effectiveness of antioxidants in the treatment of IBD comes from animal or *in vitro* studies. Several animal studies in rodent models of IBD (mainly experimental colitis and models of intestinal inflammation) have shown that vitamin E or selenium supplementation alone or in combination can significantly reduce markers of disease activity or severity, inflammation, and/or oxidative damage (Ademoglu et al. 2004; Tirosh et al. 2007; Bitiren et al. 2010; Tahan et al. 2011). In addition, there is much evidence that pure polyphenol molecules, such as quercetin, apigenin, genistein, resveratrol, and epigallocatechin-3-gallate, as well as natural polyphenolic extracts, such as extracts from green tea leaves and red wine, are capable of attenuating IBD severity and activity, by reducing immune cell infiltration in the intestine, intestinal inflammation, and oxidative stress markers (Romier et al. 2009). Interesting enough are the beneficial effects of curcumin on IBD treatment, shown in several *in vivo* studies (Jian et al. 2005; Camacho-Barquero et al. 2007; Deguchi et al. 2007; Mouzaoui et al. 2012), while only two of the aforementioned human trials have reproduced these data (Holt et al. 2005; Hanai et al. 2006). In brief, the main mechanisms proposed behind the observed effects of curcumin include free radical scavenging, the increase in the antioxidant enzymes, the suppression of proinflammatory enzymes (e.g., COX-2) and inflammatory cytokines (e.g., TNF-α, like INF-γ), and the modulation of signal transduction and transcription factors, including NF-κB. In addition, apart from curcumin's potent anti-inflammatory properties, its potential chemopreventive effects on carcinogenesis are currently being investigated (Baliga et al. 2012). Subsequently, limited *in vitro* studies also indicate that pure polyphenols and plant polyphenolic extracts could exert anti-inflammatory properties via the modulation of intracellular signaling cascades in the intestinal cell. However, other *in vitro* studies have produced contradictory results, making it difficult to draw definite conclusions (Romier et al. 2009).

Undoubtedly, further research is needed through well-designed human randomized controlled trials to elucidate the applicability of antioxidants in IBD treatment. In addition, more *in vitro* and *in vivo* studies are also required to understand the complex mechanisms regarding the actions of antioxidants on IBD pathogenesis and progression.

CONCLUSIONS

Although mounting evidence supports the involvement of oxidative stress in IBD pathogenesis and progression, data regarding the role of specific antioxidants on IBD risk and management remain thus far limited and do not allow the development of evidence-based recommendations on dietary antioxidant intake for these diseases. Nevertheless, given that current dietary guidelines for patients with both CD and UC suggest vitamin and mineral supplementation for all patients, or at least in those with malnutrition or those exhibiting reduced oral intake (Brown et al. 2011), the selection of supplements that also contain antioxidant compounds should be considered, to improve patients' nutritional and blood antioxidant status.

REFERENCES

Abraham, C., and J. H. Cho. 2009. Inflammatory bowel disease. *N Engl J Med* 21:2066–78.

Ademoglu, E., Y. Erbil, B. Tam et al. 2004. Do vitamin E and selenium have beneficial effects on trinitrobenzenesulfonic acid-induced experimental colitis? *Dig Dis Sci* 1:102–8.

Aghdassi, E., B. E. Wendland, A. H. Steinhart et al. 2003. Antioxidant vitamin supplementation in Crohn's disease decreases oxidative stress. A randomized controlled trial. *Am J Gastroenterol* 2:348–53.

Andersen, V., A. Olsen, F. Carbonnel et al. 2012. Diet and risk of inflammatory bowel disease. *Dig Liver Dis* 3:185–94.

Assadsangabi, A., and A. J. Lobo. 2013. Diagnosing and managing inflammatory bowel disease. *Practitioner* 1763:13–8, 2.

Baliga, M. S., N. Joseph, M. V. Venkataranganna et al. 2012. Curcumin, an active component of turmeric in the prevention and treatment of ulcerative colitis: Preclinical and clinical observations. *Food Funct* 11:1109–17.

Bernardo, D., B. Martinez-Abad, S. Vallejo-Diez et al. 2012. Ascorbate-dependent decrease of the mucosal immune inflammatory response to gliadin in coeliac disease patients. *Allergol Immunopathol (Madr)* 1:3–8.

Bitiren, M., A. Z. Karakilçik, M. Zerin et al. 2010. Protective effects of selenium and vitamin E combination on experimental colitis in blood plasma and colon of rats. *Biol Trace Elem Res* 1:87–95.

Bousvaros, A., D. Zurakowski, C. Duggan et al. 1998. Vitamins A and E serum levels in children and young adults with inflammatory bowel disease: Effect of disease activity. *J Pediatr Gastroenterol Nutr* 2:129–35.

Brown, A. C., S. D. Rampertab, and G. E. Mullin. 2011. Existing dietary guidelines for Crohn's disease and ulcerative colitis. *Expert Rev Gastroenterol Hepatol* 3:411–25.

Calder, P. C., R. Albers, J. M. Antoine et al. 2009. Inflammatory disease processes and interactions with nutrition. *Br J Nutr* 101(Suppl 1):S1–45.

Camacho-Barquero, L., I. Villegas, J. M. Sanchez-Calvo et al. 2007. Curcumin, a *Curcuma longa* constituent, acts on MAPK p38 pathway modulating COX-2 and iNOS expression in chronic experimental colitis. *Int Immunopharmacol* 3:333–42.

Ciclitira, P. J., D. J. Evans, N. L. Fagg et al. 1984. Clinical testing of gliadin fractions in coeliac patients. *Clin Sci (Lond)* 3:357–64.

Deguchi, Y., A. Andoh, O. Inatomi et al. 2007. Curcumin prevents the development of dextran sulfate sodium (DSS)-induced experimental colitis. *Dig Dis Sci* 11:2993–8.

De Paolo, R. W., V. Abadie, F. Tang et al. 2011. Co-adjuvant effects of retinoic acid and IL-15 induce inflammatory immunity to dietary antigens. *Nature* 7337:220–4.

De Stefano, D., M. C. Maiuri, B. Iovine et al. 2006. The role of NF-kappaB, IRF-1, and STAT-1alpha transcription factors in the iNOS gene induction by gliadin and IFN-gamma in RAW 264.7 macrophages. *J Mol Med (Berl)* 1:65–74.

De Stefano, D., M. C. Maiuri, V. Simeon et al. 2007. Lycopene, quercetin and tyrosol prevent macrophage activation induced by gliadin and IFN-gamma. *Eur J Pharmacol* 1–3:192–9.

D'Odorico, A., S. Bortolan, R. Cardin et al. 2001. Reduced plasma antioxidant concentrations and increased oxidative DNA damage in inflammatory bowel disease. *Scand J Gastroenterol* 12:1289–94.

Engel, M. A., and M. F. Neurath. 2010. New pathophysiological insights and modern treatment of IBD. *J Gastroenterol* 6:571–83.

Ferretti, G., T. Bacchetti, S. Masciangelo et al. 2012. Celiac disease, inflammation and oxidative damage: A nutrigenetic approach. *Nutrients* 4:243–57.

Filippi, J., R. Al-Jaouni, J. B. Wiroth et al. 2006. Nutritional deficiencies in patients with Crohn's disease in remission. *Inflamm Bowel Dis* 3:185–91.

Fries, W., and S. Comunale. 2011. Ulcerative colitis: Pathogenesis. *Curr Drug Targets* 10:1373–82.

Geerling, B. J., A. Badart-Smook, R. W. Stockbrugger et al. 1998. Comprehensive nutritional status in patients with long-standing Crohn disease currently in remission. *Am J Clin Nutr* 5:919–26.

Geerling, B. J., A. Badart-Smook, R. W. Stockbrugger et al. 2000a. Comprehensive nutritional status in recently diagnosed patients with inflammatory bowel disease compared with population controls. *Eur J Clin Nutr* 6:514–21.

Geerling, B. J., A. Badart-Smook, C. van Deursen et al. 2000b. Nutritional supplementation with N-3 fatty acids and antioxidants in patients with Crohn's disease in remission: Effects on antioxidant status and fatty acid profile. *Inflamm Bowel Dis* 2:77–84.

Hall, N. J., G. Rubin, and A. Charnock. 2009. Systematic review: Adherence to a gluten-free diet in adult patients with coeliac disease. *Aliment Pharmacol Ther* 4:315–30.

Hanai, H., T. Iida, K. Takeuchi et al. 2006. Curcumin maintenance therapy for ulcerative colitis: Randomized, multicenter, double-blind, placebo-controlled trial. *Clin Gastroenterol Hepatol* 12:1502–6.

Hart, A. R., R. Luben, A. Olsen et al. 2008. Diet in the aetiology of ulcerative colitis: A European prospective cohort study. *Digestion* 1:57–64.

Holt, P. R., S. Katz, and R. Kirshoff. 2005. Curcumin therapy in inflammatory bowel disease: A pilot study. *Dig Dis Sci* 11:2191–3.

Hou, J. K., B. Abraham, and H. El-Serag. 2011. Dietary intake and risk of developing inflammatory bowel disease: A systematic review of the literature. *Am J Gastroenterol* 4: 563–73.

Jena, G., P. P. Trivedi, and B. Sandala. 2012. Oxidative stress in ulcerative colitis: An old concept but a new concern. *Free Radic Res* 11:1339–45.

Jian, Y. T., G. F. Mai, J. D. Wang et al. 2005. Preventive and therapeutic effects of NF-kappaB inhibitor curcumin in rats colitis induced by trinitrobenzene sulfonic acid. *World J Gastroenterol* 12:1747–52.

Kawakami, Y., H. Okada, Y. Murakami et al. 2007. Dietary intake, neutrophil fatty acid profile, serum antioxidant vitamins and oxygen radical absorbance capacity in patients with ulcerative colitis. *J Nutr Sci Vitaminol (Tokyo)* 2:153–9.

Koutroubakis, I. E., N. Malliaraki, P. D. Dimoulios et al. 2004. Decreased total and corrected antioxidant capacity in patients with inflammatory bowel disease. *Dig Dis Sci* 9:1433–7.

Kumagai, T., N. Matsukawa, Y. Kaneko et al. 2004. A lipid peroxidation-derived inflammatory mediator: Identification of 4-hydroxy-2-nonenal as a potential inducer of cyclooxygenase-2 in macrophages. *J Biol Chem* 46:48389–96.

Lomer, M. C. 2011. Dietary and nutritional considerations for inflammatory bowel disease. *Proc Nutr Soc* 3:329–35.

Meplan, C., and J. Hesketh. 2012. The influence of selenium and selenoprotein gene variants on colorectal cancer risk. *Mutagenesis* 2:177–86.

Mirbagheri, S. A., B. G. Nezami, S. Assa et al. 2008. Rectal administration of d-alpha tocopherol for active ulcerative colitis: A preliminary report. *World J Gastroenterol* 39:5990–5.

Molodecky, N. A., I. S. Soon, D. M. Rabi et al. 2012. Increasing incidence and prevalence of the inflammatory bowel diseases with time, based on systematic review. *Gastroenterology* 1:46–54.e42; quiz e30.

Mouzaoui, S., I. Rahim, and B. Djerdjouri. 2012. Aminoguanidine and curcumin attenuated tumor necrosis factor (TNF)-alpha-induced oxidative stress, colitis and hepatotoxicity in mice. *Int Immunopharmacol* 1:302–11.

Ramakrishna, B. S., R. Varghese, S. Jayakumar et al. 1997. Circulating antioxidants in ulcerative colitis and their relationship to disease severity and activity. *J Gastroenterol Hepatol* 7:490–4.

Reif, S., I. Klein, F. Lubin et al. 1997. Pre-illness dietary factors in inflammatory bowel disease. *Gut* 6:754–60.

Rezaie, A., R. D. Parker, and M. Abdollahi. 2007. Oxidative stress and pathogenesis of inflammatory bowel disease: An epiphenomenon or the cause? *Dig Dis Sci* 9:2015–21.

Ringstad, J., S. Kildebo, and Y. Thomassen. 1993. Serum selenium, copper, and zinc concentrations in Crohn's disease and ulcerative colitis. *Scand J Gastroenterol* 7:605–8.

Romier, B., Y. J. Schneider, Y. Larondelle et al. 2009. Dietary polyphenols can modulate the intestinal inflammatory response. *Nutr Rev* 7:363–78.

Rosman-Urbach, M., Y. Niv, Y. Birk et al. 2006. Relationship between nutritional habits adopted by ulcerative colitis relevant to cancer development patients at clinical remission stages and molecular–genetic parameters. *Br J Nutr* 1:188–95.

Sakamoto, N., S. Kono, K. Wakai et al. 2005. Dietary risk factors for inflammatory bowel disease: A multicenter case–control study in Japan. *Inflamm Bowel Dis* 2:154–63.

Seidner, D. L., B. A. Lashner, A. Brzezinski et al. 2005. An oral supplement enriched with fish oil, soluble fiber, and antioxidants for corticosteroid sparing in ulcerative colitis: A randomized, controlled trial. *Clin Gastroenterol Hepatol* 4:358–69.

Shepherd, S. J., and P. R. Gibson. 2013. Nutritional inadequacies of the gluten-free diet in both recently-diagnosed and long-term patients with coeliac disease. *J Hum Nutr Diet* 4:349–58.

Sousa Guerreiro, C., M. Cravo, A. R. Costa et al. 2007. A comprehensive approach to evaluate nutritional status in Crohn's patients in the era of biologic therapy: A case–control study. *Am J Gastroenterol* 11:2551–6.

Stazi, A. V., and B. Trinti. 2010. Selenium status and over-expression of interleukin-15 in celiac disease and autoimmune thyroid diseases. *Ann Ist Super Sanita* 4:389–99.

Stojiljkovic, V., A. Todorovic, N. Radlovic et al. 2007. Antioxidant enzymes, glutathione and lipid peroxidation in peripheral blood of children affected by coeliac disease. *Ann Clin Biochem* 44(Pt 6):537–43.

Stojiljkovic, V., A. Todorovic, S. Pejic et al. 2009. Antioxidant status and lipid peroxidation in small intestinal mucosa of children with celiac disease. *Clin Biochem* 13–14:1431–7.

Suzuki, T., and H. Hara. 2011. Role of flavonoids in intestinal tight junction regulation. *J Nutr Biochem* 5:401–8.

Szaflarska-Poplawska, A., A. Siomek, M. Czerwionka-Szaflarska et al. 2010. Oxidatively damaged DNA/oxidative stress in children with celiac disease. *Cancer Epidemiol Biomarkers Prev* 8:1960–5.

Tahan, G., E. Aytac, H. Aytekin et al. 2011. Vitamin E has a dual effect of anti-inflammatory and antioxidant activities in acetic acid-induced ulcerative colitis in rats. *Can J Surg* 5:333–8.

Thomson, A., D. Hemphill, and K. N. Jeejeebhoy. 1998. Oxidative stress and antioxidants in intestinal disease. *Dig Dis* 3:152–8.

Tirosh, O., E. Levy, and R. Reifen. 2007. High selenium diet protects against TNBS-induced acute inflammation, mitochondrial dysfunction, and secondary necrosis in rat colon. *Nutrition* 11–12:878–86.

Trebble, T. M. 2005. Bone turnover and nutritional status in Crohn's disease: Relationship to circulating mononuclear cell function and response to fish oil and antioxidants. *Proc Nutr Soc* 2:183–91.

Trebble, T. M., N. K. Arden, S. A. Wootton et al. 2004. Fish oil and antioxidants alter the composition and function of circulating mononuclear cells in Crohn disease. *Am J Clin Nutr* 5:1137–44.

Trebble, T. M., M. A. Stroud, S. A. Wootton et al. 2005. High-dose fish oil and antioxidants in Crohn's disease and the response of bone turnover: A randomised controlled trial. *Br J Nutr* 2:253–61.

Trevisani, M., J. Siemens, S. Materazzi et al. 2007. 4-Hydroxynonenal, an endogenous aldehyde, causes pain and neurogenic inflammation through activation of the irritant receptor TRPA1. *Proc Natl Acad Sci U S A* 33:13519–24.

Troncone, R., R. Auricchio, and V. Granata. 2008a. Issues related to gluten-free diet in coeliac disease. *Curr Opin Clin Nutr Metab Care* 3:329–33.

Troncone, R., A. Ivarsson, H. Szajewska et al. 2008b. Review article: Future research on coeliac disease—A position report from the European multistakeholder platform on coeliac disease (CDEUSSA). *Aliment Pharmacol Ther* 11:1030–43.

Wierdsma, N. J., M. A. van Bokhorst-de van der Schueren, M. Berkenpas et al. 2013. Vitamin and mineral deficiencies are highly prevalent in newly diagnosed celiac disease patients. *Nutrients* 10:3975–92.

Wiese, D. M., B. A. Lashner, E. Lerner et al. 2011. The effects of an oral supplement enriched with fish oil, prebiotics, and antioxidants on nutrition status in Crohn's disease patients. *Nutr Clin Pract* 4:463–73.

Yuce, A., H. Demir, I. N. Temizel et al. 2004. Serum carnitine and selenium levels in children with celiac disease. *Indian J Gastroenterol* 3:87–8.

Zallot, C., D. Quilliot, J. B. Chevaux et al. 2013. Dietary beliefs and behavior among inflammatory bowel disease patients. *Inflamm Bowel Dis* 1:66–72.

Zhang, Y. Z., and Y. Y. Li. 2014. Inflammatory bowel disease: Pathogenesis. *World J Gastroenterol* 1:91–9.

Zhu, H., and Y. R. Li. 2012. Oxidative stress and redox signaling mechanisms of inflammatory bowel disease: Updated experimental and clinical evidence. *Exp Biol Med (Maywood)* 5:474–80.

13 Antioxidants in Obesity and Inflammation

Chrysi Koliaki, Alexander Kokkinos,
and Nicholas Katsilambros

CONTENTS

Introduction 233
Obesity as an Inflammatory Condition 234
Association of Obesity with Oxidative Stress 234
Defective Antioxidant Defense in Obesity 235
Clinical and Experimental Evidence on the Effects of Exogenous
Antioxidants in Obesity 236
    Green Tea Catechins 237
    Anthocyanins and Blueberries 239
    Curcumin 239
    Resveratrol 240
    Coenzyme Q 241
    α-Lipoic Acid 241
    Fruits, Legumes, and Nuts 241
Safety Concerns and Open Questions 242
Recommendations 243
Concluding Remarks and Perspectives 243
References 244

INTRODUCTION

The development of obesity is characterized by an increased number and size of fat cells due to enhanced processes of adipocyte proliferation and differentiation, which are regulated by interacting genetic, metabolic, pharmacological, environmental, and nutritional factors. The key abnormality in obesity is an energy imbalance promoting excess energy storage in adipose tissue, which becomes progressively hypertrophic, hyperplastic, and dysfunctional, and is characterized by severe metabolic stress and disrupted energy metabolism.

Obesity is strongly associated with increased risk for type 2 diabetes mellitus (T2DM) and cardiovascular disease (CVD), mainly due to concomitant chronic subclinical inflammation and oxidative stress (Dali-Youcef et al., 2013; Vincent and Taylor, 2006), providing the rationale for testing the short- and long-term effectiveness of several antioxidant and anti-inflammatory pharmacological and dietary interventions for the prevention and treatment of obesity and its cardiometabolic complications. Experimental data from animal and *in vitro* studies as well as small-scale observational studies in humans suggest beneficial effects of specific antioxidant compounds on obesity-related conditions. However, it is important to note that randomized controlled clinical trials assessing the long-term safety and efficacy of antioxidant supplementation in obese humans are currently limited, inconsistent, and raise a number of methodological issues that warrant a cautious interpretation and critical appraisal of their findings.

OBESITY AS AN INFLAMMATORY CONDITION

Low-grade systemic inflammation is a prominent characteristic of obesity and is defined as a modest upregulation of circulating indicators of inflammation such as leukocyte count and concentrations of acute-phase proteins, pro-inflammatory cytokines, chemokines, soluble adhesion molecules, and prothrombotic mediators. In obese humans, systemic concentrations of pro-inflammatory mediators are consistently higher than in lean individuals, and promote cardiometabolic dysregulation by increasing the risk for insulin resistance and atherosclerosis (Calder et al., 2011). Obesity has been mechanistically linked to low-grade inflammation through the concept that adipose tissue synthesizes and secretes into the circulation a number of biologically active molecules such as hormones, growth factors, inflammatory mediators, and immune system effectors. White adipose tissue is no longer viewed as an inert energy storage organ, but is rather perceived as the largest endocrine gland of the human body. The secretory products of adipose tissue are collectively termed adipokines, and represent the mediating link between local and systemic inflammation in the context of obesity (Tilg and Moschen, 2006). Some adipokines are produced exclusively by adipocytes (leptin, adiponectin), while others are produced by both adipocytes and other cell populations of the stromovascular fraction of adipose tissue, predominantly the resident macrophages that infiltrate the hypertrophic adipose tissue (Weisberg et al., 2003). The anatomical localization of adipose tissue is of paramount importance for determining its physiological function, especially with regard to lipid handling (lipolysis and lipogenesis), gene expression patterns, insulin sensitivity, and profile of secreted adipokines. Central fat accumulation in the thorax and abdomen has been associated with increased systemic inflammation and cardiometabolic risk, whereas peripheral fat distribution is considered metabolically benign (Peppa et al., 2013). Obesity-related chronic low-grade inflammation can be further aggravated by hyperglycemia, which is commonly prevalent in obese humans owing to their concomitant peripheral insulin resistance (Calder et al., 2011).

ASSOCIATION OF OBESITY WITH OXIDATIVE STRESS

Oxidative stress is one of the unifying mechanisms underlying the development of obesity-related comorbidities, mainly T2DM and CVD. In obesity, multiple contributing factors may promote increased oxidative stress, including hyperglycemia, hyperleptinemia, increased tissue lipid availability leading to lipotoxicity, inadequate antioxidant capacity, and chronic subclinical inflammation (Vincent and Taylor, 2006). Data from cross-sectional studies provide solid evidence for increased systemic oxidative stress in obesity. Markers of systemic lipid peroxidation (plasma malondialdehyde levels, thiobarbituric acid reactive substances) are increased in obese humans, and low-density lipoprotein (LDL) cholesterol is oxidized much faster, promoting atherosclerosis (Van Gaal et al., 1998). Urinary isoprostane excretion rates are higher in obese subjects and correlate positively with body mass index (BMI), as shown in the Framingham offspring cohort (Keaney et al., 2003). Plasma isoprostane levels have been also shown to correlate positively with BMI and total and visceral fat mass (Urakawa et al., 2003). Biomarkers of oxidative stress are present in several tissues of obese humans, including plasma, skeletal muscle, and erythrocytes. The strong association between obesity and oxidative stress is highlighted by the finding that measures targeted at reducing body weight, such as physical activity, caloric restriction, and surgical interventions, have been shown to substantially improve biomarkers of oxidative stress in obese humans (Vincent and Taylor, 2006).

DEFECTIVE ANTIOXIDANT DEFENSE IN OBESITY

Antioxidants can be either nonenzymatic (dietary antioxidants and endogenous coenzyme Q) or enzymatic (antioxidant enzymes). Dietary antioxidants mainly comprise vitamins (C, E, β-carotene), antioxidant minerals (zinc, copper, selenium, manganese), and phytochemicals (phenols, flavonoids, lycopene, hydroxytyrosol), while the major antioxidant enzymes include superoxide dismutase (SOD), glutathione peroxidase (GPX), and catalase. The collective antioxidant capacity can be measured by total antioxidant status, representing free radical inhibition attained by all the antioxidants listed above in a tissue sample such as serum or plasma (Vincent and Taylor, 2006).

In the healthy state, endogenous and exogenous antioxidants work cooperatively to maintain the pro-oxidant/antioxidant balance and prevent tissue damage. An adequate combination of enzymatic and nonenzymatic antioxidants is indeed critical to secure cellular homeostasis. In obesity, total antioxidant defense from both endogenous and exogenous (dietary) sources is insufficient (Figure 13.1). A low dietary intake of protective antioxidants and phytochemicals has been reported in obese humans, since these individuals tend to consume relatively low amounts of antioxidant-rich foods such as fruit, vegetables, whole grains, legumes, wine, olive oil, seeds, and nuts (Vincent et al., 2010). This distinct dietary behavior leads to reduced serum levels of vitamins (C, E, β-carotene) and trace minerals such as selenium and zinc, which are important cofactors for proper antioxidant enzyme function (Ozata et al., 2002; Wallström et al., 2001). As a result of poor antioxidant intake, obese humans face an antioxidant deficit, independent of the external metabolic stressors imposed on their body. Beyond that, it has been suggested that dietary antioxidants are more rapidly depleted in obese humans to effectively combat the excessive pro-oxidant processes, leaving them ultimately less defended against free radical toxicity (Vincent and Taylor, 2006). Furthermore, the activity of all major antioxidant enzymes appears to be impaired in obesity. In obese humans, erythrocyte antioxidant enzyme activities (SOD, GPX) are markedly lower compared with their lean counterparts (Olusi, 2002). Of note, all the above data refer to long-standing obesity. Interestingly, it has been proposed that in the early stages of obesity, there might be a transient upregulation of total radical–scavenging capacity to counteract increased

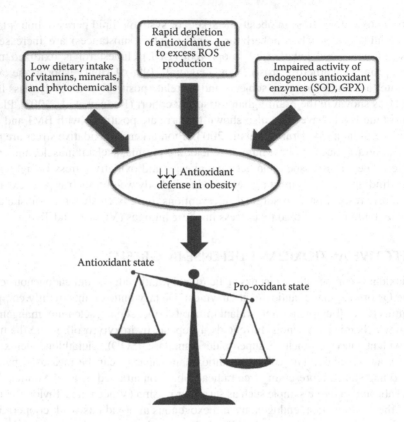

FIGURE 13.1 Mechanisms for reduced antioxidant defense capacity in human long-standing obesity. Low dietary intake of protective antioxidants (vitamins, trace minerals, phytochemicals), rapid depletion of available antioxidants to confront excessive radical production, and impaired activity of antioxidant enzymes all contribute to insufficient antioxidant defense mechanisms in chronically obese humans, shifting the pro-oxidant/antioxidant balance toward increased oxidative stress. GPX, glutathione peroxidase; ROS, reactive oxygen species; SOD, superoxide dismutase.

oxidative stress, which is, however, followed by progressive depletion of all available antioxidants, a process induced by prolonged obesity (Vincent et al., 2001).

In summary, the combination of inadequate dietary and enzymatic antioxidants with increased production of reactive oxygen species (ROS) leads to an imbalance that favors lipid and protein oxidation in obesity. The available antioxidant capacity is "overpowered" by excessive uncontrolled ROS formation in obese humans, shifting the pro-oxidant/antioxidant balance toward oxidative stress.

CLINICAL AND EXPERIMENTAL EVIDENCE ON THE EFFECTS OF EXOGENOUS ANTIOXIDANTS IN OBESITY

The term phytochemicals is used to describe naturally occurring, plant-derived, bioactive compounds that exert beneficial effects in the prevention and treatment of chronic metabolic and inflammatory disorders, including obesity. Dietary polyphenols are considered the leading phytochemicals and comprise catechins, anthocyanins, curcumin, and resveratrol, which are discussed in detail below. These compounds may modulate physiological and molecular pathways involved in energy metabolism, and their antiobesity effects have been demonstrated in cell cultures, animal models of obesity, and clinical/epidemiological studies (Meydani and Hasan, 2010).

GREEN TEA CATECHINS

Green tea has been extensively studied for its putative disease-preventing effects and is rich in polyphenolic flavonoids known as catechins (Sae-tan et al., 2011). A typical brewed green tea beverage (2.5 g green tea in 250 mL hot water) contains 240–320 mg catechins, including epicatechin (EC), epigallocatechin (EGC), epicatechin-3-gallate (ECG), and epigallocatechin-3-gallate (EGCG), which is considered the most abundant and well-studied green tea polyphenol, accounting for approximately 30–50% of total green tea catechin (GTC) content. As summarized in Table 13.1, the main mechanisms suggested to be involved in the antiobesity effects of GTCs have been demonstrated in *in vitro* studies and include (Moon et al., 2007) (i) inhibition of dietary fat absorption resulting in increased fecal lipid excretion due to inhibition of pancreatic lipase and changes in lipid emulsification properties of gastric and duodenal fluids, leading to impaired capacity of pancreatic lipase to digest dietary fat (Nakai et al., 2005); (ii) modulation of lipid metabolism in liver and adipose tissue in the direction of decreased *de novo* lipogenesis and enhanced fat oxidation and thermogenesis in brown adipose tissue (Lee et al., 2009; Park et al., 2011); (iii) activation of the nutrient-sensing enzyme adenosine monophosphate (AMP)-dependent protein kinase (AMPK), which prevents fat accumulation and favors fat oxidation and glucose utilization (Murase et al., 2009); and (iv) modulation of mitogenic, endocrine, and metabolic function of adipocytes (Lin and Lin-Shiau, 2006).

TABLE 13.1

Main Mechanisms Suggested to Be Involved in the Antiobesity Effects of Dietary Polyphenols such as Green Tea Catechins, Resveratrol, and Curcumin

Reduced dietary fat digestion, absorption, and transportation

Decreased lipogenesis in liver and adipose tissue

Increased catecholamine-mediated thermogenesis in brown adipose tissue

Activation of adenosine monophosphate-dependent protein kinase (AMPK)

Increased fat oxidation in the liver and muscle

Inhibition of adipocyte proliferation and differentiation

Suppressed angiogenesis in adipose tissue

Improvement of peripheral glucose uptake

Reduced inflammation in liver and adipose tissue

In more detail, EGCG or EGCG-containing green tea extracts have been shown to reduce food intake, lipid digestion, absorption and transportation, and increase energy expenditure by stimulating thermogenesis in brown adipose tissue through a synergistic interaction with norepinephrine, enhancing fatty acid oxidation in liver and muscle, increasing muscle glucose uptake through glucose transporter-4 (GLUT4) translocation, and promoting fecal lipid excretion (Bose et al., 2008; Klaus et al., 2005). In adipose tissue, EGCG exerts antimitogenic and antilipogenic effects. The antimitogenic effects of EGCG on preadipocytes are mediated by downregulated activities of cell cycle control kinases such as extracellular signal-regulated kinases 1/2 (ERK 1/2) and cyclin-dependent kinase 2 (CDK2), leading to suppressed adipocyte proliferation and differentiation (Lin and Lin-Shiau, 2006). Beyond inhibiting preadipocyte maturation, EGCG may also induce apoptosis in mature adipocytes (Lin et al., 2005). EGCG exerts its antilipogenic effects through inhibited expression and activity of multiple lipogenic enzymes such as acetyl-coA carboxylase (rate-limiting step in fatty acid synthesis), fatty acid synthase, glycerol-3-phosphate dehydrogenase (rate-limiting step in triglyceride biosynthesis), and stearoyl-coA-desaturase 1 (rate-limiting enzyme in monounsaturated fatty acid synthesis) (Ahmad and Mukhtar, 1999; Ikeda et al., 2005; Lee et al., 2009).

Animal data suggest that supplementation of a high-fat diet (HFD) with EGCG results in lower weight gain due to reduced fat absorption from the gut (Bose et al., 2008). In addition to decreasing intestinal fat absorption, EGCG may prevent diet-induced obesity in mice by enhancing fat oxidation and augmenting norepinephrine-mediated sympathetic stimulation of thermogenesis in brown adipose tissue (Klaus et al., 2005). It has been also suggested that long-term green tea supplementation in animal models of obesity may exert beneficial metabolic effects, leading to a significant decline in fasting glucose and insulin levels and improved insulin sensitivity (Wu et al., 2004).

With regard to clinical data, not all epidemiological studies provide clear-cut evidence that green tea consumption is linked to body weight. A cross-sectional study conducted in Taiwan reported an association of habitual green tea consumption with lower body fat mass (Wu et al., 2003), in line with a longitudinal study from the Netherlands showing that green tea consumption is associated with lower BMI (Hughes et al., 2008). However, other studies found no association of green tea with adiposity measures, but only with an improved lipoprotein profile, which is beneficial for the overall obesity-associated atherosclerotic risk. In one of these studies, green tea consumption was associated with reduced total and LDL cholesterol but not with body weight (Tokunaga et al., 2002). In another study performed in male subjects over the age of 40 years, green tea consumption again displayed no correlation with body weight, but was associated with increased high-density lipoprotein (HDL) cholesterol and decreased LDL cholesterol and triglycerides (Imai and Nakachi, 1995). Thus, the epidemiological (cross-sectional and prospective) data remain inconsistent. Similarly controversial are the data regarding the effects of GTCs on energy expenditure and fat oxidation in humans. In one study comparing an EGCG-containing green tea extract enriched with 50 mg caffeine against caffeine alone, the green tea extract formulation was significantly more potent in stimulating 24-h energy expenditure, fat oxidation, and urinary norepinephrine excretion in healthy male humans (Dulloo et al., 1999). In contrast with these data, in another study in overweight and moderately obese male and female subjects, green tea extracts rich in EGCG and caffeine consumed for 13 weeks were not associated with maintenance of body weight lost after a very-low-calorie diet, indicating no effects of GTCs on fat oxidation and energy homeostasis (Kovacs et al., 2004). With regard to controlled clinical intervention trials, they suggest overall that long-term consumption of green tea at high doses may be effective in reducing body weight and fat mass in humans (Saetan et al., 2011), particularly when combined with physical activity (Venables et al., 2008). In a clinical study, it was shown that an EGCG-rich green tea extract reduced body weight and waist circumference by 4.5% in moderately obese patients after 3 months of treatment (Chantre and Lairon, 2002). In the same direction, daily ingestion of one bottle of tea rich in GTCs (690 mg) for 12 weeks resulted in lower body weight, waist circumference, and total and subcutaneous fat, compared with a bottle of tea with a lower amount of GTCs (22 mg) (Nagao et al., 2005). The heterogeneity of data presented above must be acknowledged and is possibly related to differences in the treatment protocols employed, the purity of extracts tested, the percentage of concomitant caffeine enrichment, the duration of intervention, and the distinct physiological characteristics of the studied participants.

ANTHOCYANINS AND BLUEBERRIES

Anthocyanins are the major active component of blueberries, which are fruit rich in bioactive polyphenolic compounds such as hydroxycinnamic acid, flavonoids, proanthocyanidines, and anthocyanins. Blueberry juice can be biotransformed within the gut by *Serratia vaccinii* bacteria, increasing its polyphenolic content and quadrupling its antioxidant activity (Meydani and Hasan, 2010).

In animal studies, it has been shown that supplementation of an HFD with purified anthocyanins extracted from blueberries has no marked effects on body weight, hepatic steatosis, and food intake, but exerts beneficial metabolic effects on serum lipids, fasting glucose, leptin levels, and β-cell function (Prior et al., 2009). Of note, the same effects are not accomplished with administration of blueberry extracts, suggesting that the absorption and bioavailability of anthocyanins from the gut may be hindered by the concomitant presence of carbohydrates and lipids contained in whole blueberry extracts (Prior et al., 2008). In a mouse model of obesity and diabetes, chronic administration of anthocyanins failed to reduce body weight, but decreased fasting glucose and increased adiponectin (Vuong et al., 2009). In another animal study, supplementation of an HFD with whole blueberry powder again showed no effects on body weight, but improved insulin sensitivity and glucose homeostasis due to inhibition of macrophage infiltration in adipose tissue (DeFuria et al., 2009).

In summary, anthocyanins and blueberry extracts seem to have no beneficial effects on obesity per se, but may favorably impact obesity-associated conditions such as insulin resistance and inflammation, thus promoting cardiometabolic health.

CURCUMIN

Curcumin is the major, low-molecular, bioactive polyphenol found in the spice turmeric and possesses a great number of biological properties such as antioxidant, anti-inflammatory, anticancer, antiangiogenetic, chemopreventive, and chemotherapeutic effects. Cell culture and animal studies suggest that curcumin may modulate energy metabolism, ameliorate inflammation, and suppress angiogenesis, which might also account for its anticancer effects (Strimpakos and Sharma, 2008). With regard to obesity, curcumin has been shown to inhibit the expression of several growth factors in adipose tissue such as vascular endothelial growth factor, fibroblast growth factor, epidermal growth factor, and angiopoietin, leading to reduced angiogenesis in adipose tissue and thus preventing its expansion (antiadipogenic effect) (Gururaj et al., 2002). Of note, the antiobesity effects of curcumin have been mainly studied in animal experiments, whereas intervention studies in humans are mainly focused on its anti-inflammatory and anticancer properties.

In HFD-fed mice, curcumin supplementation reduced the density of microvessels in adipose tissue, providing direct evidence for suppressed angiogenesis (Ejaz et al., 2009). In addition, it activated AMPK, downregulated lipogenic gene expression, and enhanced fat oxidation. In hamsters, supplementation of an HFD with curcumin reduced blood lipids, leptin levels, and insulin resistance (Jang et al., 2008). Furthermore, in a mouse model of obesity and insulin resistance, a generous amount of curcumin in the diet significantly improved glycemic control and reduced hepatic and adipose tissue inflammation, in addition to lowering body weight and fat mass as measured by magnetic resonance imaging (Weisberg et al., 2008).

RESVERATROL

Resveratrol is a well-studied polyphenol, which is present, among other foods, in grapes, red wine, peanuts, and ground nuts, and is considered protective against CVD, T2DM, aging, cancer, and obesity through its pluripotent antioxidant and anti-inflammatory properties. Studies in animal models have shown that resveratrol induces biological effects similar to those observed after caloric restriction, such as increased longevity and prevention of age-associated cardiometabolic abnormalities (Barger et al., 2008). It acts by stimulating AMPK activity, thus leading to enhanced fat oxidation and peripheral glucose uptake through GLUT4 translocation (Zang et al., 2006). It has also been suggested that it may upregulate sirtuin 1 activity, which deacetylates and activates a critical transcription factor related to mitochondrial biogenesis (peroxisome proliferator-activated receptor γ co-activator 1a), leading to increased oxidative phosphorylation capacity and reduced lipid accumulation (Lagouge et al., 2006). *In vitro* data from cell cultures and gene microarray analyses have shown that resveratrol inhibits adipogenesis and enhances lipolysis in isolated human adipocytes, and downregulates the expression of lipogenic genes in hepatic tissue (Ahn et al., 2008). Through its potent antioxidant activity, resveratrol may also prevent oxidative damage related to impaired glucose metabolism, thus preventing the pathogenesis of diabetic complications.

Resveratrol treatment has been shown to significantly reduce total and regional body fat in both genetic and diet-induced animal models of adiposity (Meydani and Hasan, 2010). In humans, a double-blinded, placebo-controlled, randomized, cross-over clinical trial showed that resveratrol treatment for 30 days (150 mg/day) improved adipose tissue function in healthy obese men, by decreasing adipocyte size and upregulating intracellular pathways related to lysosomal and phagosomal processes, suggesting autophagy as an alternative mechanism of resveratrol-induced lipid breakdown (Konings et al., 2013).

Despite compelling evidence from molecular, cell culture, and animal studies that resveratrol may contribute to the prevention of obesity, epidemiological and randomized clinical trials are needed to substantiate its effects on humans.

COENZYME Q

Coenzyme Q (CoQ) is the only nonenzymatic antioxidant synthesized by humans and the single lipid component of the mitochondrial electron transport chain, regulating mitochondrial membrane permeability and activity of uncoupling proteins at a subcellular level (Turunen et al., 2004). CoQ is at the crossroad between oxidative stress and mitochondria, which are thought to play a crucial role in adipocyte differentiation and energy metabolism in obesity. A strong negative correlation between CoQ content in adipose tissue and obesity markers in rodents and humans has been found. In mice, HFD-induced obesity depletes CoQ from subcutaneous adipose tissue, whereas a long-term increase in CoQ content by gene overexpression related to its synthesis inhibits adipogenesis, suggesting CoQ as a potent antiadipogenic factor (Bour et al., 2011). In obese humans, adipose tissue CoQ levels are markedly reduced and a critical threshold of CoQ content in adipose tissue has been identified, below which all rodents and humans develop an obese phenotype (species-conserved threshold value) (Bour et al., 2011). In the clinical setting, CoQ treatment for 8–9 weeks has been associated with a clear body weight reduction in obese humans (Van Gaal et al., 1984).

α-LIPOIC ACID

α-Lipoic acid (ALA) is a naturally occurring short-chain fatty acid, which serves as an essential cofactor for enzymes of the mitochondrial respiratory chain. It is a powerful antioxidant and widely used as a nutrient supplement due to its antioxidant properties. It has been shown that ALA supplementation may prevent lipid peroxidation and oxidative DNA damage in obese rats, suppress *ad libitum* food intake, increase whole-body energy expenditure, reduce body weight and visceral fat mass, and additionally decrease blood glucose and insulin levels (Kim et al., 2004). Since ALA was effective after both intraperitoneal and intracerebrovascular administration in animal studies, the central nervous system appears as the primary site of its anorexigenic effects, which are particularly mediated by suppressed hypothalamic AMPK activity (Kim et al., 2004). In humans, the antiobesity effects of ALA supplementation are less prominent. In a double-blinded, placebo-controlled, randomized clinical trial in a large number of overweight and obese subjects with comorbidities, ALA treatment for 20 weeks led to minimal weight loss (2.1%) only at the highest dosage (1800 mg/day) (Koh et al., 2011).

FRUITS, LEGUMES, AND NUTS

A nutritional intervention study in obese men and women comparing two energy-restricted diets enriched or not in fruits for 8 weeks showed that both diets led to significant weight loss, but only the fruit-enriched diet resulted in an additional decrease of oxidized LDL cholesterol and increase of total serum antioxidant capacity (Crujeiras et al., 2006). Legumes are also a significant dietary source of polyphenolic compounds, including flavonoids, isoflavones, phenolic acids, and lignans. In a nutritional intervention study, soya consumption increased total plasma antioxidant capacity in obese postmenopausal women (Azadbakht et al., 2007), while more common legumes such as beans, lentils, and chickpeas have been shown to improve cardiovascular risk factors and biomarkers of oxidative stress in obese humans. Consumption of four servings of legumes per week within a weight reduction program followed for 8 weeks led to more significant weight loss compared with a diet without frequent legume consumption, and furthermore improved plasma antioxidant capacity and decreased circulating proatherogenic cholesterol levels (Crujeiras et al., 2007). Additional metabolic benefits of legumes are their satiety-promoting effects and their potential to alleviate the negative effects induced by hypocaloric diets on lean body mass and basal metabolic rate (Abete et al., 2008).

Nuts represent one more "functional" food with multiple bioactive compounds. The American Heart Association has recommended regular nut consumption since 2000 (Krauss et al., 2000). Their mono- and polyunsaturated fat content relates to their lipid-lowering effects, while their rich concentration of copper, magnesium, tocopherols, squalene, and phytosterols accounts for their strong antioxidant capacity (Alexiadou and Katsilambros, 2011). The concern that they might promote weight gain due to their high energy density is not evidence-based, since it has been shown that subjects who consume nuts more than 2 times per week have a lower risk of prospective weight gain than those who eat rarely or no nuts, after adjusting for several obesity-related factors (Bes-Rastrollo et al., 2007).

SAFETY CONCERNS AND OPEN QUESTIONS

In observational and laboratory studies, high doses of EGCG have been associated with hepatotoxicity (hepatic necrosis and inflammation) (Lambert et al., 2010). In humans, a limited number of controlled clinical trials have been conducted to determine the maximum tolerated dose of GTCs administered via diet or in alternative formulations such as pills or capsules. To date, no large-scale human intervention study has reported any serious adverse effects with GTCs. Mild adverse effects have been reported in a few cases of resveratrol treatment in humans (Cottart et al., 2009), while in animal studies high doses of resveratrol supplementation have been associated with anemia, nephrotoxicity, hepatotoxicity, increased homocysteine, and reduced HDL cholesterol levels (Crowell et al., 2004; Noll et al., 2009).

Beyond the underexplored safety issues related to long-term antioxidant supplementation in humans, there is also a number of aspects that have not been adequately addressed yet. The primary molecular and cellular targets of action of dietary antioxidants, their dose-response relationships, their threshold dose, and, most important, the translation of animal and *in vitro* data to human intervention studies remain relevant unresolved questions. Of note, the major proposed mechanisms of action are based on *in vitro* studies and occur only at high concentrations of the tested compounds. Owing to the absence of compelling *in vivo* evidence supporting these mechanisms, their *in vivo* relevance still remains uncertain. Furthermore, it has been intriguingly suggested that antioxidant supplements beyond critical concentrations may not only fail to accomplish the desired effects but also lead to opposite results from those anticipated (Spanou et al., 2010). For all the above reasons, the positive study findings with antioxidant supplementation in humans should be viewed and interpreted with caution.

RECOMMENDATIONS

At present, there is no sufficient evidence to support the long-term use of exogenous antioxidant supplements as a safe and effective measure for the prevention and treatment of obesity and its concomitant state of low-grade inflammation. The routine supplementation of diet with antioxidants and vitamins is therefore not considered necessary (Katsilambros et al., 2006). Nevertheless, the integration of healthy foods containing bioactive compounds in the context of a balanced energy-restricted dietary pattern can help maintain a normal body weight and prevent obesity-related cardiometabolic complications.

Finally, coffee, which also possesses antioxidant properties, may also be included as part of a healthy, heart-friendly diet. A recent review of the currently available evidence on the effects of habitual coffee intake on cardiometabolic outcomes has clearly demonstrated that a moderate daily consumption of two to three cups of coffee (300 mg caffeine) is safe, harmless, and associated with neutral to beneficial health outcomes for the general public (O'Keefe et al., 2013). In the same lines, there is evidence that green coffee extract may also exert a beneficial effect on weight, although the existing data are still not unequivocal (Onakpoya et al., 2011).

CONCLUDING REMARKS AND PERSPECTIVES

Despite uncertainties, nutritional intervention remains the safest and most cost-effective treatment and prevention option for obesity and the metabolic syndrome. Although antioxidant supplementation should be viewed with caution, consumption of foods with anti-inflammatory and antioxidant properties should be considered an important component of a dietary approach against obesity and CVD. A diet rich in antioxidant compounds may enhance the benefits of weight loss, especially in patients with metabolic syndrome and high cardiovascular risk.

Further *in vivo* studies examining the primary molecular and cellular mechanisms of action of dietary antioxidants, and their temporal and dose-response relationships, are warranted. As to safety issues, the therapeutic index of all suggested antioxidant agents must be established, not only when these compounds are delivered through the diet, but especially when they are converted to a bolus formulation such as a pill or capsule (pharmacokinetic studies). Only with complete understanding of all possible effects and side effects of antioxidant interventions can their potential benefits for the prevention and treatment of obesity and obesity-related comorbidities be fully unraveled and critically appraised.

REFERENCES

Abete, I., Parra, D., Martinez, J.A. 2008. Energy-restricted diets based on a distinct food selection affecting the glycemic index induce different weight loss and oxidative response. *Clin Nutr* 27:545–51.

Ahmad, N., Mukhtar, H. 1999. Green tea polyphenols and cancer: Biologic mechanisms and practical implications. *Nutr Rev* 57:78–83.

Ahn, J., Cho, I., Kim, S., Kwon, D., Ha, T. 2008. Dietary resveratrol alters lipid metabolism-related gene expression of mice on an atherogenic diet. *J Hepatol* 49:1019–28.

Alexiadou, K., Katsilambros, N. 2011. Nuts: Anti-atherogenic food? *Eur J Intern Med* 22:141–6.

Azadbakht, L., Kimiagar, M., Mehrabi, Y., Esmaillzadeh, A., Hu, F.B., Willett, W.C. 2007. Dietary soya intake alters plasma antioxidant status and lipid peroxidation in postmenopausal women with the metabolic syndrome. *Br J Nutr* 98:807–13.

Barger, J.L., Kayo, T., Vann, J.M., Arias, E.B., Wang, J., Hacker, T.A., Wang, Y., Raederstorff, D., Morrow, J.D., Leeuwenburgh, C., Allison, D.B., Saupe, K.W., Cartee, G.D., Weindruch, R., Prolla, T.A. 2008. A low dose of dietary resveratrol partially mimics caloric restriction and retards aging parameters in mice. *PLoS One* 3:e2264.

Bes-Rastrollo, M., Sabaté, J., Gómez-Gracia, E., Alonso, A., Martínez, J.A., Martínez-González, M.A. 2007. Nut consumption and weight gain in a Mediterranean cohort: The SUN study. *Obesity (Silver Spring)* 15:107–16.

Bose, M., Lambert, J.D., Ju, J., Reuhl, K.R., Shapses, S.A., Yang, C.S. 2008. The major green tea polyphenol, (–)-epigallocatechin-3-gallate, inhibits obesity, metabolic syndrome, and fatty liver disease in high-fat-fed mice. *J Nutr* 138:1677–83.

Bour, S., Carmona, M.C., Galinier, A., Caspar-Bauguil, S., Van Gaal, L., Staels, B., Pénicaud, L., Casteilla, L. 2011. Coenzyme Q as an antiadipogenic factor. *Antioxid Redox Signal* 14:403–13.

Calder, P.C., Ahluwalia, N., Brouns, F., Buetler, T., Clement, K., Cunningham, K., Esposito, K., Jönsson, L.S., Kolb, H., Lansink, M., Marcos, A., Margioris, A., Matusheski, N., Nordmann, H., O'Brien, J., Pugliese, G., Rizkalla, S., Schalkwijk, C., Tuomilehto, J., Wärnberg, J., Watzl, B., Winklhofer-Roob, B.M. 2011. Dietary factors and low-grade inflammation in relation to overweight and obesity. *Br J Nutr* 106 Suppl 3:S5–78.

Chantre, P., Lairon, D. 2002. Recent findings of green tea extract AR25 (Exolise) and its activity for the treatment of obesity. *Phytomedicine* 9:3–8.

Cottart, C.H., Nivet-Antoine, V., Laguillier-Morizot, C., Beaudeux, J.L. 2009. Resveratrol bioavailability and toxicity in humans. *Mol Nutr Food Res* 54:7–16.

Crowell, J.A., Korytko, P.J., Morrissey, R.L., Booth, T.D., Levine, B.S. 2004. Resveratrol-associated renal toxicity. *Toxicol Sci* 82:614–9.

Crujeiras, A.B., Parra, M.D., Rodríguez, M.C., Martínez de Morentin, B.E., Martínez, J.A. 2006. A role for fruit content in energy-restricted diets in improving antioxidant status in obese women during weight loss. *Nutrition* 22:593–9.

Crujeiras, A.B., Parra, D., Abete, I., Martínez, J.A. 2007. A hypocaloric diet enriched in legumes specifically mitigates lipid peroxidation in obese subjects. *Free Radic Res* 41:498–506.

Dali-Youcef, N., Mecili, M., Ricci, R., Andrès, E. 2013. Metabolic inflammation: Connecting obesity and insulin resistance. *Ann Med* 45:242–53.

DeFuria, J., Bennett, G., Strissel, K.J., Perfield, J.W. 2nd, Milbury, P.E., Greenberg, A.S., Obin, M.S. 2009. Dietary blueberry attenuates whole-body insulin resistance in high fat-fed mice by reducing adipocyte death and its inflammatory sequelae. *J Nutr* 139:1510–6.

Dulloo, A.G., Duret, C., Rohrer, D., Girardier, L., Mensi, N., Fathi, M., Chantre, P., Vandermander, J. 1999. Efficacy of a green tea extract rich in catechin polyphenols and caffeine in increasing 24-h energy expenditure and fat oxidation in humans. *Am J Clin Nutr* 70:1040–5.

Ejaz, A., Wu, D., Kwan, P., Meydani, M. 2009. Curcumin inhibits adipogenesis in 3T3-L1 adipocytes and angiogenesis and obesity in C57/BL mice. *J Nutr* 139:919–25.

Gururaj, A.E., Belakavadi, M., Venkatesh, D.A., Marmé, D., Salimath, B.P. 2002. Molecular mechanisms of anti-angiogenic effect of curcumin. *Biochem Biophys Res Commun* 297:934–42.

Hughes, L.A., Arts, I.C., Ambergen, T., Brants, H.A., Dagnelie, P.C., Goldbohm, R.A., van den Brandt, P.A., Weijenberg, M.P.; Netherlands Cohort Study. 2008. Higher dietary flavone, flavonol, and catechin intakes are associated with less of an increase in BMI over time in women: A longitudinal analysis from the Netherlands Cohort Study. *Am J Clin Nutr* 88:1341–52.

Ikeda, I., Hamamoto, R., Uzu, K., Imaizumi, K., Nagao, K., Yanagita, T., Suzuki, Y., Kobayashi, M., Kakuda, T. 2005. Dietary gallate esters of tea catechins reduce deposition of visceral fat, hepatic triacylglycerol, and activities of hepatic enzymes related to fatty acid synthesis in rats. *Biosci Biotechnol Biochem* 69:1049–53.

Imai, K., Nakachi, K. 1995. Cross sectional study of effects of drinking green tea on cardiovascular and liver diseases. *BMJ* 310:693–6.

Jang, E.M., Choi, M.S., Jung, U.J., Kim, M.J., Kim, H.J., Jeon, S.M., Shin, S.K., Seong, C.N., Lee, M.K. 2008. Beneficial effects of curcumin on hyperlipidemia and insulin resistance in high-fat-fed hamsters. *Metabolism* 57:1576–83.

Katsilambros, N., Liatis, S., Makrilakis, K. 2006. Critical review of the international guidelines: What is agreed upon—What is not? *Nestle Nutr Workshop Ser Clin Perform Programme* 11:207–18; discussion 218.

Keaney, J.F. Jr., Larson, M.G., Vasan, R.S., Wilson, P.W., Lipinska, I., Corey, D., Massaro, J.M., Sutherland, P., Vita, J.A., Benjamin, E.J.; Framingham Study. 2003. Obesity and systemic oxidative stress: Clinical correlates of oxidative stress in the Framingham Study. *Arterioscler Thromb Vasc Biol* 23:434–9.

Kim, M.S., Park, J.Y., Namkoong, C., Jang, P.G., Ryu, J.W., Song, H.S., Yun, I Y., Namgoong, I.S., Ha, J., Park, I.S., Lee, I.K., Viollet, B, Youn, J.H., Lee, H.K., Lee, K.U. 2004. Antiobesity effects of alpha-lipoic acid mediated by suppression of hypothalamic AMP-activated protein kinase. *Nat Med* 10:727–33.

Klaus, S., Pültz, S., Thöne-Reineke, C., Wolfram, S. 2005. Epigallocatechin gallate attenuates diet-induced obesity in mice by decreasing energy absorption and increasing fat oxidation. *Int J Obes (Lond)* 29:615–23.

Koh, E.H., Lee, W.J., Lee, S.A., Kim, E.H., Cho, E.H., Jeong, E., Kim, D.W., Kim, M.S., Park, J.Y., Park, K.G., Lee, H.J., Lee, I.K., Lim, S., Jang, H.C., Lee, K.H., Lee, K.U. 2011. Effects of alpha-lipoic acid on body weight in obese subjects. *Am J Med* 124:85.e1–8.

Konings, E., Timmers, S., Boekschoten, M.V., Goossens, G.H., Jocken, J.W., Afman, L.A., Müller, M., Schrauwen, P., Mariman, E.C., Blaak, E.E. 2013. The effects of 30 days resveratrol supplementation on adipose tissue morphology and gene expression patterns in obese men. *Int J Obes (Lond)* 38:470–3.

Kovacs, E.M., Lejeune, M.P., Nijs, I., Westerterp-Plantenga, M.S. 2004. Effects of green tea on weight maintenance after body-weight loss. *Br J Nutr* 91:431–7.

Krauss, R.M., Eckel, R.H., Howard, B., Appel, L.J., Daniels, S.R., Deckelbaum, R.J., Erdman, J.W. Jr., Kris-Etherton, P., Goldberg, I.J., Kotchen, T.A., Lichtenstein, A.H., Mitch, W.E., Mullis, R., Robinson, K., Wylie-Rosett, J., St. Jeor, S., Suttie, J., Tribble, D.L., Bazzarre, T.L. 2000. AHA Dietary Guidelines: Revision 2000: A statement for healthcare professionals from the Nutrition Committee of the American Heart Association. *Circulation* 102:2284–99.

Lagouge, M., Argmann, C., Gerhart-Hines, Z., Meziane, H., Lerin, C., Daussin, F., Messadeq, N., Milne, J., Lambert, P., Elliott, P., Geny, B., Laakso, M., Puigserver, P., Auwerx, J. 2006. Resveratrol improves mitochondrial function and protects against metabolic disease by activating SIRT1 and PGC-1alpha. *Cell* 127:1109–22.

Lambert, J.D., Kennett, M.J., Sang, S., Reuhl, K.R., Ju, J., Yang, C.S. 2010. Hepatotoxicity of high oral dose (−)-epigallocatechin-3-gallate in mice. *Food Chem Toxicol* 48:409–16.

Lee, M.S., Kim, C.T., Kim, Y. 2009. Green tea (−)-epigallocatechin-3-gallate reduces body weight with regulation of multiple genes expression in adipose tissue of diet-induced obese mice. *Ann Nutr Metab* 54:151–7.

Lin, J.K., Lin-Shiau, S.Y. 2006. Mechanisms of hypolipidemic and anti-obesity effects of tea and tea polyphenols. *Mol Nutr Food Res* 50:211–7.

Lin, J., Della-Fera, M.A., Baile, C.A. 2005. Green tea polyphenol epigallocatechin gallate inhibits adipogenesis and induces apoptosis in 3T3-L1 adipocytes. *Obes Res* 13:982–90.

Meydani, M., Hasan, S.T. 2010. Dietary polyphenols and obesity. *Nutrients* 2:737–51.

Moon, H.S., Lee, H.G., Choi, Y.J., Kim, T.G., Cho, C.S. 2007. Proposed mechanisms of (−)-epigallocatechin-3-gallate for anti-obesity. *Chem Biol Interact* 167:85–98.

Murase, T., Misawa, K., Haramizu, S., Hase, T. 2009. Catechin-induced activation of the LKB1/AMP-activated protein kinase pathway. *Biochem Pharmacol* 78:78–84.

Nagao, T., Komine, Y., Soga, S., Meguro, S., Hase, T., Tanaka, Y., Tokimitsu, I. 2005. Ingestion of a tea rich in catechins leads to a reduction in body fat and malondialdehyde-modified LDL in men. *Am J Clin Nutr* 81:122–9.

Nakai, M., Fukui, Y., Asami, S., Toyoda-Ono, Y., Iwashita, T., Shibata, H., Mitsunaga, T., Hashimoto, F., Kiso, Y. 2005. Inhibitory effects of oolong tea polyphenols on pancreatic lipase *in vitro*. *J Agric Food Chem* 53:4593–8.

Noll, C., Hamelet, J., Ducros, V., Belin, N., Paul, J.L., Delabar, J.M., Janel, N. 2009. Resveratrol supplementation worsens the dysregulation of genes involved in hepatic lipid homeostasis observed in hyperhomocysteinemic mice. *Food Chem Toxicol* 47:230–6.

O'Keefe, J.H., Bhatti, S.K., Patil, H.R., DiNicolantonio, J.J., Lucan, S.C., Lavie, C.J. 2013. Effects of habitual coffee consumption on cardiometabolic disease, cardiovascular health, and all-cause mortality. *J Am Coll Cardiol* 62:1043–51.

Olusi, S.O. 2002. Obesity is an independent risk factor for plasma lipid peroxidation and depletion of erythrocyte cytoprotectic enzymes in humans. *Int J Obes Relat Metab Disord* 26:1159–64.

Onakpoya, I., Terry, R., Ernst, E. 2011. The use of green coffee extract as a weight loss supplement: A systematic review and meta-analysis of randomised clinical trials. *Gastroenterol Res Pract* pii:382852.

Ozata, M., Mergen, M., Oktenli, C., Aydin, A., Sanisoglu, S.Y., Bolu, E., Yilmaz, M.I., Sayal, A., Isimer, A., Ozdemir, I.C. 2002. Increased oxidative stress and hypozincemia in male obesity. *Clin Biochem* 35:627–31.

Park, H.J., DiNatale, D.A., Chung, M.Y., Park, Y.K., Lee, J.Y., Koo, S.I., O'Connor, M., Manautou, J.E., Bruno, R.S. 2011. Green tea extract attenuates hepatic steatosis by decreasing adipose lipogenesis and enhancing hepatic antioxidant defenses in ob/ob mice. *J Nutr Biochem* 22:393–400.

Peppa, M., Koliaki, C., Hadjidakis, D.I., Garoflos, E., Papaefstathiou, A., Katsilambros, N., Raptis, S.A., Dimitriadis, G.D. 2013. Regional fat distribution and cardiometabolic risk in healthy postmenopausal women. *Eur J Intern Med* 24:824–31.

Prior, R.L., Wu, X., Gu, L., Hager, T.J., Hager, A., Howard, L.R. 2008. Whole berries versus berry anthocyanins: Interactions with dietary fat levels in the C57BL/6J mouse model of obesity. *J Agric Food Chem* 56:647–53.

Prior, R.L., Wu, X., Gu, L., Hager, T., Hager, A., Wilkes, S., Howard, L. 2009. Purified berry anthocyanins but not whole berries normalize lipid parameters in mice fed an obesogenic high fat diet. *Mol Nutr Food Res* 53:1406–18.

Sae-tan, S., Grove, K.A., Lambert, J.D. 2011. Weight loss and prevention of metabolic syndrome by green tea. *Pharmacol Res* 64:146–54.

Spanou, C., Stagos, D., Aligiannis, N., Kouretas, D. 2010. Influence of potent antioxidant Leguminosae family plant extracts on growth and antioxidant defense system of Hep2 cancer cell line. *J Med Food* 13:149–55.

Strimpakos, A.S., Sharma, R.A. 2008. Curcumin: Preventive and therapeutic properties in laboratory studies and clinical trials. *Antioxid Redox Signal* 10:511–45.

Tilg, H., Moschen, A.R. 2006. Adipocytokines: Mediators linking adipose tissue, inflammation and immunity. *Nat Rev Immunol* 6:772–83.

Tokunaga, S., White, I.R., Frost, C., Tanaka, K., Kono, S., Tokudome, S., Akamatsu, T., Moriyama, T., Zakouji, H. 2002. Green tea consumption and serum lipids and lipoproteins in a population of healthy workers in Japan. *Ann Epidemiol* 12:157–65.

Turunen, M., Olsson, J., Dallner, G. 2004. Metabolism and function of coenzyme Q. *Biochim Biophys Acta* 1660:171–99.

Urakawa, H., Katsuki, A., Sumida, Y., Gabazza, E.C., Murashima, S., Morioka, K., Maruyama, N., Kitagawa, N., Tanaka, T., Hori, Y., Nakatani, K., Yano, Y., Adachi, Y. 2003. Oxidative stress is associated with adiposity and insulin resistance in men. *J Clin Endocrinol Metab* 88:4673–6.

Van Gaal, L., De Leeuw, I., Vadhanavikit, S., Folkers, K. 1984. *Exploratory Study of Coenzyme Q10 in Obesity. Biomedical and Clinical Aspects of Coenzyme Q.* Martinsried, Munich: FRG, pp. 369–72.

Van Gaal, L.F., Vertommen, J., De Leeuw, I.H. 1998. The *in vitro* oxidizability of lipoprotein particles in obese and non-obese subjects. *Atherosclerosis* 137 Suppl:S39–44.

Venables, M.C., Hulston, C.J., Cox, H.R., Jeukendrup, A.E. 2008. Green tea extract ingestion, fat oxidation, and glucose tolerance in healthy humans. *Am J Clin Nutr* 87:778–84.

Vincent, H.K., Powers, S.K., Dirks, A.J., Scarpace, P.J. 2001. Mechanism for obesity-induced increase in myocardial lipid peroxidation. *Int J Obes Relat Metab Disord* 25:378–88.

Vincent, H.K., Taylor, A.G. 2006. Biomarkers and potential mechanisms of obesity-induced oxidant stress in humans. *Int J Obes (Lond)* 30:400–18.

Vincent, H.K., Bourguignon, C.M., Taylor, A.G. 2010. Relationship of the dietary phytochemical index to weight gain, oxidative stress and inflammation in overweight young adults. *J Hum Nutr Diet* 23:20–9.

Vuong, T., Benhaddou-Andaloussi, A., Brault, A., Harbilas, D., Martineau, L.C., Vallerand, D., Ramassamy, C., Matar, C., Haddad, P.S. 2009. Antiobesity and antidiabetic effects of biotransformed blueberry juice in KKA(y) mice. *Int J Obes (Lond)* 33:1166–73.

Wallström, P., Wirfält, E., Lahmann, P.H., Gullberg, B., Janzon, L., Berglund, G. 2001. Serum concentrations of beta-carotene and alpha-tocopherol are associated with diet, smoking, and general and central adiposity. *Am J Clin Nutr* 73:777–85.

Weisberg, S.P., McCann, D., Desai, M., Rosenbaum, M., Leibel, R.L., Ferrante, A.W. Jr. 2003. Obesity is associated with macrophage accumulation in adipose tissue. *J Clin Invest* 112:1796–808.

Weisberg, S.P., Leibel, R., Tortoriello, D.V. 2008. Dietary curcumin significantly improves obesity-associated inflammation and diabetes in mouse models of diabesity. *Endocrinology* 149:3549–58.

Wu, C.H., Lu, F.H., Chang, C.S., Chang, T.C., Wang, R.H., Chang, C.J. 2003. Relationship among habitual tea consumption, percent body fat, and body fat distribution. *Obes Res* 11:1088–95.

Wu, L.Y., Juan, C.C., Ho, L.T., Hsu, Y.P., Hwang, L.S. 2004. Effect of green tea supplementation on insulin sensitivity in Sprague–Dawley rats. *J Agric Food Chem* 52:643–8.

Zang, M., Xu, S., Maitland-Toolan, K.A., Zuccollo, A., Hou, X., Jiang, B., Wierzbicki, M., Verbeuren, T.J., Cohen, R.A. 2006. Polyphenols stimulate AMP-activated protein kinase, lower lipids, and inhibit accelerated atherosclerosis in diabetic LDL receptor-deficient mice. *Diabetes* 55:2180–91.

14 Modulation of Immune Response by Antioxidants

Kathrin Becker, Florian Überall,
Dietmar Fuchs, and Johanna M. Gostner

CONTENTS

Introduction 249
Small Redox Molecules and Redox Homeostasis 250
Production of Cellular ROS/RNS 251
Antioxidant Systems 252
TH1-Type Immune Response 254
Monitoring Immune Response *In Vitro* 256
Antioxidants—A Two-Edged Sword 257
Conclusion 258
References 258

INTRODUCTION

Healthy living is the best way to prevent disease. Environmental pollution, sunlight exposure, and many other influences favor radical stress, leading to an increasing number of oxidative stress–associated inflammatory diseases. Cardiovascular disease, cancer, neurological disorders, diabetes, ischemia/reperfusion, or even normal aging processes are characterized by an imbalance between radical generation and neutralization (Dalle-Donne et al., 2006; Dhalla et al., 2000; Jenner, 2003). Free radicals, like reactive oxygen species (ROS) or reactive nitrogen species (RNS), lead to oxidation and nitration of biomolecules, which can subsequently result in destruction of whole cellular compartments (Kovacic and Jacinto, 2001). To protect from radical damage, cells are equipped with a variety of enzymatic and nonenzymatic antioxidant systems. Exogenous antioxidants derived from diet or medications are suggested to support these protective mechanisms; however, excessive antioxidant intake may also lead to adverse effects. In this chapter, we will focus on the interference of antioxidants with immune response and discuss possible consequences of unconsidered high-dose antioxidant supplementation.

SMALL REDOX MOLECULES AND REDOX HOMEOSTASIS

In a redox reaction, electrons are transferred from one molecule to another. One agent becomes reduced by receiving electrons from the reaction partner, which will be oxidized. Such reactions are crucial for life; however, aberrant or excessive oxidation of biomolecules can become damaging for the cell (Davies, 1995).

Free radicals are defined as molecules with one or more unpaired electrons. An unpaired electron extremely raises the reactivity of a molecule. Among the many small redox-active molecules, in particular ROS and RNS, were intensively investigated because of their important roles as both deleterious and beneficial molecules (Valko et al., 2006). Cells continuously produce radicals such as superoxide anion ($O_2^{\bullet-}$) or nitric oxide ($NO^{\bullet}$), which react to a variety of ROS/RNS, such as hydroxyl radical ($HO^{\bullet}$), hydrogen peroxide (H_2O_2), hypochlorite (OCl^-), and peroxynitrite ($ONOO^-$) or nitrogen dioxide ($NO_2^{\bullet}$) (Dröge, 2002; Wink et al., 2011).

Despite the variable structure of redox molecules, they share common mechanisms that harm cells and tissues through damage of proteins, DNA, or lipids (Valko et al., 2007). All components of the DNA, the purine and pyrimidine bases as well as the deoxyribose backbone, were shown to be targets of, e.g., $HO^{\bullet}$ (Halliwell and Gutteridge, 1999). Polyunsaturated fatty acid residues of phospholipids are extremely sensitive to oxidation and are easily attacked by ROS (Siems et al., 1995). Also, the side chains of all amino acid residues of proteins, in particular cysteine and methionine residues, are susceptible to RNS/ROS attacks (Stadtman et al., 2004).

Various mechanisms to counteract ROS have been described: (i) endogenous antioxidant enzymes such as catalase (CAT), glutathione reductase (GSR), or superoxide dismutase (SOD), as well as (ii) nonenzymatic systems such as glutathione (GSH), urate, and coenzyme Q. In addition, other various free amino acids, peptides, and proteins serve as low molecular weight antioxidants (Valko et al., 2006). All these enzymes and molecules have the ability to transform ROS/RNS into more stable, and thus harmless, compounds via redox-based mechanisms.

Production of high levels of ROS/RNS during respiratory burst reaction is an important strategy in the defense against invading pathogens (Decoursey et al., 2005). However, at such high concentrations, free radicals can be hazardous and damage not only target cells but also host cells in the inflamed tissue. Thus, ROS/RNS generation, release, and neutralization has to be tightly regulated during immune response. At low concentrations, ROS/RNS play an important role in many signaling processes as regulatory mediators. Stress response signaling, detoxification, and several immunobiochemical pathways can be activated by ROS/RNS-derived signals in a dose-dependent manner (Gostner et al., 2013; Valko et al., 2007; Wink et al., 2011). Small redox molecules are also involved in the induction and maintenance of cell growth and differentiation. Thus, the cellular redox status is an intrinsic indicator of cellular and systemic homeostasis.

Normally, redox reactions are balanced and a dynamic equilibrium of radical generation and scavenging free radicals exists, called "redox homeostasis." A disturbed equilibrium of pro-oxidant/antioxidant reactions, misbalance between enzymatic and nonenzymatic antioxidant systems in the body, but also an overdose of antioxidant intake, can be reasons for a shift of the redox state, possibly leading to pathological consequences.

There are numerous studies that extrapolate the potential of ROS to trigger specific disease conditions and, in these, immune responses play a major role. An imbalanced redox homeostasis and oxidative stress was described to be associated with diseases that are accompanied by chronic immune activation such as infections, allergies, autoimmune disorders, neurodegenerative diseases, several malignancies, or the normal aging process (Dalle-Donne et al., 2006; Murr et al., 2005; Sayre et al., 2001). Elevated oxidative stress levels are suggested to be involved in the development and progression of chronic diseases. To support the cellular antioxidant machinery in detoxification and neutralization of ROS/RNS, uptake of antioxidant therapeutics and supplements, but also an antioxidant-rich diet, was suggested to be beneficial.

However, for several pathologies, it is questionable if oxidative stress is causative for disease onset or if it is an accompanying factor due to sustained inflammation. Thus, antioxidant treatment would only be helpful in reducing symptoms, but not the disease causes. Unreflected neutralization of reactive species may even cause shortage of RNS/ROS within the cell, which means that no more free radicals can perform their regulatory mechanisms of redox-regulated pathways and further pathologies could develop. Poor or even adverse outcomes of an antioxidant therapy in clinical studies support the view that further/other therapeutic approaches should be considered for such diseases (Bjelakovic et al., 2004; Dotan et al., 2009; Gerss and Köpcke, 2009; Kris-Etherton et al., 2004).

PRODUCTION OF CELLULAR ROS/RNS

Under normal conditions, the main intracellular source of ROS is $O_2^{\cdot-}$, resulting as a by-product from the mitochondrial respiratory chain (Dröge 2002; LeBras et al., 2005); however, xanthine oxidase (McNally et al., 2003), lipid peroxidases (Zhang et al., 2002), cytochrome P450 enzymes (Fleming et al., 2001), and uncoupled NO synthases (Vásquez-Vivar et al., 1998) also produce ROS as secondary products.

NADPH oxidases (NOX) produce ROS as their primary and sole function. NOX are membrane-bound enzyme complexes composed of a catalytic transmembrane spanning subunit and several regulatory proteins (Altenhöfer et al., 2012). The main reaction of NOX is to reduce molecular oxygen to $O_2^{\cdot-}$ (Altenhöfer et al., 2012; Rossi and Zatti, 1964). Phagocyte NOX was first identified to be responsible for the high amounts of $O_2^{\cdot-}$ and H_2O_2 released during the respiratory burst reaction. Excessive stimulation of NOX can become a major source of free radicals (Keisari et al., 1983).

Oxygenation of L-arginine in the presence of NADPH by nitric oxide synthase (NOS) leads to the formation of NO$^{\cdot}$, NADP+, and L-citrulline (McNeill and Channon, 2012). NO$^{\cdot}$ is commonly known to be a regulator of the vasomotor tone. NO$^{\cdot}$ is able to diffuse through cell membranes and can initiate a variety of signaling cascades in a dose-dependent manner (Vignais, 2002; Wink et al., 2011). There exist three types of NOS isoforms: (i) neuronal NOS (nNOS), (ii) endothelial NOS (eNOS), and (iii) inducible NOS (iNOS). nNOS is involved, e.g., in the regulation of synaptic signaling and in the control of muscle contractility and local blood flow, while eNOS is involved in vasodilation, inhibition of platelet aggregation, and leukocyte adhesion, and controls vascular smooth muscle proliferation and endothelial progenitor cell activation (Förstermann and Sessa, 2012). iNOS has effects on vascular functions under conditions of sepsis, and is an important mediator of inflammation. nNOS and eNOS are calcium dependent, while iNOS can act independently. Many tissues express one or more of these isoforms. Low amounts of NO$^\bullet$, at nanomolar concentrations, are normally produced by the constitutively expressed eNOS and nNOS (Mariotto et al., 2004), while iNOS expression is inducible in macrophages, after stimulation with, e.g., lipopolysaccharide (LPS), cytokines like interferon-gamma (IFN-γ), or other proinflammatory stimuli, and NO$^\bullet$ levels can increase up to micromolar concentrations (Thomas et al., 2008). Such large amounts of NO$^\bullet$ can have cytostatic effects. Excessive NO$^\bullet$ production by iNOS can also contribute to chronic inflammatory pathologies and plays a crucial role in septic shock (Förstermann and Sessa, 2012).

ROS and RNS production during the respiratory burst reaction is conducted in the phagosome to minimize damage to cells. The regulation of phagosomal pH and $O_2^{\bullet-}$ production in neutrophils, macrophages, and dendritic cells follows distinct programs due to differences in NOX localization and phagosomal NO$^\bullet$ concentrations (Savina and Amigorena, 2007). The interaction of NO$^\bullet$ and $O_2^{\bullet-}$/ROS can lead to the formation of nitrite (NO$_2^-$), nitrogen dioxide (NO$_2^\bullet$), and also nitrogen trioxide (N$_2$O$_3$). The ROS/RNS balance is important in orchestrating immunomodulatory mechanisms. However, both oxidative and nitrosative stress can interfere with intracellular redox buffer systems and thus result in a decrease of antioxidant ability (Wink et al., 2011).

ANTIOXIDANT SYSTEMS

Various enzymatic and nonenzymatic antioxidant defense systems protect cells against ROS/RNS attacks (Cadenas, 1997), and further preventive and repair mechanisms contribute to the overall protection.

SOD, CAT, and glutathione peroxidase (GPX) are the primary antioxidant enzymes that counteract ROS damage. SODs dismutate $O_2^{\bullet-}$ to H$_2$O$_2$ or molecular oxygen. CAT catalyzes the composition of H$_2$O$_2$ to water and molecular oxygen. GPX requires GSH as an electron donor and converts H$_2$O$_2$ very efficiently to water (Valko et al., 2007).

The primary intracellular nonenzymatic systems are GSH, cysteine/cystine (Cys/CySS) couples, and thioredoxins (TRXs). GSH is the major intracellular redox buffer in mammalian cells. GSH acts as a cofactor for several detoxifying enzymes and as a free radical scavenger. It is able to regenerate important antioxidants, like vitamins, back into their active forms. The capacity to regenerate important antioxidants is linked with the redox state of the glutathione/glutathione-disulfide couple (GSH/GSSH). GSH/GSSH couples are located in the cytoplasm, nucleus, mitochondria, plasma, or other organelles, but at different concentrations and different redox potentials (Kemp et al., 2008). Upon secretion of GSH, most of it is cleaved into its components and the resulting cysteines will fill the extracellular Cys/CySS pool, which is the major thiol/disulfide extracellular redox buffer system (Kemp et al., 2008). The GSH/GSSG ratio is a good measure to detect oxidative stress within the cell (Jones et al., 2000; Nogueira et al., 2004). TRXs are low molecular weight proteins that contain a conserved dithiol at the active site. They are mostly found in the cytoplasm and nuclei in mammalian cells, and possess cytokine-like properties (Kemp et al., 2008). All thiol/disulfide buffers share similarities in their mode of action; however, each system has its own and unique function and is able to support the reduction of different subsets of proteins (Kemp et al., 2008; Lillig and Holmgren, 2007).

The intracellular redox balance is primarily held by the thiol/disulfide buffers. Under oxidative stress, not only the GSSG content increases but, in parallel, the content of protein mixed disulfides also augments (Valko et al., 2007). Thiol-containing signaling proteins such as receptors, protein kinases, and some transcription factors can be altered in their function by the formation of mixed disulfides. Thus, thiol/disulfide buffers represent an important element for various signal transduction networks, e.g., for the activation and differentiation of T cells but also for several other immunological mechanisms (Kesarwani et al., 2013).

Besides cellular antioxidant systems, antioxidant substances can be absorbed from dietary intake. Many food compounds exhibit antioxidative properties such as vitamins; phytochemicals can also be potential antioxidants, e.g., carotenoids like lutein and zeaxanthin, polyphenols, and flavonoids or stilbenes such as resveratrol have been shown to modulate redox homeostasis *in vitro* (Butt and Sultan, 2009; Santhakumar et al., 2014; Zaknun et al., 2012). Many of these compounds are contained in so-called healthy food, especially in fruits or vegetables or in beverages such as red and white wine, cacao and tea, and they are considered to play a major role in preventing disease and improving health (Heidemann et al., 2008). Thus, in the last years, ascorbic acid (vitamin C), carotenes (vitamin A), melatonin, glutathione, tocopherols, and tocotrienols (vitamin E) were in the focus of research because of their antioxidant capacities as potent agents for nutritional supplementation (Balsano and Alisi, 2009; Zaknun et al., 2012).

Although a clear demonstration of beneficial effects of the use of antioxidant supplements in disease prevention is not yet available (Stanner et al., 2006), such preparations are already widely used, sometimes also without any medical indication. Besides that many clinical trials could not associate a connection between antioxidant supplementation and disease prevention, high-dose (single) antioxidants could even increase the risk of disease as was reported, e.g., for age-related diseases or cardiovascular disorders (Bjelakovic et al., 2007; Jha et al., 1995; Myung et al., 2013; Zheng Selin et al., 2013). There is also evidence accumulating that high vitamin supplementation in early life increases the risk of an allergy later in life (Hyppönen et al., 2004; Milner et al., 2004). Furthermore, excess of vitamin uptake can cause neurotoxicity; however, vitamin deficiency may lead to neurological defects (Lanska, 2010; Snodgrass, 1992).

Of note, in daily life antioxidant uptake is often not recognized as such and many people do not even know which substances can act as antioxidants, as it is the case for several food additives such as preservatives and colorants but also for vitamins. Addition of antioxidants to food or beverage has increased, to stabilize them for transport and storage, to maintain color, or because of potential beneficial health implications, and an overexposure is not easy to avoid.

Extra-high-dose antioxidant uptake might not only support the development of allergy but could also disturb the successful execution of an immune response. Cytocidal products like ROS or RNS are necessary as a defense strategy, and their shortage may not only counteract pathogen eradication but also interfere with negative feedback loops of antiproliferative mechanisms, which regulate control and limit immune reactions. Thus far, several studies have investigated the influence of antioxidants on Th1-type immune response by focusing on tryptophan breakdown (Jenny et al., 2011).

TH1-TYPE IMMUNE RESPONSE

Various cell types act in cooperation for an effective immune response, whereby they cross-regulate each other. A coordinated interplay between innate and adaptive immune system is necessary for an efficient defense.

If an antigen enters the body, it will be presented on major histocompatibility complexes of antigen-presenting cells to T cells. There it will be recognized by the T-cell receptor and the presence of additional costimulatory signals such as protein ligand B7 and cluster of differentiation 28 (CD28) interaction ensures that T cells get activated (Balakrishnan and Adams, 1995). Antigen-mediated signals and stimuli from the microenvironment, such as cytokines, are critically involved in T cell differentiation into different effector subtypes.

Activated Th1-type cells secrete cytokines and thus activate T effector cells, like cytotoxic T cells or nonspecific effector cells such as natural killer cells and macrophages. They represent an important subpopulation of T helper cells that are characterized by the release of interleukin (IL)-2 and IFN-γ. Other cytokines like IL-4, IL-5, IL-6, and IL-13 are secreted by the subpopulation Th2-type cells and favor the Th2-type immune response (Romagnani, 2006). The classical division of Th1- and Th2-type cells has been extended as additional Th cell subtypes were identified in recent years. T-cell differentiation into Th1- and Th2-type cells is suggested to crucially depend on the redox environment, where oxidative conditions favor Th1 development and "antioxidative stress" leads to a shift in allergic Th2 responses (Gostner et al., 2013; Zaknun et al., 2012) (Figure 14.1).

Th17-type cells, which combine the innate and adaptive immunity, were found to be involved in the defense against extracellular fungi or bacteria (Yu and Gaffen, 2008). The Th9-type subset controls growth and activation (Schmitt et al., 2014), and follicular helper T (Tfh) cells are involved in B-cell maturation (Zhou et al., 2009). Another type of T-helper cells—the regulatory T (Treg) cells—are responsible for the maintenance of self-tolerance (Hori et al., 2003) and can limit the potential of collateral tissue damage (Hori et al., 2003; Zhou et al., 2009).

During defense against intracellular pathogens, Th1-type cells release the most prominent pro-inflammatory cytokine, IFN-γ. It is probably the most important inducer of antimicrobial and antitumoral defenses, and stimulates the production of ROS in macrophages (Nathan et al., 1983; Nathan, 1987). These high amounts of ROS further triggers redox-sensitive signaling cascades, e.g., mitogen-activated protein kinase, transcription factor nuclear factor-κB (NF-κB), and activator protein (AP)-1-dependent signaling cascades. NF-κB is a central inflammation mediator that

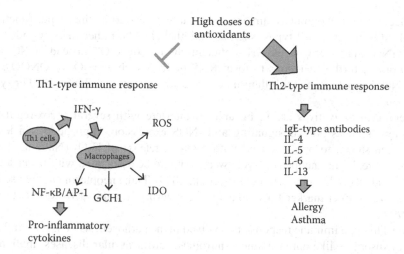

FIGURE 14.1 Owing to the cross-regulation between Th1- and Th2-type immune responses, high doses of antioxidants can suppress Th1-type responses and favor the development of allergy or asthma. During Th1-type immune response, macrophages produce large amounts of reactive oxygen species (ROS) to protect the cell against pathogens. In parallel, signaling cascades such as transcription factor nuclear factor-κB (NF-κB) and activator protein (AP)-1-dependent pathways are induced. Antioxidants can exhibit anti-inflammatory properties by suppressing ROS production. Excessive antioxidants shift the balance towards Th2-type reactions that are associated with a risk for allergy development.

regulates the expression of pro-inflammatory cytokines, chemokines, and adhesion molecules (Aggarwal, 2004). Morever, NF-κB coordinates the expression of different subsets of genes; thus, NF-κB signaling is not only involved in the initiation but also in the maintenance and resolution of immune responses.

IFN-γ induces biochemical pathways such as GTP-cyclohydrolase (GCH1), indoleamine 2,3-dioxygenase 1 (IDO1), and iNOS (Werner et al., 2011; Widner et al., 2000). IDO is the rate-limiting enzyme in the conversion of the essential amino acid tryptophan into kynurenine. IDO1 is expressed in various cells such as macrophages, microglia, neurons, and astrocytes (Guillemin et al., 2007), and its activation plays an essential role as an antiproliferative strategy for pathogens and malignant cells but also as a negative feedback loop in the control of Th1-type immune response (Samelson-Jones and Yeh, 2006). Tryptophan metabolism is implicated in a variety of physiological and pathophysiological processes like antimicrobial, antitumor defense, neuropathology, and immunoregulation. Also, antioxidant activities have been described for IDO owing to the utilization of $O_2^{\cdot-}$ both as a substrate and as cofactor (Thomas and Stocker, 1999).

Activation of GCH1 leads to the formation of neopterin, a pteridine derivate, and of 5,6,7,8-tetrahydrobiopterin (BH$_4$). Neopterin has been identified as a biomarker for oxidative stress (Murr et al., 2002). BH$_4$ is an essential cofactor for several mono-oxygenases, such as iNOS (Werner et al., 2011). Of note, BH$_4$ is stabilized by several antioxidants to guarantee proper function. Owing to a relative deficiency of human macrophages in pyruvoyl tetrahydropterin synthase, high neopterin instead of BH$_4$ is produced. The NO• output in humans is probably generated by the proper function-ing of NOS in other cell types, such as endothelial cells, rather than by inducible NOS (iNOS) of macrophages. BH_4-deficient NOS produce $O_2^{•-}$ instead of NO• and can promote further reactions to form RNS or ROS such as H_2O_2 or $ONOO^-$. Of note, NO• can act as an anti-inflammatory agent by directly inhibiting IDO enzyme function.

Neopterin derivatives are to be able to interfere with several redox-regulated pathways, such as NF-κB signaling and iNOS expression. High neopterin levels have been shown to be associated with a strong release of H_2O_2 (Nathan, 1986). Furthermore, higher neopterin levels were found to be associated with lower levels of antioxidants in human serum (Murr et al., 2009). Thus, neopterin can be used as a sensitive indirect marker for oxidative stress during immune activation (Murr et al., 1999).

The Th1-type immune response is involved in the pathogenesis of several inflam-matory disorders like autoimmune syndromes, cardiovascular diseases, malignant tumor diseases, or neurodegenerative disorders (Romagnani, 2004; Schroecksnadel et al., 2006, 2007). Several *in vitro* studies confirmed the association of altered neopterin levels and IDO activity in patients with infectious disease, including HIV, cardiovascular disease, malignancies, neurodegenerative disorders, or nor-mal aging processes (Capuron et al., 2011; DeRosa et al., 2011; Fuchs et al., 1992; Schroecksnadel and Fuchs, 2006).

Neopterin is a stable biomarker that can be measured in body fluids like urine, blood, and cerebrospinal fluid with enzyme-linked immunosorbent assays (Fuchs et al., 1992; Murr et al., 2002). IDO activation can be estimated by the calculation of the kynurenine-to-tryptophan ratio, which can be measured by using high-performance liquid chromatography (Widner et al., 1997). Thus, neopterin formation and trypto-phan breakdown are robust readouts to evaluate the immune activation status.

MONITORING IMMUNE RESPONSE *IN VITRO*

Peripheral blood mononuclear cells (PBMCs) isolated via density centrifugation from blood of healthy donors can be used as *in vitro* model to measure the immuno-modulatory influences of various substances on Th1-type immune response (Jenny et al., 2011). PBMCs comprise lymphocytes, mainly T cells but also B cells and natu-ral killer cells, and monocytes/macrophages. T cells can be stimulated with mitogens such as phytohemagglutinin (PHA) to produce IFN-γ, which activates monocytes and initiates Th1-type pathways. When analyzing for GCH1 and IDO activity, neop-terin, tryptophan, and kynurenine concentrations can be measured in cell superna-tants after 2 days of incubation. With PHA stimulation, an artificial inflammatory milieu is generated, and different substances can be tested concerning whether they can influence immunobiochemical pathways (Figure 14.2).

Several drugs that are known to possess antioxidant activities, like aspirin, sali-cylic acid, atorvastatin, or vitamin A or C but also phytocompounds and botanical extracts, were shown to suppress tryptophan breakdown and neopterin produc-tion in PHA-stimulated PBMCs in a dose-dependent manner (Becker et al., 2014; Jenny et al., 2011).

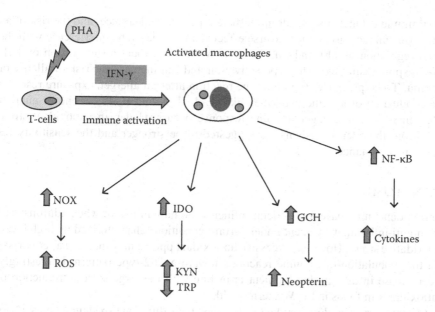

FIGURE 14.2 The *in vitro* model for cellular (Th1-type) immune response employs human peripheral blood mononuclear cells (PBMCs) and mimics the T-cell/macrophage interplay during immune activation. This model represents a convenient testing system to measure immunomodulatory effects of drugs, chemicals, and botanical extracts *in vitro*. T cells are activated upon stimulation with phytohemagglutinin (PHA) and release large amounts of the pro-inflammatory cytokine interferon-γ (IFN-γ), which induces monocyte differentiation and activates several enzymatic cascades. GTP-cyclohydrolase (GCH) produces the oxidative stress marker neopterin; in parallel, indoleamine 2,3-dioxygenase (IDO) converts tryptophan (TRP) into kynurenine (KYN). Furthermore, NADPH oxidase (NOX) produces reactive oxygen species (ROS), and the activated transcription factor nuclear factor-κB (NF-κB) induces the expression of pro-inflammatory cytokines.

A central target of antioxidants is NF-κB signaling. NF-κB is highly inducible by ROS and mediates pro-inflammatory cytokine expression (Asehnoune et al., 2004). A close relationship between NF-κB activation, production of neopterin, and degradation of tryptophan was demonstrated in the human myelomonocytic cell-line THP1-Blue *in vitro* (Schroecksnadel et al., 2010). This reporter cell line expresses an alkaline phosphatase reporter upon activation of NF-κB/AP-1 signaling, allowing a colorimetric readout of NF-κB activity in the cell supernatant.

ANTIOXIDANTS—A TWO-EDGED SWORD

The anti-inflammatory properties of antioxidants might be helpful during a situation of an overwhelming immune activation. Still, there is a question of dosage and the timepoint of intervention with antioxidant therapeutics or high-dose supplements during the course of infection or disease.

However, excessive antioxidant uptake presents a potential risk for unwanted adverse effects, especially when taken over longer periods. Too low ROS/RNS during the immune defense may result in inefficient pathogen clearance, and the risk of an infection can increase. Other adverse effects can be due to the interference with the cross-regulation of Th1 and Th2 immune responses, where a suppression of Th1-type response can favor Th2-type activation and can increase the risk of allergy or asthma. The typical Th2-type immune reaction after an allergen exposure result in the production of specific cytokines like IL-4, IL-5, and IL-13; whenever another allergen is met, a stronger immune response occurs. Under an antioxidant stress condition, the allergic response is suggested to be stronger and the sensitivity for allergens is enhanced.

CONCLUSION

Antioxidants may have a beneficial influence on human health when administered as an anti-inflammatory agent under certain conditions characterized by high levels of oxidative stress. However, excessive antioxidant uptake may increase allergy risks via the modulation of immune reactions toward a Th2-type pattern. Interestingly, the increase in allergy development is in line with the large-scale introduction of antioxidants in foods in the Western world.

Of note, for several antioxidant molecules, their direct antioxidant activity is not their sole function; the indirect effects mediated by these compounds should also be taken into consideration (Dinkova-Kostova and Talalay, 2008). The origin of the antioxidant may also play a role, especially when evaluating a high-dose uptake of single antioxidants in comparison to antioxidant-rich nutrition.

In general, a well-functioning human being does not need further supplementation of antioxidants; a balanced diet together with regular physical exercises will keep the body healthy and balanced.

REFERENCES

Aggarwal, B.B. 2004. Nuclear factor-kappaB: The enemy within. *Cancer Cell.* 6:203–8.

Altenhöfer, S., Kleikers, P.W., Radermacher, K.A., Scheurer, P., Rob Hermans, J.J., Schiffers, P., Ho, H., Wingler, K., Schmidt, H.H. 2012. The NOX toolbox: Validating the role of NADPH oxidases in physiology and disease. *Cell Mol Life Sci.* 69:2327–43.

Asehnoune, K., Strassheim, D., Mitra, S., Kim, J.Y., Abraham, E. 2004. Involvement of reactive oxygen species in Toll-like receptor 4-dependent activation of NF-kappa B. *J Immunol.* 172:2522–9.

Balakrishnan, K., Adams, L.E. 1995. The role of the lymphocyte in an immune response. *Immunol Invest.* 24:233–44.

Balsano, C., Alisi, A. 2009. Antioxidant effects of natural bioactive compounds. *Curr Pharm Des.* 15:3063–73.

Becker, K., Schroecksnadel, S., Gostner, J., Zaknun, C., Schennach, H., Uberall, F., Fuchs, D. 2014. Comparison of *in vitro* tests for antioxidant and immunomodulatory capacities of compounds. *Phytomedicine.* 21:164–71.

Bjelakovic, G., Nikolova, D., Simonetti, R.G., Gluud, C. 2004. Antioxidant supplements for prevention of gastrointestinal cancers: A systematic review and meta-analysis. *Lancet.* 364:1219–28.

Bjelakovic, G., Nikolova, D., Gluud, L.L., Simonetti, R.G., Gluud, C. 2007. Mortality in randomized trials of antioxidant supplements for primary and secondary prevention: Systematic review and meta-analysis. *JAMA.* 297:842–57.

Butt, M.S., Sultan, M.T. 2009. Green tea: Nature's defense against malignancies. *Crit Rev Food Sci Nutr.* 49:463–73.

Cadenas, E. 1997. Basic mechanisms of antioxidant activity. *Biofactors.* 6:391–7.

Capuron, L., Schroecksnadel, S., Féart, C., Aubert, A., Higueret, D., Barberger-Gateau, P., Layé, S., Fuchs, D. 2011. Chronic low-grade inflammation in elderly persons is associated with altered tryptophan and tyrosine metabolism: Role in neuropsychiatric symptoms. *Biol Psychiatry.* 70:175–82.

Dalle-Donne, I., Rossi, R., Colombo, R., Giustarini, D., Milzani, A. 2006. Biomarkers of oxidative damage in human disease. *Clin Chem.* 52:601–23.

Davies, K.J. 1995. Oxidative stress: The paradox of aerobic life. *Biochem Soc Symp.* 61:1–31.

Decoursey, T.E., Ligeti, E. 2005. Regulation and termination of NADPH oxidase activity. *Cell Mol Life Sci.* 62:2173–93.

DeRosa, S., Cirillo, P., Pacileo, M., Petrillo, G., D'Ascoli, G.L., Maresca, F., Ziviello, F., Chiariello, M. 2011. Neopterin: From forgotten biomarker to leading actor in cardiovascular pathophysiology. *Curr Vasc Pharmacol.* 9:188–99.

Dhalla, N.S., Temsah, R.M., Netticadan, T. 2000. Role of oxidative stress in cardiovascular diseases. *J Hypertens.* 18:655–73.

Dinkova-Kostova, A.T., Talalay, P. 2008. Direct and indirect antioxidant properties of inducers of cytoprotective proteins. *Mol Nutr Food Res.* 52(Suppl 1):S128–38.

Dotan, Y., Pinchuk, I., Lichtenberg, D., Leshno, M. 2009. Decision analysis supports the paradigm that in'discriminate supplementation of vitamin E does more harm than good. *Arterioscler Thromb Vasc Biol.* 29:1304–9.

Dröge, W. 2002. Free radicals in the physiological control of cell function. *Physiol Rev.* 82:47–95.

Fleming, I., Michaelis, U.R., Bredenkötter, D., Fisslthaler, B., Dehghani, F., Brandes, R.P., Busse, R. 2001. Endothelium-derived hyperpolarizing factor synthase (cytochrome P450 2C9) is a functionally significant source of reactive oxygen species in coronary arteries. *Circ Res.* 88:44–51.

Förstermann, U., Sessa, W.C. 2012. Nitric oxide synthases: Regulation and function. *Eur Heart J.* 33:829–37.

Fuchs, D., Weiss, G., Reibnegger, G., Wachter, H. 1992. The role of neopterin as a monitor of cellular immune activation in transplantation, inflammatory, infectious, and malignant diseases. *Crit Rev Clin Lab Sci.* 29:307–41.

Gerss, J., Köpcke, W. 2009. The questionable association of vitamin E supplementation and mortality—Inconsistent results of different meta-analytic approaches. *Cell Mol Biol (Noisy-le-grand)* 55:OL1111–20.

Gostner, J.M., Becker, K., Fuchs, D., Sucher, R. 2013. Redox regulation of the immune response. *Redox Rep.* 18:88–94.

Guillemin, G.J., Cullen, K.M., Lim, C.K., Smythe, G.A., Garner, B., Kapoor, V., Takikawa, O., Brew, B.J. 2007. Characterization of the kynurenine pathway in human neurons. *J Neurosci.* 27:12884–92.

Halliwell, G., Gutteridge, J.M. 1999. *Free Radicals in Biology and Medicine*, 3rd Ed. Oxford University Press, New York.

Heidemann, C., Schulze, M.B., Franco, O.H., van Dam, R.M., Mantzoros, C.S., Hu, F.B. 2008. Dietary patterns and risk of mortality from cardiovascular disease, cancer, and all causes in a prospective cohort of women. *Circulation.* 118:230–7.

Hori, S., Nomura, T., Sakaguchi, S. 2003. Control of regulatory T cell development by the transcription factor Foxp3. *Science.* 299:1057–61.

Hyppönen, E., Sovio, U., Wjst, M., Patel, S., Pekkanen, J., Hartikainen, A.L., Järvelinb, M.R. 2004. Infant vitamin D supplementation and allergic conditions in adulthood: Northern Finland birth cohort 1966. *Ann N Y Acad Sci.* 1037:84–95.

Jenner, P. 2003. Oxidative stress in Parkinson's disease. *Ann Neurol.* 53(Suppl 3):S26–36.

Jenny, M., Klieber, M., Zaknun, D., Schroecksnadel, S., Kurz, K., Ledochowski, M., Schennach, H., Fuchs, D. 2011. *In vitro* testing for anti-inflammatory properties of compounds employing peripheral blood mononuclear cells freshly isolated from healthy donors. *Inflamm Res.* 60:127–35.

Jha, P., Flather, M., Lonn, E., Farkouh, M., Yusuf, S. 1995. The antioxidant vitamins and cardiovascular disease. A critical review of epidemiologic and clinical trial data. *Ann Intern Med.* 123:860–72.

Jones, D.P., Carlson, J.L., Mody, V.C., Cai, J., Lynn, M.J., Sternberg, P. 2000. Redox state of glutathione in human plasma. *Free Radic Biol Med.* 28:625–35.

Keisari, Y., Braun, L., Flescher, E. 1983. The oxidative burst and related phenomena in mouse macrophages elicited by different sterile inflammatory stimuli. *Immunobiology.* 165:78–89.

Kemp, M., Go, Y.M., Jones, D.P. 2008. Nonequilibrium thermodynamics of thiol/disulfide redox systems: A perspective on redox systems biology. *Free Radic Biol Med.* 44:921–37.

Kesarwani, P., Murali, A.K., Al-Khami, A.A., Mehrotra, S. 2013. Redox regulation of T-cell function: From molecular mechanisms to significance in human health and disease. *Antioxid Redox Signal.* 18:1497–534.

Kovacic, P., Jacintho, J.D. 2001. Mechanisms of carcinogenesis: Focus on oxidative stress and electron transfer. *Curr Med Chem.* 8:773–96.

Kris-Etherton, P.M., Lichtenstein, A.H., Howard, B.V., Steinberg, D., Witztum, J.L.; Nutrition Committee of the American Heart Association Council on Nutrition, Physical Activity, and Metabolism. 2004. Antioxidant vitamin supplements and cardiovascular disease. *Circulation.* 110:637–41.

Lanska, D.J. 2010. Chapter 30: Historical aspects of the major neurological vitamin deficiency disorders: The water-soluble B vitamins. *Handb Clin Neurol.* 95:445–76.

LeBras, M., Clément, M.V., Pervaiz, S., Brenner, C. 2005. Reactive oxygen species and the mitochondrial signaling pathway of cell death. *Histol Histopathol.* 20:205–19.

Lillig, C.H., Holmgren, A. 2007. Thioredoxin and related molecules—From biology to health and disease. *Antioxid Redox Signal.* 9:25–47.

Mariotto, S., Menegazzi, M., Suzuki, H. 2004. Biochemical aspects of nitric oxide. *Curr Pharm Des.* 10:1627–45.

McNally, J.S., Davis, M.E., Giddens, D.P., Saha, A., Hwang, J., Dikalov, S., Jo, H., Harrison, D.G. 2003. Role of xanthine oxidoreductase and NAD(P)H oxidase in endothelial superoxide production in response to oscillatory shear stress. *Am J Physiol Heart Circ Physiol.* 285:H2290–7.

McNeill, E., Channon, K.M. 2012. The role of tetrahydrobiopterin in inflammation and cardiovascular disease. *Thromb Haemost.* 108:832–9.

Milner, J.D., Stein, D.M., McCarter, R., Moon, R.Y. 2004. Early infant multivitamin supplementation is associated with increased risk for food allergy and asthma. *Pediatrics.* 114:27–32.

Murr, C., Fuith, L.C., Widner, B., Wirleitner, B., Baier-Bitterlich, G., Fuchs, D. 1999. Increased neopterin concentrations in patients with cancer: Indicator of oxidative stress? *Anticancer Res.* 19:1721–8.

Murr, C., Widner, B., Wirleitner, B., Fuchs, D. 2002. Neopterin as a marker for immune system activation. *Curr Drug Metab.* 3:175–87.

Murr, C., Schroecksnadel, K., Winkler, C., Ledochowski, M., Fuchs, D. 2005. Antioxidants may increase the probability of developing allergic diseases and asthma. *Med Hypotheses.* 64:973–7.

Murr, C., Winklhofer-Roob, B.M., Schroecksnadel, K., Maritschnegg, M., Mangge, H., Böhm, B.O., Winkelmann, B.R., März, W., Fuchs, D. 2009. Inverse association between serum concentrations of neopterin and antioxidants in patients with and without angiographic coronary artery disease. *Atherosclerosis.* 202:543–9.

Myung, S.K., Ju, W., Cho, B., Oh, S.W., Park, S.M., Koo, B.K., Park, B.J.; Korean Meta-Analysis Study Group. 2013. Efficacy of vitamin and antioxidant supplements in prevention of cardiovascular disease: Systematic review and meta-analysis of randomised controlled trials. *BMJ.* 346:f10.

Nathan, C.F. 1986. Peroxide and pteridine: A hypothesis on the regulation of macrophage antimicrobial activity by interferon gamma. *Interferon.* 7:125–43.

Nathan, C.F. 1987. Secretory products of macrophages. *J Clin Invest.* 79:319–26.

Nathan, C.F., Murray, H.W., Wiebe, M.E., Rubin, B.Y. 1983. Identification of interferon-gamma as the lymphokine that activates human macrophage oxidative metabolism and antimicrobial activity. *J Exp Med.* 158:670–89.

Nogueira, C.W., Zeni, G., Rocha, J.B. 2004. Organoselenium and organotellurium compounds: Toxicology and pharmacology. *Chem Rev.* 104:6255–85.

Romagnani, S., 2004. Immunologic influences on allergy and the TH1/TH2 balance. *J Allergy Clin Immunol.* 113:395–400.

Romagnani, S. 2006. Regulation of the T cell response. *Clin Exp Allergy.* 36:1357–66.

Rossi, F., Zatti, M. 1964. Biochemical aspects of phagocytosis in polymorphonuclear leucosytes. NADH and NADPH oxidation by the granules of resting and phagocytizing cells. *Experientia.* 20:21–3.

Samelson-Jones, B.J., Yeh, S.R. 2006. Interactions between nitric oxide and indoleamine 2,3-dioxygenase. *Biochemistry.* 45:8527–38.

Santhakumar, A.B., Bulmer, A.C., Singh, I. 2014. A review of the mechanisms and effectiveness of dietary polyphenols in reducing oxidative stress and thrombotic risk. *J Hum Nutr Diet.* 27(1):1–21.

Savina, A., Amigorena, S. 2007. Phagocytosis and antigen presentation in dendritic cells. *Immunol Rev.* 219:143–56.

Sayre, L.M., Smith, M.A., Perry, G. 2001. Chemistry and biochemistry of oxidative stress in neurodegenerative disease. *Curr Med Chem.* 8:721–38.

Schmitt, E., Klein, M., Bopp, T. 2014. Th9 cells, new players in adaptive immunity. *Trends Immunol.* 36:61–8.

Schroecksnadel, K., Fuchs, D. 2006. Interferon-gamma for counteracting T-cell activation. *Trends Immunol.* 27:398.

Schroecksnadel, K., Wirleitner, B., Winkler, C., Fuchs, D. 2006. Monitoring tryptophan metabolism in chronic immune activation. *Clin Chim Acta.* 364:82–90.

Schroecksnadel, K., Fischer, B., Schennach, H., Weiss, G., Fuchs, D. 2007. Antioxidants suppress Th1-type immune response *in vitro. Drug Metab Lett.* 1:166–71.

Schroecksnadel, S., Jenny, M., Kurz, K., Klein, A., Ledochowski, M., Uberall, F., Fuchs, D. 2010. LPS-induced NF-kappaB expression in THP-1Blue cells correlates with neopterin production and activity of indoleamine 2,3-dioxygenase. *Biochem Biophys Res Commun.* 399:642–6.

Siems, W.G., Grune, T., Esterbauer, H. 1995. 4-Hydroxynonenal formation during ischemia and reperfusion of rat small intestine. *Life Sci.* 57:785–9.

Snodgrass, S.R. 1992. Vitamin neurotoxicity. *Mol Neurobiol.* 6(1):41–73.

Stadtman, E.R. 2004. Role of oxidant species in aging. *Curr Med Chem.* 11:1105–12.

Stanner, S.A., Hughes, J., Kelly, C.N., Buttriss, J. 2006. A review of the epidemiological evidence for the 'antioxidant hypothesis'. *Public Health Nutr.* 7:407–22.

Thomas, D.D., Ridnour, L.A., Isenberg, J.S., Flores-Santana, W., Switzer, C.H., Donzelli, S., Hussain, P., Vecoli, C., Paolocci, N., Ambs, S., Colton, C.A., Harris, C.C., Roberts, D.D.,

Wink, D.A. 2008. The chemical biology of nitric oxide: Implications in cellular signaling. *Free Radic Biol Med.* 45:18–31.

Thomas, S.R., Stocker, R. 1999. Redox reactions related to indoleamine 2,3-dioxygenase and tryptophan metabolism along the kynurenine pathway. *Redox Rep.* 4:199–220.

Valko, M., Rhodes, C.J., Moncol, J., Izakovic, M., Mazur, M. 2006. Free radicals, metals and antioxidants in oxidative stress-induced cancer. *Chem Biol Interact.* 160:1–40.

Valko, M., Leibfritz, D., Monc, J., Cronin, M.T., Mazur, M., Telser, J. 2007. Free radicals and antioxidants in normal physiological functions and human disease. *Int J Biochem Cell Biol.* 39:44–84.

Vásquez-Vivar, J., Kalyanaraman, B., Martásek, P., Hogg, N., Masters, B.S., Karoui, H., Tordo, P., Pritchard, K.A. Jr. 1998. Superoxide generation by endothelial nitric oxide synthase: The influence of cofactors. *Proc Natl Acad Sci U S A.* 95:9220–5.

Vignais, P.V. 2002. The superoxide-generating NADPH oxidase: Structural aspects and activation mechanism. *Cell Mol Life Sci.* 59:1428–59.

Werner, E.R., Blau, N., Thöny, B. 2011. Tetrahydrobiopterin: Biochemistry and pathophysiology. *Biochem J.* 438:397–414.

Widner, B., Werner, E.R., Schennach, H., Wachter, H., Fuchs, D. 1997. Simultaneous measurement of serum tryptophan and kynurenine by HPLC. *Clin Chem.* 43:2424–6.

Widner, B., Ledochowski, M., Fuchs, D. 2000. Interferon-gamma-induced tryptophan degradation: Neuropsychiatric and immunological consequences. *Curr Drug Metab.* 1:193–204.

Wink, D.A., Hines, H.B., Cheng, R.Y., Switzer, C.H., Flores-Santana, W., Vitek, M.P., Ridnour, L.A., Colton, C.A. 2011. Nitric oxide and redox mechanisms in the immune response. *J Leukoc Biol.* 89:873–91.

Yu, J.J., Gaffen, S.L. 2008. Interleukin-17: A novel inflammatory cytokine that bridges innate and adaptive immunity. *Front Biosci.* 13:170–7.

Zaknun, D., Schroecksnadel, S., Kurz, K., Fuchs, D. 2012. Potential role of antioxidant food supplements, preservatives and colorants in the pathogenesis of allergy and asthma. *Int Arch Allergy Immunol.* 157:113–24.

Zhang, R., Brennan, M.L., Shen, Z., MacPherson, J.C., Schmitt, D., Molenda, C.E., Hazen, S.L. 2002. Myeloperoxidase functions as a major enzymatic catalyst for initiation of lipid peroxidation at sites of inflammation. *J Biol Chem.* 277:46116–22.

Zheng Selin, J., Rautiainen, S., Lindblad, B.E., Morgenstern, R., Wolk, A. 2013. High-dose supplements of vitamins C and E, low-dose multivitamins, and the risk of age-related cataract: A population-based prospective cohort study of men. *Am J Epidemiol.* 177:548–55.

Zhou, L., Chong, M.M., Littman, D.R. 2009. Plasticity of CD4+ T cell lineage differentiation. *Immunity.* 30:646–55.

15 HIV/AIDS

Heike Englert and Germaine Nkengfack

CONTENTS

Introduction...263
　Epidemiology..263
　Types of HIV Infection..264
　HIV Transmission..264
Pathomechanism of HIV..265
　CD4 Cells and HIV..265
　Viral Load and HIV...266
HIV/AIDS and Malnutrition..266
HIV and Nutrition..267
HIV/AIDS and Oxidative Stress..267
Antioxidants and HIV/AIDS..268
　Vitamin A..268
　β-Carotene...269
　Vitamin C..269
　Vitamin E..269
　Selenium..270
　Zinc..270
　Polyphenols...271
　N-Acetyl Cysteine (NAC)...271
Factors Affecting Antioxidant Level in HIV/AIDS Patients...............................272
　Opportunistic Condition..272
　Medication Intake..272
　Combination Therapy (HAARTS)...272
　Dietary Intake..272
　Socioeconomic Status...273
Adverse Effects of Supplementation of Antioxidants on HIV/AIDS Patients.......273
　HIV Prevention..274
References...274

INTRODUCTION

EPIDEMIOLOGY

Human immunodeficiency virus/acquired immunodeficiency syndrome (HIV/AIDS) remains one of the most important public health challenges worldwide, especially in low- and middle-income countries. According to the World Health Organization (WHO) and UNAIDS (Joint United Nations Programme on HIV/AIDS), 34 million people globally were living with the HIV infection in 2010. Also in the same year, 2.7 million new HIV infections, including 390,000 among children less than 15 years old, and an annual death rate of 1.8 million people was reported [1]. In sub-Sahara Africa, where two-third (22.6 million) of the HIV-infected people live, more than 6800 new infections and more than 5700 persons were dying from HIV in 2010 [2,3]. After sub-Sahara Africa, the regions with the highest rate of infection are the Caribbean, Eastern Europe, and Central Asia [3].

TYPES OF HIV INFECTION

Two types of HIV infections are known, HIV-1 and HIV-2. Both strains of HIV are retroviruses and causative agents of AIDS. Although both viruses are similar in terms of basic gene arrangement, mode of transmission, intracellular replication pathway, and clinical consequence, important differences exist between infections caused by both viruses (Table 15.1; Refs. [4–6]).

HIV TRANSMISSION

HIV can be transmitted through a multitude of routes. In Africa, about 90% of HIV transmission in adults occurs through sexual contact. In industrialized countries, it has been observed that the prevalence of HIV among men who have sex with men is consistently higher than that in the general population [7]. Another path for HIV transmission is HIV from mother-to-child transmission (MTCT). MTCT

TABLE 15.1

Differences between HIV-1 and HIV-2

Characteristic	HIV-1	HIV-2
Origin	SIV cpz	SIV smm
Epidemiology	Extends worldwide	Largely confined in West Africa and communities in Europe with socioeconomic links to West Africa, e.g., Portugal
Clinical progression	Progression to immunodeficiency is faster	Progression to immunodeficiency is slower; hence, individuals are mostly long-term nonprogressors
Pathological processes	Progression occurs at lower CD4 counts	Progression occurs at higher CD4 counts
Virology	Rate of DNA replication is higher, leading to higher viral load	Rate of DNA replication about 100-fold lower, leading to lower viral load
Cellular response	Less polyfunctional and produce less IL-2	More polyfunctional and produce more IL-2

Source: Nyamweya S et al., *Rev. Med. Virol.*, 23, 221, 2013; Martinez-Steele E et al., *AIDS*, 21, 317, 2007; Sharp PM and Hahn BH, *Cold Spring Harbor Perspect. Med.*, 1, a006841, 2011.

is responsible for about 630,000 pediatric infection annually, with more than 90% of these children living in sub-Sahara Africa [1,8]. HIV can also be transmitted through contaminated blood during blood transfusion or objects. Chen and coworkers discovered that the natural history of AIDS was caused by blood transfusion [9].

PATHOMECHANISM OF HIV

CD4 CELLS AND HIV

The HIV virus affects various cells of the immune system. Besides mononuclear phagocytes (monocytes and macrophages), studies *in vivo* show that CD4 lymphocytes are the most affected by HIV-1. To measure the state of the immune system and the degree of immune suppression due to HIV infection, the concentration of CD4 (cluster of differentiation 4) cells in plasma is used. The higher the CD4 cell count, the better the condition and prognosis of the individual (Table 15.2; Ref. [10]).

CD4 cells act as receptors for the entry of HIV virus into the cells. CCR5 (human C–C chemokine receptor 5), expressed on immune receptor cells and antigen-presenting cells, together with CD4 cells, are the primary receptors used by HIV for viral entry. Specific molecules that bind to CCR5 include MIP-1α, MIP-1β, and RANTES. These molecules play an important role in the homing and migration of effector and memory T cells during acute infections. Activation of CCR5 cells

TABLE 15.2

HIV Indicators and Measure of HIV Progression

Clinical Parameter	Level	Stage of Infection	Significance	Common Infections
CD4 cell count	500–1400 cells/μl		Average counts in healthy, HIV-negative individuals	
	<500 cells/μl	Early symptomatic phase	Immune system is damaged	Oral thrush, pneumonia, tuberculosis
	<350 cells/μl	Late symptomatic phase	Damage is severe and patient is officially diagnosed as an AIDS patient	Weight loss, diarrhea, chronic fatigue
	<50 cells/μl		Infection is advanced and damage may be irreparable	
Viral load	>100.000 copies of HIV/ml of blood	Symptomatic phase		Tuberculosis, *Mycobacterium avium* complex

Source: Nielsen K and Bryson YJ, *Pediatr. Clin. North Am.*, 47, 39, 2000.

by chemokine leads to T-cell migration to the site of inflammation and immune response to antigen [11].

VIRAL LOAD AND HIV

HIV viral load is one of the main surrogate indicators used for monitoring and managing HIV disease progression and treatment success in adults and children worldwide [12]. Viral load represents the number of copies of HIV virus per milliliter of blood and measures the speed with which the infection is progressing. The higher the viral load, the faster the progression. HIV patients are required to test their CD4 count and viral load regularly since these values will help the clinician determine the appropriate time to initiate the antiretroviral therapy. However, in many resource-limited areas, it is difficult to systematically monitor HIV progression through HIV viral load. This difficulty is due to the high cost of testing in big cities and the lack of equipment and technology in rural areas, where most of the infected persons live. For this reason, CD4 count or CD4% are now frequently used to monitor HIV-1 disease progression in both children and adults.

The progressive depletion of CD4 and increase in viral load are the hallmarks for HIV infection. Although the mechanism by which the HIV virus causes CD4 depletion is not well known, evidence exist that the depletion of CD4 is caused by an indirect mechanism. The most acceptable mechanism, supported by *in vivo* studies, includes the consequences of HIV interaction with resting CD4 lymphocytes, which cannot support viral replication. The binding of the HIV virus to resting CD4 cells in the lymphoid tissues leads to the upregulation of the lymph node homing receptors (L-selectin and Fas) [12]. When these HIV-signaled CD4 cells return to the blood, they home very rapidly back to peripheral lymph nodes and axial bone marrow. Their disappearance from the blood is likely due to their leaving the circulatory system. Most of the cells that have been induced by HIV to home on lymph nodes are subsequently induced into apoptosis during the process of trans-endothelial migration when secondary signals are received through various homing receptors [13]. The more CD4 cells are being activated, the higher the number of homing receptors (signs of CD4 destruction by apoptosis), and consequently the higher the HIV-1 viral load.

HIV/AIDS AND MALNUTRITION

Despite the major advances in understanding the biology of the HIV infection and important progress in the HIV/AIDS therapy, the basic role of the patients' nutrition in the pathogenesis of HIV infection is still a subject of great interest. Malnutrition and HIV are intricately interrelated with one another. Evidence exists that malnutrition increases the rate of disease progression as well as the rate of transmission of infection from mother to child. Also, HIV infection enhances malnutrition through its impact on nutrient intake, absorption, and utilization. However, it is still unclear which specific nutritional deficiencies contribute to poor clinical outcomes. With the increased global HIV/AIDS pandemic, coupled with the limited HIV drug availability, especially in developing countries, nutritional strategies to correct micronutrient deficiencies are gaining interest. Micronutrient deficiency during an HIV infection is provoked by body metabolism changes and opportunistic conditions such as mouth sores, pain in the mouth, swallowing problems, anorexia, fever, diarrhea, vomiting, or loss of appetite, which, in turn, lead to reduced food intake and visible weight loss. These conditions lead to deficiencies of vitamins and minerals (vitamins A, C, and E; selenium; zinc, etc.) that are required to enhance the immune system [14,15]. Studies indicate that micronutrient supplements reduce plasma HIV RNA viral load, improve CD4+ cell counts, and reduce the incidence of opportunistic infections [16].

HIV AND NUTRITION

Recently, the importance of nutrition in human health is receiving increasing attention. Also, the assessment and improvement of the nutritional status in HIV infection has been recognized as an important part of comprehensive care of HIV-infected persons [17]. The use of nutritional supplements as well as natural food has been used to investigate its effects in various health conditions, including HIV/AIDS.

During an HIV infection, a long-term practice of adequate nutrition would compensate for energy lost due to HIV infection and would help the body resist further infections. To achieve this goal, the body has to be fed with relevant nutrients that can boost the immune system. Examples of such nutrients are micronutrients, including antioxidants such as vitamins A, C, and E; selenium; zinc; etc. These antioxidants are known in clinical interventions to positively influence the nutritional status and immunological parameters of HIV/AIDS patients. Besides nutritional supplements, a wide range of natural foods such as fruits, vegetables, cereals, etc., are rich sources of micronutrients [18,19]. The WHO recommends the "five-a-day" intake of fruits and vegetables, which can cover the required daily allowance of antioxidants. Environmental and epidemiological studies indicate that a high intake of fruit and vegetables is associated with a reduced risk of cancer, cardiovascular diseases, and oxidative stress [20]. Meanwhile, the health benefits of a high fruit and vegetable intake has been attributed to their high antioxidant content.

HIV/AIDS AND OXIDATIVE STRESS

During HIV infection, oxidative stress occurs through the activation of reactive oxygen species (ROS), produced after the activation of phagocytic cells (macrophages and neutrophils). ROS are also produced as by-products during electron mitochondrial transport of aerobic respiration, oxidoreductase catalysis, and metal-catalyzed oxidation. ROS are thus highly reactive and capable of causing significant damages to cell structure and function. Common ROS are the hydroxyl radical, hydrogen peroxide, and superoxide anion. ROS are known to play a critical role in the induction of oxidative stress and the degradation of immune cells [21]. Excess production of ROS can attack double bonds in polyunsaturated fatty acids, inducing lipid peroxidation that may result in more oxidative cellular stress. Oxidative stress is a condition when the balance between pro-oxidants and antioxidants is upset, causing an overproduction of ROS [22]. Oxidative stress promotes the replication of the virus by upregulating the activation of NF-kappa B (NF-κB), a transcriptional promoter of proteins involved in the inflammatory and acute-phase response. NF-κB is bound to I-κB in the cytoplasm in its inactive form. However, tumor necrosis factor-α and ROS can cause the activation of NF-κB from I-κB. NF-κB then translocates to the nucleus and binds to the DNA, promoting transcription of HIV-1 [23,24]. To prevent such damages, adequate amounts of neutralizing antioxidants to act as scavenger of free radicals are required.

ANTIOXIDANTS AND HIV/AIDS

Antioxidants are nutrients who protect cells and tissues against ROS, produced as a result of immune activation to eradicate pathogens. Antioxidants occur endogenously in the body and also naturally in foods such as fruits and vegetables [25]. Common endogenous antioxidants include superoxide dismutase (catalyzes the conversion of two superoxide anions into a molecule each of hydrogen peroxide and oxygen), catalase (catalyzes the conversion of hydrogen peroxide to water and oxygen), and glutathione peroxidase (catalyzes the degradation of hydrogen peroxides and other organic peroxides to alcohols). They are known for their beneficial effects on free radicals in biological systems, reducing oxidative stress on immune cells and reducing the replication of the HIV virus [26]. Common exogenous antioxidants include ascorbic acid, α-tocopherol, carotenoids, polyphenolic flavonoids, selenium, and zinc, which can be obtained directly from the diet.

VITAMIN A

Of all the known vitamins, the role of vitamin A has been studied most extensively. Studies show that vitamin A has an effect on the immune system through the action of *all-trans* retinoic acid, which supports robust antibody responses by promoting Th_2 (type 2 helper) cell development [27]. Th_2 produces cytokines (IL-4, IL-5, and IL-10) that are responsible for strong antibody production as well as activation of eosinophils and inhibition of several macrophage functions, hence providing a phagocyte-independent protective response [28]. Hoag et al. observed a profound reduction in Th_2 cells in vitamin A–deficient mice, accounting for their depressed T-dependent antibody responses [29]. Providing vitamin A or its active metabolites reversed this defect. Vitamin A deficiency is a result of a low serum level of vitamin A due to reduced dietary intake following the HIV-related conditions already mentioned [30]. Vitamin A deficiency can also be a result of increased urinary excretion due to acute infections [31]. Visser and coworkers also observed, in resource-poor settings in South Africa, an association between advanced disease and/or weight loss and lowered blood concentrations of vitamin A [32]. Vitamin A deficiency can lead to pathological changes in the mucosal surfaces, impaired antibody responses, decreased CD4 cell population, and altered T- and B-cell functions.

Previous studies have shown that low vitamin A levels are also associated with increased risk of transmission of HIV from mother to child [33]. Fawzi and coworkers proposed that advanced HIV disease may suppress the release of vitamin A from the liver, leading to low levels of vitamin A in the plasma (despite the body having enough vitamin A liver stores) and, correspondingly, an increase in the risk of MTCT [34].

Recently, another researcher observed no improvement in vitamin A level, CD4 counts, and viral load after supplementing HIV-positive patients with a fortified sorghum meal. The conclusion was made that the major differences between these trials of multiple micronutrient supplements in HIV-infected adults—including: variations in the characteristics of study participants, composition and doses of the supplements, study duration, and other differences—could explain these contradictory findings [35].

β-Carotene

Carotenoids are among the most important dietary antioxidants found in human plasma. Their concentrations in plasma are considered to be the most accurate indicator of dietary carotenoid intake. Many epidemiologic studies have associated high carotenoid intake with a decrease in the incidence of chronic disease. However, the biological mechanisms for such protection are currently unclear. β-Carotene, among other carotenoids, is known to have antioxidant properties; however, the antioxidant activity of these compounds can shift into a pro-oxidant effect, depending on factors such as oxygen tension or carotenoid concentration. Mixtures of carotenoids alone or in association with other antioxidants can increase their activity against lipid peroxidation [36]. Although some clinical trials found no benefit of supplementing β-carotene on CD4 counts [37], others indicate its beneficial effects on HIV disease progression [38]. Baeten and coworkers observed in a multivariate analysis that β-carotene concentrations below the median were associated with elevated C-reactive protein (>10 mg/l) and higher HIV-1 plasma viral load. The authors suggest that low β-carotene concentrations primarily reflect a more active HIV infection, rather than true deficiency amenable to intervention [39].

Vitamin C

Vitamin C, also known as ascorbic acid, is synthesized in the liver of most mammalian species but not by humans. Like most antioxidants, studies indicate an increased utilization of vitamin C in HIV-infected persons compared with healthy controls [31,40]. Increased use coupled with low dietary intake of vitamin C can lead to vitamin deficiency during HIV infection. Previous studies already confirmed that massive doses of vitamin C can suppress the symptoms of HIV disease and significantly reduce the occurrence of secondary infections [41]. Later, Fawzi and coworkers observed that supplementation of vitamin C in combination with vitamin E may provide protection to red blood cells against being destroyed by free radicals [34]. Recent studies indicate that increased intakes of vitamin C during HIV infection can lead to mild increase of CD4 counts, help prevent oxidative damage, and enhance normal immune function and survival [42].

Vitamin E

Studies disclose the presence of low vitamin E levels in the plasma of HIV-infected persons [31,43]. This can be a result of increased utilization of vitamin E in quenching free radicals, thus reducing the peroxidation of polyunsaturated fatty acids [44].

Vitamin E deficiency in HIV patients can also be due to poor dietary intake, poor absorption, diarrhea, and impairment of the recycling mechanism of vitamin E through vitamin C [45]. Studies have shown an association between higher vitamin E intake and lower risk of progression to AIDS [32,43]. Other studies indicate the possibility for the supplementation of vitamin E to influence the production of RANTES, an important antiviral chemokine. In a small supplementation study, 500 mg α-tocopherol given once daily for 2 months reduced RANTES production and increased the expression of CCR5 on the surface of CD4 cells of HIV-1-infected persons. Endogenous production of antiviral factors like RANTES may significantly affect HIV-1 replication and the pace of disease progression.

SELENIUM

Selenium is an important part of glutathione peroxidase, which is a very important enzyme in the metabolism of erythrocytes. Selenium plays an important role in the selenoenzyme glutathione peroxidase, which protects cells against free radical damage and oxidative stress [46]. Evidence exists that the utilization of selenium increases in HIV patients, leading to low plasma selenium levels. Low serum selenium level exacerbates the oxidative stress induced by HIV, increasing the risk of mortality and the occurrence of AIDS-related opportunistic infections [30,47]. Previous studies showed an increase in lipid peroxidation (oxidative stress) in HIV-positive individuals with lower plasma concentrations of selenium. Further studies illustrated that supplementation with selenium in HIV-positive patients led to higher glutathione peroxidase levels [48]. These studies do not indicate an improvement in CD4 cells. Meanwhile, Hurwitz and coworkers observed a suppression of the viral load in HIV patients after supplementation with selenium. However, since most studies on selenium are small and observational studies, confounding could be a possible justification for conflicting results [15].

ZINC

Zinc is a vital mineral known to affect a multitude of enzymes involved in the synthesis and metabolism of carbohydrates, lipids, proteins, nucleic acids, alcohol and membrane stabilization, etc. Zinc deficiency in humans could be a result of the intake of diets poor in zinc and animal proteins, and rich in inhibitors of zinc absorption such as phytic acid and inorganic calcium salts. Studies indicate an association between zinc deficiency and impaired immune function and increasing infection risk [49,50]. Zinc is involved in the growth, development, and function of neutrophils, macrophages, natural killer cells, and T and B lymphocytes. Studies also show that zinc supplementation can reduce the rate of diarrheal diseases, reduce acute lower respiratory tract infections, and increase CD4 cells [51]. Abrams and coworkers, in a related study, also indicated a positive relationship between CD4 counts and dietary intake of zinc, although no relation between dietary intake of zinc and HIV disease progression was evident [52]. However, the reported relationships of zinc and HIV-related outcomes have not been consistent across studies. A possible explanation for this contradictory observation could be confounding due to the small size of studies and study design, as already mentioned above.

POLYPHENOLS

Polyphenols are a class of bioactive secondary plant substances that are widespread in plants, including sorghum, millet, barley, dry beans, peas, and other legumes; fruits such as apples, blackberries, cranberries, grapes, oranges, pears, plums, raspberries, and strawberries; and vegetables such as cabbage, celery, onion, and parsley. Phenolic compounds are also present in tea and wine. They are known to exert strong antioxidant and antiinflammatory effects *in vitro* [24,53]. Polyphenols are known to boost immune function in HIV-infected persons by their ability to counteract oxidative stress [54]. Some studies, however, show no effect of polyphenols on CD4 and viral load after supplementation with fruit juices, although plasma antioxidant capacity is increased [55]. Both previous and recent studies indicate increased antioxidant capacity and increased intracellular glutathione in T cells (an indication of reduced intracellular oxidative stress), increased proliferation of CD4 cell count, decreased viral load in the subgroups with advanced immunodeficiency, after treatment with polyphenol-rich antioxidants [26,56]. Despite the positive effects of polyphenols on lymphocyte proliferation and apoptosis, it will be profitable to further research in this area, considering larger sample sizes and longer duration. Also, a variety of polyphenols should be taken into consideration.

N-ACETYL CYSTEINE (NAC)

NAC has been in clinical practice for several years and has been used for the treatment of several disorders, including HIV/AIDS. NAC has been proven beneficial in patients with the autoimmune disorder systemic lupus erythematosus. In these patients, the mechanism underlying NAC activity was ascribed to a blockade of the mammalian target of rapamycin (mTOR) in T lymphocytes. Activation of mTOR occurs upon glutathione (GSH) depletion or after exposure to nitric oxide (NO), which causes mitochondrial hyperpolarization. This can lead to a downregulation of the transcription factor for knead box P3 and, subsequently, to a decline in CD4. NAC blocks the activation of mTOR and increases the number of T lymphocytes [57]. NAC can cross the epithelial cell membrane and sustain the synthesis of glutathione (GSH), which is the ubiquitous source of the thiol pool in the body and an important antioxidant involved in numerous physiological processes. These include detoxification of electrophilic xenobiotic modulation of redox-regulated signal transduction, regulation of immune response, prostaglandin and leukotriene metabolism, antioxidant defense, neurotransmitter signaling, and modulation of cell proliferation [58]. NAC reacts relatively slowly with superoxide, hydrogen peroxide, and peroxynitrite, which casts some doubt on the importance of these reactions under physiological conditions. Finally, Samuni and coworkers made the major conclusion that the antioxidative activity of NAC, as of other thiols, can be attributed to its fast reactions with OH, NO_2, CO_3 (−), and thiyl radicals, as well as to restitution of damaged targets in vital cellular components [59].

FACTORS AFFECTING ANTIOXIDANT LEVEL IN HIV/AIDS PATIENTS

Opportunistic Condition

Opportunistic conditions such as thrush, vomiting, and tuberculosis often lead to a lack of appetite, which further leads to reduced food intake or malabsorption and consequently micronutrient and antioxidant deficiencies.

Medication Intake

The intake of a series of drugs such as diuretics, laxatives, bile acid, etc., often leads to increased loss of nutrient accompanied by micronutrients such as vitamin A, vitamin B, zinc, etc.

Combination Therapy (HAARTS)

Besides the effects of the medication mentioned above, the therapy (HAARTS) used for HIV/AIDS treatment also affects antioxidant levels. Standard HAARTS is a combination of at least three antiretroviral drugs, mostly made up of one protease inhibitor combined with at least two nucleoside analogue reverse transcriptase inhibitors. ART/HAARTS cannot cure HIV, but its effectiveness in the suppression of plasma HIV-1 RNA to undetectable concentrations has been shown in several clinical trials [60,61]. In the above-mentioned studies, the introduction of HAART resulted to about a 50% decline in AIDS mortality, decreased MTCT rate, as well as reduced incidence rate of opportunistic infections. Although limited studies have found a reduction in antiretroviral concentration due to supplementation with antioxidants, evidence exists that high concentrations of vitamin C may significantly reduce indinavir (a protease inhibitor used in the treatment of HIV patients) plasma concentration [62,63]. Merenstein et al., after supplementing with vitamin C, observed an increased rate of adherence to HAARTS; however, its effects on CD4 and viral load were not ascertaining [40]. Previous research by Ngondi and coworkers, in an attempt to observe the effects of combination therapy on oxidative stress markers, found that the combination treatment therapy I [stavudine (80 mg) + lamivudin (600 mg) + nevirapine + (400 mg) + zidovudine (600 mg)] brought about a significant reduction in the plasma concentration of protein sulfhydryl groups, thiobarbituric acid reactive substances, and vitamin C levels compared with therapy II [stavudine (80 mg) + lamivudin (300 mg) + nevirapin (400 mg)] or with a combination therapy III [zidovudine (600 mg) + lamivudin (300 mg) with efavirenz (600 mg)] [64].

Regardless of the type of combination therapy, intake of HAARTS has always been linked with adverse effects such as nausea, vomiting, etc., which indirectly leads to reduced nutrient intake and micronutrient deficiencies (Table 15.3; Ref. [65]).

Dietary Intake

Low dietary intake of micronutrient antioxidants through fruits and vegetables and/ or antioxidant supplements will eventually lead to micronutrient deficiency, especially including vitamins A, C, and E; zinc; and selenium.

TABLE 15.3

Adverse Effects of ARV/HAARTS on Nutrition

Medication	Adverse Effects
Zidovudin (Retrovir)	Nausea
Didanosin (Videx)	Nausea, diarrhea, loss of taste
141 W94 (Glaxo Wellcome)	Nausea, diarrhea
Abacanir (Glaxo Wellcome)	Nausea
Saquinavir (Invirase)	Nausea
Indinavir (Crixivan)	Kidney stones (>21 days drinking)
Ritonavir (Norvir)	Nausea, diarrhea
Adefovir	Lack of appetite, diarrhea, nausea
Nelfinavir (Viracept)	Diarrhea

Source: Biesalski H-K et al., *Medikamente mit Einfluss auf die Ernaehrung. Ernährungsmedizin*, 3rd Ed. p. 495, 2004.

SOCIOECONOMIC STATUS

Micronutrient deficiency is not only limited to poor countries but also extends to high-income nations—especially in people with low economic and educational status. However, micronutrient deficiencies in HIV/AIDS patients are highly prevalent in developing countries, where expensive high-quality animal-derived products are often not affordable to the poor, and associated with important negative biomedical consequences. Furthermore, studies show that vitamin A deficiency has been associated with a lack of knowledge rather than with low income, contrary to iron deficiency whose main cause was mainly economically determined [66].

ADVERSE EFFECTS OF SUPPLEMENTATION OF ANTIOXIDANTS ON HIV/AIDS PATIENTS

Previous studies have shown positive effects of antioxidant supplements and/or an antioxidant-rich diet on standard biological markers such as CD4 cells and viral load [32,34]. Meanwhile, some studies demonstrate the adverse effect of antioxidant supplementation on the immune system. The supplementation of vitamin E, for example, has been shown to increase the expression of CCR5 (the major cell entry coreceptor for T-cell line–tropic and macrophage-tropic strains of HIV-1), hence an increased infection of CD4 cells and whence an increased viral load [11]. Meanwhile, other researchers suggest that high doses of supplemented antioxidants could cause fluctuating CD4 concentrations, which could indirectly increase the rate of oxidative stress, deteriorating the health condition [20,67].

Besides the adverse effect of supplements on health, they are often very expensive and unaffordable for the majority of HIV/AIDS patients in resource-limited settings [68].

HIV PREVENTION

Besides the provision of antiretroviral medication and counseling on adequate nutrition, HIV/AIDS prevention is one of the most important aspects of comprehensive care of HIV/AIDS-infected people. Addressing prevention in comprehensive care is vital and will go a long way to reduce the number of HIV new infection rates, as well as delay the onset of AIDS for already infected individuals. Strategies to assure effective prevention of HIV infection among children and adults include providing free HIV testing campaigns, strengthening the capacities of HIV prevention services, providing contraceptives and counseling, and providing HIV care and treatment to infected persons timely. Other prevention strategies include promoting behavior change. Behavior change will help promote safer individual behavior and change in social customs, and consequently healthier forms of sexual behavior, e.g., correct and consistent use of condoms. Also, providing behavior change programs for sex workers and men who have sex with men will help reduce the prevalence of HIV in this group of individuals [69].

REFERENCES

1. UNAIDS. 2010. *2010 Report on the Global AIDS Epidemic*. Geneva: UNAIDS.
2. WHO. 2011. *World Health Statistics Report*. Media center. Geneva: WHO.
3. UNAIDS, UNICEF. 2011. *Global HIV/AIDS Response: Epidemic Update and Health Sector Progress towards Universal Access*. Switzerland: Villars-sous-Yens; Progress Report 2011.
4. Nyamweya S, Hegedus A, Jaye A, Rowland-Jones S, Flanagan KL and Macallan DC. 2013. Comparing HIV-1 and HIV-2 infection: Lessons for viral immunopathogenesis. *Rev. Med. Virol.* 23(4):221–240. doi: 10.1002/rmv.1739.
5. Martinez-Steele E, Awasana AA, Corrah T, Sabally S, van der Sande M, Jaye A, Togun T, Sarge-Njie R, McConkey SJ, Whittle H and Schim van der Loeff MF. 2007. Is HIV-2-induced AIDS different from HIV-1-associated AIDS? Data from a West African clinic. *AIDS* 21:317–324.
6. Sharp PM and Hahn BH. 2011. Origins of HIV and the AIDS pandemic. *Cold Spring Harbor Perspect. Med.* 1:a006841.
7. Silan V, Kant S, Haldar P, Goswami K, Rai SK and Misra P. 2013. HIV risk behavior among men who have sex with men. *N. Am. J. Med. Sci.* 5(9):515–522. doi: 10.4103/1947-2714.118931.
8. Noubiap JJN, Bongoe A and Demanou SA. 2013. Mother-to-child transmission of HIV: Findings from an Early Infant Diagnosis program in Bertoua, Eastern Cameroon. *Pan Afr. Med. J.* 15:65. doi: 10.11604/pamj.2013.15.65.2551.
9. Chen SL, Zhao HR, Zhang YQ, Zhao CY, Li BJ, Bai GY, Liang L, Chen ZQ, Hui YL, Wang W and Lu XL. 2012. [A retrospective cohort study on the natural history of AIDS caused by blood transfusion]. *Zhonghua Liu Xing Bing Xue Za Zhi* 33(7):658–662.
10. Nielsen K and Bryson YJ. 2000. Diagnosis of HIV infection in children. *Pediatr. Clin. North Am.* 47(1):39–63.
11. Portales P, Guerrier T, Clot J, Corbeau P, Mettling C, Lin YL, Baillat V, de Boever CM, Le Moing V, Tramoni C, Reynes J and Segondy M. 2004. Vitamin E supplementation increases the expression of the CCR5 coreceptor in HIV-1 infected subjects. *Clin. Nutr.* 23:1244–1245.
12. Poonia B, Pauza CD and Salvato MS. 2009. Role of the Fas/FasL pathway in HIV or SIV disease. *Retrovirology* 6:91.

13. Ikomey G, Assoumou MC, Atashili J, Mesembe M, Mukwele B, Lyonga E, Eyoh A, Kafando A and Ndumbe PM. 2013. The potentials of Fas receptors and ligands in monitoring HIV-1 disease in children in Yaounde, Cameroon. *J. Int. Assoc. Provid. AIDS Care.* doi: 10.1177/2325957413488202.

14. Paton NI, Sangeetha S, Earnest A and Bellamy R. 2006. The impact of malnutrition on survival and the CD4 count response in HIV-infected patients starting anti-retrovirals. *HIV Med.* 7(5):323–330.

15. Hurwitz BE, Klaus JR, Llabre MM, Gonzalez A, Lawrence PJ, Maher KJ, Greeson JM, Baum MK, Shor-Posner G, Skyler JS and Schneiderman N. 2007. Suppression of human immunodeficiency virus type 1 viral load with selenium supplementation: A randomized controlled trial. *Arch. Intern. Med.* 167(2):148–154.

16. Nigel R. 2007. Food insecurity—A risk factor for HIV infection. *PLoS Med.* 4(10):e301.

17. Singhal N and Austin J. 2002. A clinical review of micronutrients in HIV infection. *J. Int. Assoc. Physicians AIDS Care* 1(2):63–75.

18. Benadé AJ. 2003. A place for palm fruit oil to eliminate vitamin A deficiency. *Asia Pac. J. Clin. Nutr.* 12(3):369–372.

19. van Jaarsveld PJ, Faber M, Tanumihardjo SA, Nestel P, Lombard CJ and Benadé AJ. 2009. β-Carotene–rich orange-fleshed sweet potato improves the vitamin A status of primary school children assessed with the modified-relative-dose-response test. *Am. J. Clin. Nutr.* 81(5):1080–1087.

20. Birringer M and Ristow M. 2012. Efficacy and risks of supplementation with antioxidants. *Ernaerungs Umschau* 59:10–14. doi: 10.4455/eu.2012.018.

21. Meydani SN and Benarko AA. 1998. Recent developments in Vitamin E and the immune response. *Nutr. Rev.* 56(Suppl. 2):49–58.

22. Baruchel S and Wainberg MA. 1992. The role of oxidative stress in disease progression in individuals infected by the human immunodeficiency virus. *J. Leukoc. Biol.* 52:111–114.

23. Schreck R, Rieber P and Baeuerle PA. 1991. Reactive oxygen intermediates as apparently widely used messengers in the activation of NF-kappa B transcription factor and HIV-1. *EMBO J.* 10:2247–2258.

24. Gil L, Lewis L, Martinez G, Tarinas A, Gonzalez I, Alvarez A, Tapanes R, Guiliani A, Leon OS and Perez J. 2005. Effect of dietary micronutrient intake on oxidative stress indicators in HIV/AIDS patients. *Int. J. Vitam. Nutr. Res.* 75(1):19–27.

25. Arendt BM, Boetzer AM, Lemoch H, Winkler P, Rockstroh JK, Berthold HK, Spengler U and Goerlich R. 2001. Plasma antioxidant capacity of HIV-seropositive and healthy subjects during long-term ingestion of fruit juice or a fruit–vegetable concentrate containing antioxidant polyphenols. *Eur. J. Clin. Nutr.* 55:786–792.

26. Holt EM, Stephen LM, Moran A, Basu S, Steinberger L, Ross JA, Hong CP and Sinaiko AR. 2009. Fruit and vegetable consumption and its relation to markers of inflammation and oxidative stress in adolescents. *J. Am. Diet. Assoc.* 109(3):414–421.

27. Duriancik DM, Lackey DE and Hoag KA. 2010. Vitamin A as a regulator of antigen presenting cells. *J. Nutr.* 140:1395–1399.

28. Romagnani S. 1999. Th₁/Th₂ cells. *Inflamm. Bowel Dis.* 5:285–294.

29. Hoag K, Nashold FE, Goverman J and Hayes CE. 2002. Retinoic acid enhances T helper 2 cell development that is essential for robust antibody responses through its action on antigen presenting cells. *J. Nutr.* 132:3736–3739.

30. Baum MK, Shor-Posner G, Zhang G, Lai H, Quesada JA, Campa A, Jose-Burbano M, Fletcher MA, Sauberlich H and Page JB. 1997. HIV-1 infection in women is associated with severe nutritional deficiencies. *J. Acquir. Immune Defic. Syndr. Hum. Retrovirol.* 16:272–278.

31. Stephensen CB, Marquis GS, Jacob RA, Kruzich LA, Douglas SD and Wilson CM. 2006. Vitamins C and E in adolescents and young adults with HIV infection. *Am. J. Clin. Nutr.* 83:870–879.

32. Visser ME, Maartens G, Kossew G and Hussey GD. 2003. Plasma vitamin A and zinc levels in HIV-infected adults in Cape Town, South Africa. *Br. J. Nutr.* 89(4):475–482.

33. Castetbon K, Kadio A, Bondurand A, Yao AB, Barouan C, Coulibaly Y, Anglaret X, Msellati P, Malvy D and Dabis F. 1997. Nutritional status and dietary intakes in human immunodeficiency virus (HIV)-infected outpatients in Abidjan, Côte D'Ivoire, 1995. *Eur. J. Clin. Nutr.* 51:81–86.

34. Fawzi WW, Msamanga GI, Spiegelman D, Wei R, Kapiga S, Villamor E, Mwakagile D, Mugusi F, Hertzmark E, Essex M, Hunter DJ. 2004. A randomized trial of multivitamin supplements and HIV disease progression and mortality. *N Engl J Med.* 351:23–32.

35. Motswagole BS, Mongwaketse TC, Mokotedi M, Kobue-Lekalake RI, Bulawayo BT, Thomas TS, Kurpad AV and Kwape LD. 2013. The efficacy of micronutrient-fortified sorghum meal in improving the immune status of HIV-positive adults. *Ann. Nutr. Metab.* 62:323–330.

36. Woodall AA, Britton G and Jackson MJ. 1997. Carotenoids and protection of phospholipids in solution or in liposomes against oxidation by peroxyl radicals: Relationship between carotenoid structure and protective ability. *Biochim. Biophys. Acta* 1336:575–586.

37. Nimmagadda AP, Burri BJ, Neidlinger T, O'Brien WA and Goetz MB. 1998. Effect of β-carotene supplementation on plasma human immunodeficiency virus (HIV) RNA levels and CD4+ cell counts in HIV-infected patients. *Clin. Infect. Dis.* 27:1311–1313.

38. Fawzi WW, Msamanga GI, Kupka R, Spiegelman D, Villamor E, Mugusi F, Wei R and Hunter D. 2007. Multivitamin supplementation improves hematologic status in HIV-infected women and their children in Tanzania. *Am. J. Clin. Nutr.* 85:1335–1343.

39. Baeten JM, McClelland RS, Wener MH, Bankson DD, Lavreys L, Mandaliya K, Bwayo JJ and Kreiss JK. 2007. Relationship between markers of HIV-1 disease progression and serum β-carotene concentrations in Kenyan women. *Int. J. STD AIDS* 18:202–206.

40. Merenstein D, Wang C, Gandhi M, Robison E, Levine AM, Schwartz RM, Weber KM and Liu C. 2012. An investigation of the possible interaction between the use of vitamin C and highly active antiretroviral therapy (HAART) adherence and effectiveness in treated HIV+ women. *Complement Ther. Med.* 20(4):222–227.

41. Robert F and Cathcart III, MD. 1984. Vitamin C in the treatment of acquired immune deficiency syndrome (AIDS). *Med. Hypotheses* 14(4):423–433.

42. Suttajit M. 2007. Advances in nutrition support for quality of life in HIV+/AIDS. *Asia Pac. J. Clin. Nutr.* 16(Suppl. 1):318–322.

43. Graham SM, Baete JM, Richardson BA, Bankson DD, Lavreys L, Ndinya-Achola JO, Mandaliya K, Overbaugh J and McClelland RS. 2007. Higher pre-infection vitamin E levels are associated with higher mortality in HIV-1-infected Kenyan women: A prospective study. *BMC Infect. Dis.* 7:63.

44. Olaniyi JA and Arinola OG. 2007. Essential trace elements and antioxidant status in relation to severity of HIV in Nigerian patients. *Med. Princ. Pract.* 16:420–425.

45. Bilbis LS, Idowu DB, Saidu Y, Lawal M and Njoku CH. 2010. Serum levels of antioxidant vitamins and mineral elements of human immunodeficiency virus positive subjects in Sokoto, Nigeria. *Ann. Afr. Med.* 9:235–239.

46. Gill H and Walker G. 2008. Selenium, immune function and resistance to viral infections. *Nutr. Diet.* 65(Suppl. 3):S41–S47.

47. Akinboro AO, Mejiuni DA, Onayemi O, Ayodele OE, Atiba AS and Bamimore GM. 2013. Serum selenium and skin diseases among Nigerians with human immunodeficiency virus/acquired immune deficiency syndrome. *HIV/AIDS (Auckl.)* 5:215–221.

48. Delmax-Beauieux MC, Peuchant E, Couchouron A, Constans J, Sergeant C, Simonoff M, Pellegrin JL, Leng B, Conri C and Clerc M. 1996. The enzymatic antioxidant system in blood and glutathione status in human immunodeficiency syndrome (HIV)-infected patients. Effects of supplementation with selenium or beta-carotene. *Am. J. Clin. Nutr.* 64:101–107.

49. Isa L, Lucchini A, Lodi S and Giachetti M. 1992. Blood zinc status and zinc treatment in human immunodeficiency virus-infected patients. *Int. J. Clin. Lab. Res.* 22:45–47.

50. Suter PM. 2002. Zink—Interaktionen. *Checkliste Ernährung.* Thieme, Stuttgart, Germany, p. 172.

51. Zinc Investigators' Collaborative Group. 1999. Prevention of diarrhoea and pneumonia by Zinc supplementation in Children from developing countries: Pooled analysis of randomised controlled trials. *J. Pediatr.* 135:689–697.

52. Abrams B, Duncan D and Hertz-Picciotto I. 1993. A prospective study of dietary intake and acquired immune deficiency syndrome in HIV-seropositive homosexual men. *J. Acquir. Immune Defic. Syndr.* 6(8):949–958.

53. Castilla P, Echarri R, Davalos A, Cerato F, Orega H, Teruel JL, Lucas MF, Gomez. Coronado D, Ortuno J and Lasuncion MA. 2006. Concentrated red grape juice exerts antioxidant, hypolipidemic, and anti-inflammatory effects in both hemodialysis patients and healthy subjects. *Am. J. Clin. Nutr.* 84:252–262.

54. Greenspan HC and Aruoma OI. 1994. Oxidative stress and apoptosis in HIV infection: A role for plants derived metabolites with synergetic antioxidant activity. *Immunol. Today* 15:209–213.

55. Winkler P, Ellinger S, Boetzer AM, Arendt BM, Berthold HK, Rockstroh JK, Spengler U and Goerlich R. 2004. Lymphocyte proliferation and apoptosis in HIV-seropositive and healthy subjects during long-term ingestion of fruit juices or a fruit–vegetable–concentrate rich in polyphenols and antioxidant vitamins. *Eur. J. Clin. Nutr.* 58:317–325.

56. Müller F, Svardal AM, Nerday I, Berge RK, Aukrust P and Freland SS. 2000. Virological and immunological effects of antioxidants treatment in patients with HIV infection. *Eur. J. Clin. Invest.* 30:905–914.

57. Lai ZW, Hanczko R, Bonilla E, Caza TN, Clair B, Bartos A, Miklossy G, Jimah J, Doherty E, Tily II, Francis L, Garcia R, Dawood M, Yu J, Ramos I, Coman I, Faraone SV, Phillips PE and Perl A. 2012. *N*-acetylcysteine reduces disease activity by blocking mammalian target of rapamycin in T cells from systemic lupus erythematosus patients. A randomized, double-blind, placebo-controlled trial. *Arthritis Rheum.* 64:2937–2946.

58. Dickinson DA, Moellering DR, Iles KE, Patel RP, Levonen AL, Wigley A, Darley-Usmar VM and Forman HJ. 2003. Cytoprotection against oxidative stress and the regulation of glutathione synthesis. *Biol. Chem.* 384:527–537.

59. Samuni Y, Goldstein S, Dean OM, Berk M. 2013. The chemistry and biological activities of N-acetylcysteine. *Biochim Biophys Acta.* 1830:4117-29. doi: 10.1016/j.bbagen.2013 .04.016.

60. Marston B and DeCock KM. 2004. Multivitamins, nutrition, and antiretroviral therapy for HIV disease in Africa. *N. Engl. J. Med.* 351(1):78–80.

61. *AIDS Epidemic Update.* 2007. Available at: http://data.unaids.org/pub/EPISlides/2007 /2007_epiupdate_en.pdf.

62. Slain D, Amsden JR, Khakoo RA, Fisher MA, Lalka D and Hobbs GR. 2005. Effect of high-dose Vitamin C on the steady-state pharmacokinetics of the protease inhibitor indinavir in healthy volunteers. *Pharmacotherapy* 25:165–170.

63. Lee LS, Andrade AS and Flexner C. 2006. Interactions between natural health products and antiretroviral drugs: Pharmacokineticand pharmacodynamic effects. *Clin. Infect. Dis.* 43:1052–1059.

64. Ngondi JL, Oben J, Forkah DM, Etame LH and Mbanya D. 2006. The effect of different combination therapies on oxidative stress markers in HIV infected patients in Cameroon. *AIDS Res. Ther.* 3:19.

65. Biesalski H-K, Furst P, Heinrich K, Kluthe R, Pölert W, Puchstein C and Stehelin HB. 2004. *Medikamente mit Einfluss auf die Ernaehrung. Ernährungsmedizin*, 3rd Ed., Thieme, Stuttgart, Germany, p. 495.

66. Darnton-Hill I, Webb P, Harvey PWJ, Hunt JM, Dalmiya N, Chopra M, Ball MJ, Bloem MW and de Benoist B. 2005. Micronutrient deficiencies and gender: Social and economic costs. *Am. J. Clin. Nutr.* 81(5):1198S–1205S.
67. Rolina DG and Lindi MW. 2009. Reconciling conflicting clinical studies of antioxidant supplementation as HIV therapy: A mathematical approach. *BMC Public Health* 9(1):12.
68. Lunney KM, Jenkins AL, Tavengwa NV, Majo F, Chidhanguro D, Iliff P, Strickland GT, Piwoz E, Iannotti L and Humphrey JH. 2008. HIV-positive poor women may stop breast-feeding early to protect their infants from HIV infection although available replacement diets are grossly inadequate. *J. Nutr.* 138(2):351–357.
69. Hankins CA and de Zalduondo BO. 2010. Combination prevention: A deeper understanding of effective HIV prevention. *AIDS* 24(Suppl. 4):S70–S80.

Section IV

Role of Herbs

16 Role of Herbs and Spices
In Health and Longevity and in Disease

Krishnapura Srinivasan

CONTENTS

Introduction 281
Antioxidant Effects of Spices and Herbs 283
    Turmeric (*Curcuma longa*) and Curcumin...284
    Garlic (*Allium sativum*) and Onion (*Allium cepa*) 284
    Ginger (*Zingiber officinale*) 288
    Clove (*Eugenia caryophyllus*) and Eugenol..289
Antiatherogenic and Cardioprotective Effect..290
Cancer-Preventive Property 291
Amelioration of Oxidative Stress in Diabetes..293
Anticataractogenesis 294
Neuroprotective Potential 294
Anti-Inflammatory Effect..294
Hepatoprotective and Renal-Protective Effects 295
Other Nutraceutical Properties of Herbs and Spices..296
Conclusions..296
References..297

INTRODUCTION

Herbs and spices have a long history of both culinary and medicinal use. Ayurvedic traditional medicine evolved more than 5000 years ago, and uses herbs and spices for health, including tumeric, basil, mace, cinnamon, and ginger (Govindarajan et al. 2005). Traditionally, the Chinese have integrated food, nutrition, and health, including herbs and spices in specially prepared dishes for both sustenance and for purported health benefits (Bellamy and Pfister 1992). Ginseng and ginkgo biloba are reportedly used to improve stamina and cognitive performance, respectively. Herbs and spices can be regarded as among the first "functional foods." Asian and Indian diets, which are high in vegetables and fruits, also generally include a large amount and considerable variety of herbs and spices (Sinha et al. 2003). The health-promoting effect of these foods are attributable not only to the general nutritional profile (high in dietary fiber; low in fat and salt; low energy density; and high in vitamins A, C, and folate) but also to a wide range of nonnutrient bioactives and phytochemicals such as flavonoids and other phenolics, which are found in herbs and spices. Herbs and spices add flavor to foods without salt, thus assisting to meet the reduced daily intake of sodium. Herbs and spices add flavor to foods without fat, thus assisting to meet healthy fat intake. Inclusion of herbs and spices in diets promotes intake of plant-based foods that increase the nutritional quality of the daily diet. Herbs and spices, while providing flavor and aroma to our diets, also contribute diverse bioactives that may have a role in improving human health. Herbs and spices are hence a desirable integral part of daily diet.

Oxidative stress has been implicated in the etiology of cardiovascular disease, type 2 diabetes, cataract, inflammatory diseases, neurodegenerative diseases, cancer, and also in the natural aging process. Reactive oxygen radicals are detrimental to cells since they induce lipid peroxidation in cellular membranes, generating lipid peroxides that cause extensive damage to membranes and membrane-mediated chromosomal damage. Endothelial cell injury is often the first stage of these disorders. The antioxidant enzymes, superoxide dismutase, catalase, and glutathione peroxidase, present intracellularly can directly scavenge these oxidants or prevent their conversion to toxic species. There is a growing interest in natural antioxidants found in plants that hinder the oxidative processes and thereby delay or suppress oxidative stress. A wide variety of phenolic compounds present in spices possess potent antioxidant, anti-inflammatory, antimutagenic, and cancer-preventive activities. This article lists a host of spice compounds that are experimentally evidenced to control cellular oxidative stress both *in vitro* and *in vivo* and their beneficial role in preventing or ameliorating oxidative stress–mediated diseases—cardiovascular disease, diabetes, cataract, and cancer.

A wide variety of phenolic compounds and flavonoids present in spices (Figure 16.1) are now experimentally documented to possess potent antioxidant, anti-inflammatory, antimutagenic, and anticarcinogenic activities. The antioxidative and anti-inflammatory properties of these bioactive compounds from spices appear to contribute to their chemopreventive or chemoprotective activity. Cyclooxygenase-2 (COX-2) has been recognized as a molecular target of many chemopreventive as well as anti-inflammatory agents. Studies have shown that COX-2 is regulated by the eukaryotic transcription factor NF-κB. The molecular mechanisms underlying the chemopreventive effects of spice ingredients in terms of their effects on intracellular signaling cascades, particularly those involving NF-κB and mitogen-activated protein kinases, are recently reviewed (Surh 2002). Antioxidants in foods may work in combination to produce synergistic effects. Plant foods, which are rich in flavonoids, have many different antioxidant compounds (Halvorsen et al. 2006). Many epidemiological studies show that consuming a diet high in antioxidant-rich fruits and vegetables is associated with a variety of other health benefits (Cao et al. 1998). Herbs and spices make an important contribution to total daily flavonoid intake (Baghurst 2006). Higher amounts of dietary antioxidants or higher plasma levels of antioxidants are associated with improved heart health and cellular function (Cao et al. 1998).

Spice bioactive compound	Chemical structure
Curcumin (*Curcuma longa*)	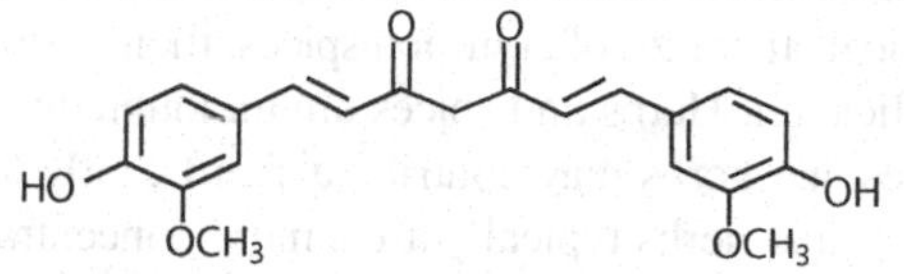
Capsaicin (*Capsicum annuum*)	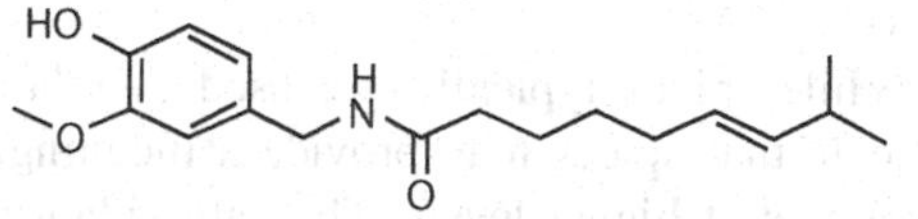
Piperine (*Piper nigrum*)	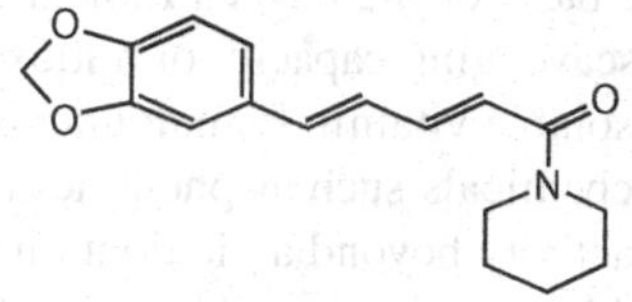
Gingerol (*Zinger officinale*)	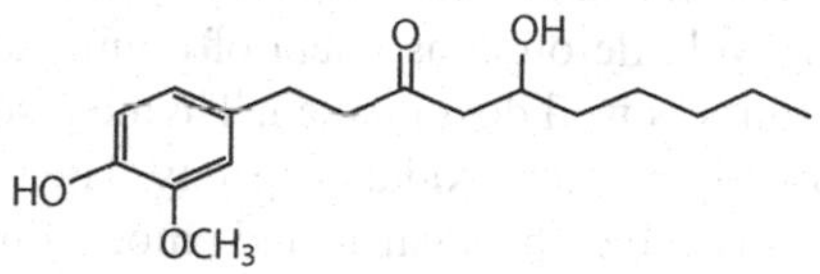
Eugenol (*Eugenia caryophyllus*)	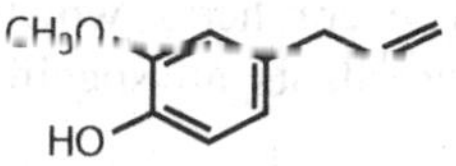
Allicin and S-allyl cysteine (*Allium sativa*)	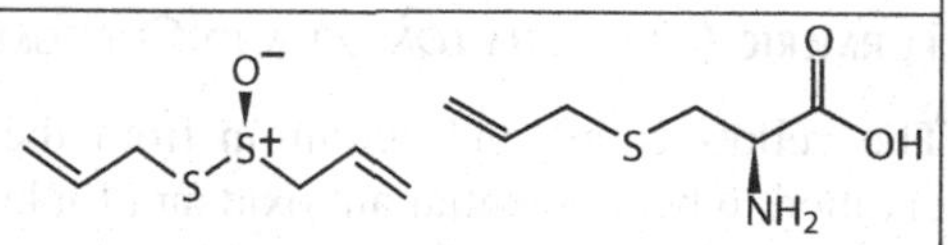
Quercetin (*Allium sativa*)	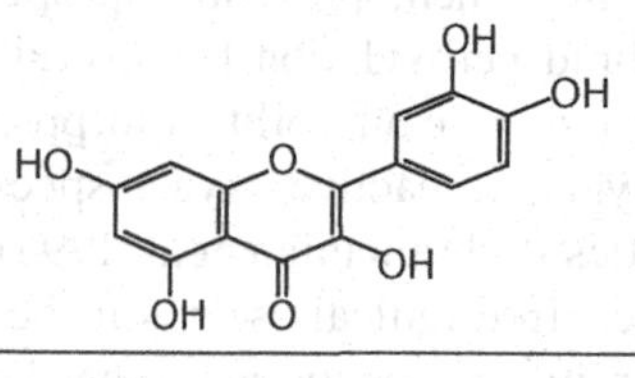

FIGURE 16.1 Spice bioactive compounds.

ANTIOXIDANT EFFECTS OF SPICES AND HERBS

In the context of the oxidative stress theory of aging and age-related degenerative diseases, dietary phenolic or thiolic antioxidants have been shown to increase the life span of laboratory animals and protect against senescent immune decline. In view of the limitations of the "lipid theory" of atherosclerosis and the current suggestion that free radical–mediated oxidation of cholesterol is a key step in atherogenesis (Duthrie and

Brown 1994), the antioxidant compounds present in spices have gained more importance for their possible role in the prevention of atherogenesis. Among the several nutraceutical attributes of common spices, their antioxidant potential has far-reaching health implication. Herbs and spices are undoubtedly a rich source of antioxidants. Culinary spices and herbs may contribute significantly to the total intake of plant antioxidants. Spices and herbs typically are a more concentrated source of dietary antioxidants than many other food groups such as fruits, berries, cereals, and vegetables (Tapsell et al. 2006).

While spices typically are used at relatively low levels in foods, these data indicate that spices may provide a meaningful level of antioxidant activity when consumed at higher levels. The antioxidant capacity of herbs and spices has been evaluated on the basis of the oxygen radical absorbance capacity, which provides a measure of the scavenging capacity of antioxidants against the peroxyl radical, and Trolox, a water-soluble vitamin E analogue, is used as a calibration standard. There are many phytochemicals such as phenolics and organosulfur compounds in spices that possess bioactivity beyond antioxidation. The volatile oil components of thyme (*Thymus vulgaris*) include carvacrol, borneol, geraniol, and thymol. Thymol is the primary volatile oil constituent of thyme, and its antioxidant protection of cellular membranes is well documented. Thyme also contains a variety of flavonoids, which increase thyme's antioxidant capacity. The antioxidative effects of spices—turmeric/curcumin (Table 16.1), garlic and onion (Table 16.2), clove/eugenol (Table 16.3), red pepper/capsaicin (Table 16.4), black pepper/piperine (Table 16.4), ginger/gingerol, and fenugreek—and of several herbs, which have been extensively studied and evidenced as potential antioxidants, are specifically discussed.

TURMERIC (*CURCUMA LONGA*) AND CURCUMIN

The yellow compound curcumin from the rhizome of *Curcuma longa* has been claimed to be a potential antioxidant (Table 16.1) and anti-inflammatory agent with bioprotective and chemopreventive properties. Curcumin is shown to be a good inhibitor of lipid peroxidation by several investigators (Reddy and Lokesh 1992). Curcumin has significant abilities to protect against single-strand breaks induced by singlet oxygen, a reactive oxygen species (ROS) with potential genotoxic/mutagenic properties (Subramanian et al. 1994). The ability of curcumin to protect DNA against oxygen free radicals seems to be related to its structure and may at least partly explain its therapeutic and other beneficial effects, including antimutagenic and anticarcinogenic properties (Figure 16.2). The antioxidant properties of turmeric and curcumin are also evidenced in animal studies (Reddy and Lokesh 1994a,b). Curcumin inhibits lipid peroxidation possibly by quenching oxygen free radicals, as inferred by *in vitro* studies, and by enhancing the activity of endogenous antioxidant enzymes.

GARLIC (*ALLIUM SATIVUM*) AND ONION (*ALLIUM CEPA*)

Diallyl sulfides and diallyl disulfides, which are active components of garlic, have known antioxidant (Table 16.2), anti-inflammatory, and antimutagenic activities.

TABLE 16.1
Antioxidant Effects of Curcumin in *In Vitro* Systems and in *In Vivo* Situations

In Vitro/Animal Model	Effect Demonstrated
In Vitro Models	
RBC membranes	Curcumin inhibited lipid peroxidation
Rat liver microsomes	Curcumin inhibited ascorbate–Fe^{2+}-induced lipid peroxidation
Xanthine–xanthine oxidase system	Curcumin inhibited superoxide anion and OH radical generation
Rat macrophages	Curcumin inhibited SO anions, H_2O_2, and nitrite radical production
Plasmid DNA	Curcumin diminished singlet oxygen–induced DNA strand damage
Rat liver microsomes	Curcumin inhibited Fe^{2+}-induced lipid peroxidation
Human LDL	Curcumin inhibited Cu^{2+}-induced lipid peroxidation
In Vivo Situations	
Mice	Curcumin lowered lipid peroxidation produced by CCl_4, paraquat
Rats	Curcumin suppressed CCl_4-induced and ^{60}Co-induced lipid peroxidation
Rats	Turmeric decreased Fe^{2+}-induced liver lipid peroxides; enhanced antioxidant enzymes
Hypercholesterolemic and high-fat fed rats	Dietary curcumin enhanced antioxidant status of red blood cells, blood, and liver
Hepatoprotective Effect	
Rats	Curcumin lowered Fe^{2+}-induced liver hepatotoxicity and lipid peroxides
Rats	Curcumin reduced alcohol-induced oxidative stress
Rats	Curumin reduced lipid peroxides in chloroquine-induced hepatotoxicity
Mice	Curcumin suppressed trichloroethylene-induced oxidative stress
Cardioprotective Effect	
Humans	Curcuminoids reduced serum lipid peroxides
Humans	*Curcuma longa* extract decreased blood lipid peroxides and LDL oxidation
Isoproterenol-treated rat	Curcumin countered lipid peroxidation in myocardial infarction
Isoprenaline-treated rat	Oral curcumin reduced oxidative stress during myocardial ischemia
Atherosclerotic rabbits	*Curcuma longa* extract decreased susceptibility LDL to lipid peroxidation
Cholesterol-fed rabbits	*Curcuma longa* reduced oxidative stress during atherosclerosis
Oxidative Stress in Diabetes	
STZ-diabetic rats	Dietary curcumin lowered lipid peroxides in plasma and urine
STZ-diabetic rats	Curcumin countered decreased enzymic/nonenzymic antioxidants
Antioxidant Effect in Cataract	
Rats	Curcumin decreased naphthalene-induced opacification of eye lens
Rats	Curcumin prevented selenium-induced oxidative damage in eye lens and delayed cataract

(Continued)

TABLE 16.1 (CONTINUED)
Antioxidant Effects of Curcumin in *In Vitro* Systems and in *In Vivo* Situations

In Vitro/Animal Model	Effect Demonstrated
STZ-diabetic rats	Curcumin/turmeric countered oxidative stress in eye lens and progression of cataract
Renal Protective Effect	
Rats	Curcumin lowered oxidative stress in induced renal toxicity
Neuroprotective Effect	
Rats	Curcumin protected lead-induced neurotoxicity
Anticancer Potential	
Mice	Curcumin increased activities of antioxidant and phase II enzymes
Mice	Curcumin showed antitumor effect in skin induced by peroxynitrite

TABLE 16.2
Antioxidant Influence of Garlic (*Allium sativum*) and Onion (*Allium cepa*)

System	Effect Observed
Garlic (*Allium sativum*) and Its Constituents	
Hamster	S-Allylcysteine suppressed the incidence of DMBA-induced buccal pouch tumors, decreased lipid peroxidation, and enhanced antioxidant enzymes
Rats	Garlic intake reduced the incidence of azoxymethane-induced colon tumor, accompanied by reduction in lipid peroxidation and higher GST activity
Rats	S-Allylcysteine administration inhibited NDA-induced liver cancer and lipid peroxidation with simultaneous increase in antioxidants
Rats	Garlic oil increased hepatic antioxidant enzyme activities
Diabetic rats	Garlic oil increased plasma total thiols and decreased lipid peroxides; higher GST activity in erythrocytes and SOD in liver and kidney
Diabetic rats	Garlic juice countered changes in lipid peroxides and activities of GST
Atherosclerotic patients	Garlic extract lowered plasma and erythrocyte malondialdehyde levels
Hypercholesterolemic subjects	Garlic extract increased blood antioxidant oxidant status, superoxide radical scavenger activity, and decreased lipid peroxides
Human subjects	Garlic supplementation increased resistance of LDL to oxidation
Rat erythrocytes	AGE prevented decrease of RBC deformability induced by lipid peroxidation and reduced lipid peroxidation
Human LDL	Garlic compounds inhibited superoxide production; suppressed copper-induced LDL oxidation

TABLE 16.2 (CONTINUED)
Antioxidant Influence of Garlic (*Allium sativum*) and Onion (*Allium cepa*)

System	Effect Observed
	Onion (*Allium cepa*) and Its Constituents
Nicotine-injected rats	Onion oil showed increased resistance to lipid peroxidation and increased tissue antioxidants and antioxidant enzymes
Alloxan diabetic rats	S-Methyl cysteine sulfoxide lowered levels of malondialdehyde, hydroperoxide, and conjugated dienes in tissues
Alloxan-diabetic rats	Onion juice countered changes in lipid peroxides and activities of GST in plasma and tissues
Rats fed with high-fat/high-sucrose diet	Onion reduced superoxide generation and increased NO availability in the aorta
Human volunteers	Ingestion of onions resulted in increased total antioxidant capacity
Human PMNL cells	Aqueous extract of onion inhibited 5'-lipoxygenase *in vitro*

Note: DMBA, dimethyl benzanthracene; GST, glutathione-S-transferase; NDA, N-nitroso diethylamine; SOD, superoxide dismutase; LDL, low-density lipoprotein; AGE, advance glycation endproducts; PMNL, polymorphonuclear leukocyte.

TABLE 16.3
Antioxidant Influence of Eugenol in *In Vitro* Systems and *In Vivo* Studies

Animal Model/*In Vitro* System	Effect Demonstrated
Human RBC	Eugenol inhibited Cu^{2+}-induced lipid peroxidation
Rat liver microsomes	Eugenol inhibited ascorbate–Fe^{2+}-induced lipid peroxidation
ROS generation in the xanthine–xanthine oxidase system	Eugenol inhibited the generation of reactive oxygen species, and prevented the oxidation of Fe^{2+} in Fenton reaction that generates OH radicals.
Peroxynitrite-induced lipid peroxidation	Eugenol decreased nitrotyrosine formation and lipid peroxidation
Human PMNL cells	Eugenol inhibited 5-lipoxygenase and formation of leukotrienes
In vitro study	Eugenol inhibited copper-induced oxidation of LDL
	Animal Models
Rats fed unsaturated fat	Dietary eugenol decreased serum and liver lipid peroxides, enhanced activities of antioxidant enzymes, and lowered lipid peroxides in liver
7,12-Dimethyl benz(α)anthracene applied mice	Eugenol inhibited the number of tumors due to radical scavenging activity
CCl_4-administered rat	Eugenol pretreatment countered hepatotoxicity
Rats	Eugenol lowered Fe^{2+}-induced lipid peroxides; lowered hepatotoxicity
Rats	Oral eugenol increased glutathione, GSH-transferase in the intestine
Swiss mice	Eugenol protected against oxidative stress caused by γ-radiation

TABLE 16.4

Antioxidant Influence of Capsaicin of Red Pepper (*Capsicum annuum*) and Piperine of Black Pepper (*Piper nigrum*)

Animal Model	Effect Demonstrated
Capsaicin of Red Pepper	
Human RBC	Capsaicin inhibited lipid peroxidation
Rat liver microsomes	Capsaicin inhibited ascorbate–Fe^{2+}-induced lipid peroxidation
Rat liver mitochondria	Capsaicin inhibited lipid peroxidation and scavenging of DPPH radicals
Human LDL	Capsaicin inhibited Cu^{2+}-induced lipid peroxidation
Human PMNL cells	Capsaicin inhibited 5′-lipoxygenase
Rats	Capsaicin reduced oxidative stress in the liver, lung, kidney, and muscle
High-fat-fed rats and hypercholesterolemic rats	Capsaicin enhanced antioxidant status of red blood cells, blood, and liver
Piperine of Black Pepper	
Rat liver	Piperine inhibited ascorbate–Fe^{2+}-induced lipid peroxidation
In vitro	Piperine inhibited/quenched superoxides and hydroxyl radicals, and inhibited lipid peroxidation
In vitro	Black pepper and piperine inhibited human PMNL 5′-lipoxygenase
Human LDL	Piperine protected Cu^{2+}-induced lipid peroxidation of human LDL
Mice	Piperine decreased mitochondrial lipid peroxidation and augmented antioxidant defense during benzo(α)pyrene-induced lung carcinogenesis
High-fat-fed rats	Black pepper/piperine reduced oxidative stress by lowering lipid peroxidation, and restored the activities of antioxidant enzymes and GSH
Rats	Piperine protected against carcinogen-induced oxidative stress in the intestinal lumen
Streptozotocin-diabetic rats	Piperine partially protected against diabetes-induced oxidative stress

Onion is a major source of flavonoids, especially the two quercetin glycosides, quercetin 4′-*o*-β-glucoside and quercetin 3,4′-*o*-β-diglucosides, which are recognized as bioactive substances. The antioxidant effect of onion oil and garlic oil (100 mg/kg for 21 days) has been reported on nicotine-induced lipid peroxidation in rat tissues (Helen et al. 1999), as inferred by countering the increased lipid peroxides in the liver, lungs, heart, and kidney tissues of nicotine-treated rats and restoration of the activities of antioxidant enzymes, which decreased in nicotine-treated rats.

GINGER (*ZINGIBER OFFICINALE*)

The antioxidant effect of the total phenols of ginger extract has been established *in vitro* (Stoilova et al. 2007). Gingerol exhibited dose-dependent inhibition of nitric oxide production and significant reduction of inducible nitric oxide synthase in lipopolysaccharide-stimulated macrophages, thus suggesting the protective ability of this

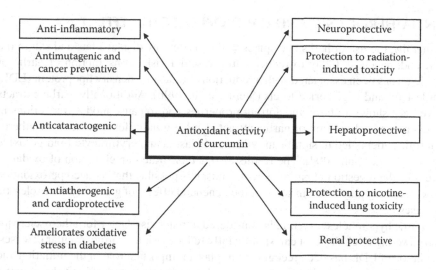

FIGURE 16.2 Diverse pharmacological activities of curcumin mediated through antioxidant potential.

compound against peroxynitrite-mediated damage (Ippoushi et al. 2003). Capsaicin (*trans*-8-methyl-*N*-vanillyl-6-nonenamide) is the major pungent and irritating ingredient of red pepper. The antioxidant property of capsaicin in terms of inhibiting lipid peroxidation in human erythrocyte membranes and in rat liver microsomes is documented (Reddy and Lokesh 1992).

CLOVE (*EUGENIA CARYOPHYLLUS*) AND EUGENOL

The antioxidant potency of eugenol, the principal flavor compound of clove (Table 16.3), is recognized by the inhibition of the generation of ROS in model systems, the inhibition of copper-induced lipid peroxidation in human erythrocyte membranes (Reddy and Lokesh 1994b), and carbon tetrachloride–induced lipid peroxidation (Nagashima 1989). Inducible COX-2 has been implicated in the processes of inflammation and carcinogenesis. Eugenol was found to potently inhibit the prostaglandin E_2 production in lipopolysaccharide-activated mouse macrophages (Kim et al. 2003), thus suggesting that eugenol might be a plausible COX-2 inhibitor, and thus acts as an anti-inflammatory or cancer chemopreventive agent. Eugenol has been investigated for its effects on the cytotoxicity and induction of apoptosis. Eugenol-treated HL-60 cells displayed features of apoptosis, including DNA fragmentation, and demonstrated that ROS plays a critical role in eugenol-induced apoptosis, and this is a possible mechanism of the anticancer effect of eugenol. The antioxidant properties of eugenol are documented in animal studies, where dietary eugenol (0.05%) significantly lowered lipid peroxidation in the serum and liver of rats and was associated with enhanced activities of antioxidant enzymes—superoxide dismutase, catalase, glutathione peroxidase, and glutathione *S*-transferase (Reddy and Lokesh 1996).

ANTIATHEROGENIC AND CARDIOPROTECTIVE EFFECT

Generally, the use of herbs and spices will considerably displace fats and salt in the diet and, hence, is likely to reduce cardiovascular risk. Consumption of garlic or garlic oil has been associated with a reduction in total/low-density lipoprotein (LDL) cholesterol and triglyceride levels (Steiner et al. 1996). Additionally, garlic extracts have been shown to have anticlotting properties and to cause modest reductions in blood pressure. Ingestion of garlic extract (1 mL/kg daily for 6 months) by atherosclerotic patients led to significantly lowered plasma and erythrocyte lipid peroxide levels (Durak et al. 2004). The results also demonstrated amelioration of oxidative stress by the ingestion of garlic extract. Thus, it is possible that reduced peroxidation processes may play a part in some of the beneficial effects of garlic in atherosclerotic diseases.

While hypercholesterolemia is considered a major risk factor for atherosclerosis, and lowering of cholesterol can significantly reduce risk for cardiovascular diseases, oxidation of LDL has been recognized to play an important role in the initiation and progression of atherosclerosis. Several garlic compounds can effectively suppress LDL oxidation *in vitro* (Lau 2001). Short-term supplementation of garlic in human subjects has demonstrated an increased resistance of LDL to oxidation; suppressed LDL oxidation may be one of the powerful mechanisms accounting for the antiatherosclerotic properties of garlic.

Intake of lemongrass (*Cymbopogon citrates*) oil (140 mg/day) by hypercholesterolemic subjects produced a drop in cholesterol concentrations up to 38 mg/dL (Huang et al. 1994). There are a large number of studies concerning the potential cardiovascular health benefits of antioxidants such as flavonoids of tea (Carnesecchi et al. 2001). Herbs and spices make an important contribution to total daily flavonoid intake. Basil (*Ocimum basilicum*) is a very good source of β-carotene (provitamin A), a powerful antioxidant that not only protects epithelial cells from free radical damage but also helps prevent free radicals from oxidizing cholesterol in the bloodstream leading to arteriosclerosis. Spice components such as zingiber, capsaicin, and curcumin have been associated with a decrease in LDL cholesterol and an increase in high-density lipoprotein (HDL) cholesterol levels in rat studies (Lantry et al. 1997).

Daily intake of curcuminoids (0.5 g) by healthy human volunteers produced a 33% reduction in blood lipid peroxide levels (Soni and Kuttan 1992). Curcumin administration (500 mg/day for 7 days) was accompanied by an increase in HDL cholesterol and a decrease in total serum cholesterol (Quiles et al. 2002). Reduction in serum lipid peroxides and cholesterol suggests the potential of curcumin as a preventive substance against arterial diseases. Supplementation with turmeric reduced oxidative stress (reduced plasma lipid peroxides and restored α-tocopherol and coenzyme-Q levels) and attenuated the development of fatty streaks in rabbits fed on a high-cholesterol diet (Quiles et al. 2002).

Oxidation of LDL plays an important role in the development of atherosclerosis. Turmeric extract decreased the susceptibility of LDL to lipid peroxidation in atherosclerotic rabbits, thus suggesting its value in the management of cardiovascular disease (Ramirez-Tortosa et al. 1999). In healthy humans, the daily intake of 200 mg turmeric extract resulted in a decrease in blood lipid peroxides as well as in HDL and LDL lipid peroxidation (Miquel et al. 2002). Dietary curcumin and capsaicin significantly inhibited the *in vivo* iron-induced LDL oxidation in rats and copper-induced oxidation of LDL *in vitro* (Manjunatha and Srinivasan 2006). Piperine of black pepper (*Piper nigrum*) has been demonstrated in *in vitro* experiments to protect against oxidative damage by inhibiting or quenching free radicals and ROS, and inhibit lipid peroxidation (Mittal and Gupta 2000). Piperine is shown to be an effective antioxidant and offer protection against oxidation of human LDL, as evaluated by copper ion–induced lipid peroxidation of human LDL (Naidu and Thippeswamy 2002) (Table 16.4).

Orally administered curcumin effectively countered the changes in the endogenous antioxidant molecules and enzymes accompanying myocardial infarction induced by *iso*-proterenol in rats (Nirmala and Puvanakrishnan 1996). Curcumin treatment was found to protect the rat myocardium against ischemic insult, and the protective effect could be attributed to its antioxidant properties as well as its inhibitory effects on xanthine dehydrogenase–xanthine oxidase conversion and resultant superoxide anion production (Manikandan et al. 2004).

CANCER-PREVENTIVE PROPERTY

Animal and *in vitro* studies suggest that certain herbs help protect against oxidative stress and inflammation, both of which are risk factors for cancer initiation and promotion (Surh 1999). Anti-inflammatory compounds of spices—curcumin, gingerol, and capsaicin—appear to act by inhibiting one or more steps in the pro-inflammatory pathway. The natural anti-inflammatory compounds quercetin, curcumin, and silymarin have been shown to be as effective as indomethacin, a nonsteroidal anti-inflammatory drug, in inhibiting the formation of aberrant crypt foci in the rat (Volate et al. 2005). Herbs and spices with known anticarcinogenic properties in animal models of carcinogenesis include tumeric, garlic, ginger, basil, rosemary, mint, and lemongrass (Table 16.5).

Methanol extract of the leaves of rosemary (*Rosmarinus officinalis*) and its constituent carnosol (a phenolic diterpene) can inhibit tumor promotion in mouse skin (Elson et al. 1989). Geraniol (an acyclic monoterpene alcohol) of *Cymbopogon citratus* (lemon grass) has been shown to inhibit growth and polyamine biosynthesis in human colon cancer cells (Hertog et al. 1993). Perillyl alcohol (a monoterpene) found in lavender and mint has been shown to reduce tumor incidence and tumor multiplicity in a mouse lung tumor (Gujaral et al. 1978). Aqueous extract of spearmint as drinking fluid during treatment with a colon carcinogen showed lower numbers of colonic aberrant crypt foci in rats (Yu et al. 2004). Myristicin of parsley has been shown to inhibit tumor multiplicity in a rodent lung cancer model and induce glutathione *S*-transferase in the liver and small intestinal mucosa (Zheng et al. 1992).

Turmeric or its constituent curcumin is found to have chemopreventive effects against cancers of the skin, forestomach, liver, and colon, and oral cancer in mice (Chuang et al. 2000; Volate et al. 2005). The effect of dietary curcumin on the activities of antioxidant and phase II–metabolizing enzymes involved in detoxification and production of ROS has been evaluated in mice (Srinivasan 2014). Induction of detoxifying enzymes by curcumin suggests the potential of this compound as a

TABLE 16.5
Potential Health Effects of Various Culinary Herbs Indicated in Scientific Literature

Herb	Bioactive Compound/ Tested Sample	Perceived Health Effects
Basil (*Ocimum basilicum*)	Eugenol and flavonoids	Anti-inflammation in cancer development; inhibition of lipid peroxidation; antimicrobial effects
Ginseng	Herb extract	Hypoglycemic effect
Lemongrass (*Cymbopogon citratus*)	Citral, limonene	Anti-inflammation and inhibition of polyamine biosynthesis in human colon cancer development
Oregano (*Poliomintha longiflora*)	Herb extract	Antimicrobial effects
Parsley (*Petroselinum crispum*)	Myristicin/herb extract	Inhibition of lung carcinogenesis; antimicrobial effects
Rosemary (*Rosmarinus officinalis*)	Flavonoids, rosmarinate	Inhibition of carcinogenesis; anti-inflammation in cancer development
Sage (*Salvia officinalis*)	Essential oil	Inhibition of bone resorption; improvement in memory retention
Spearmint (*Mentha spicata*)	Herb extract	Antimutagenic effect
Thyme (*Thymus vulgaris*)	Thymol	Inhibition of bone resorption; antimicrobial effects

protective agent against chemical carcinogenesis and other forms of electrophilic toxicity. *In vitro* and animal cancer models have shown that diallyl sulfide of garlic is effective in the detoxification of carcinogens through its effects on phase I and phase II enzymes (Wargovich et al. 2001).

The incidence of cancer at different sites may be related to oxidative damage to host genome by genotoxicants. Curcumin, which possesses antimutagenic property, appears to be a promising chemopreventive agent. The antioxidant properties of curcumin explain the diverse pharmacological potential of this phytochemical or the parent spice, turmeric (Figure 16.2). The antioxidant property is also implicated in the cancer chemopreventive effects of curcumin against the induction of tumors in various target organs. *S*-Allylcysteine of garlic modulated 7,12-dimethyl-benz[α] anthracene-induced buccal pouch carcinogenesis by decreasing the susceptibility of the buccal pouch to lipid peroxidation in Syrian hamsters, while simultaneously enhancing activities of antioxidant enzymes in the liver and circulation (Balasenthil et al. 2001). Dietary garlic (2%) has a protective effect on azoxymethane-induced colon carcinogenesis in Sprague–Dawley rats, which is mediated by modulation of oxidative stress during carcinogenesis (Sengupta et al. 2003). The phenolic compounds 6-gingerol and 6-paradol present in ginger also have antitumor promotional and antiproliferative effects. The chemopreventive and chemoprotective effects exerted by 6-gingerol are often associated with their antioxidative and anti-inflammatory activities.

Eugenol pretreatment was found to inhibit the number of tumors produced by the application of 7,12-dimethyl benz(α-)anthracene as initiator and croton oil as promoter in mice (Sukumaran et al. 1994), wherein eugenol inhibited superoxide formation and lipid peroxidation, suggesting that the radical scavenging activity may be responsible for its chemopreventive action. The ability of piperine to inhibit or reduce the oxidative changes induced by chemical carcinogens has been studied in a rat intestinal model (Khajuria et al. 1998). Carcinogenesis was initiated in intestinal lumen of rats with 7,12-dimethyl benzanthracene, dimethyl aminomethyl azobenzene, and 3-methyl cholanthrene. A protective role of piperine against the oxidative alterations by the carcinogen was indicated by the observed inhibition of lipid peroxides, a significant increase in the glutathione levels, and restoration in the activity of marker enzymes. Oral supplementation of piperine (50 mg/kg) effectively suppressed experimental lung carcinogenesis by B(α)p in mice, as revealed by a decrease in the extent of mitochondrial lipid peroxidation and concomitant increase in the activities of enzymatic antioxidant levels (Selvendiran et al. 2004). This suggests that piperine may extend its chemopreventive effect by modulating lipid peroxidation and augmenting the antioxidant defense system.

AMELIORATION OF OXIDATIVE STRESS IN DIABETES

Increasing evidence in both experimental and clinical studies suggests that oxidative stress plays a major role in the pathogenesis of diabetes mellitus. Streptozotocin-induced diabetic rats maintained on curcumin diet showed lowered lipid peroxidation in plasma and urine (Babu and Srinivasan 1995). Oral administration of curcumin (10 or 30 mg/kg) for 45 days ameliorated hyperglycemia, along with near-normalization of the antioxidant enzyme activities and the levels of lipid peroxidative markers (Mahesh et al. 2005). The efficacy of piperine treatment (10 mg/kg/day for 14 days) in diabetes-induced oxidative stress in rats has been reported (Rauscher et al. 2000). Treatment with piperine reversed the disturbances in antioxidant defense in nonhepatic tissues.

Fenugreek (*Trigonella foenum-graecum*) seed is reported to counter the increased lipid peroxidation and alterations in the content of circulating antioxidant molecules—glutathione, β-carotene, and α-tocopherol—in alloxan-induced diabetic rats (Ravikumar and Anuradha 1999). Oxygen free radicals are presumably responsible for the severity and complications of diabetes. Fenugreek administration to diabetic animals reversed the disturbed antioxidant levels and peroxidative damage, thus suggesting that fenugreek seeds have a beneficial antioxidant property that can be exploited for the treatment/reversal of the complications of diabetes (Genet et al. 2002).

Garlic oil (10 mg/kg for 15 days) is shown to effectively normalize the impaired antioxidant status (circulatory total thiols and ceruloplasmin), and activities of glutathione S-transferase and superoxide dismutase in the liver and kidney in streptozotocin-induced diabetes (Anwar and Meki 2003). The effects of this antioxidant may be useful in delaying the complicated effects of diabetes such as retinopathy, nephropathy, and neuropathy due to imbalance between free radicals and antioxidant systems.

ANTICATARACTOGENESIS

Oxidative stress has been implicated in cataractogenesis. Dietary curcumin showed a preventive role on naphthalene-induced opacification of rat lens (Pandya et al. 2000). This study demonstrated that curcumin attenuates the apoptotic effect of naphthalene in rat lens. Wistar rat pups treated with curcumin being administered with selenium showed no opacities in the lens (Padmaja and Raju 2004). Curcumin cotreatment seemed to prevent oxidative damage and delay the development of cataract induced by selenium. Dietary curcumin (0.002% and 0.01%) and turmeric (0.5%) were found to be effective against the development of diabetic cataract in streptozotocin-induced diabetic rats (Suryanarayana et al. 2005). Curcumin and turmeric supplements delayed the progression and maturation of cataract by countering the hyperglycemia-induced oxidative stress, as indicated by reversal of changes with respect to lipid peroxidation, glutathione, protein carbonyl content, and activities of antioxidant enzymes. Aggregation and insolubilization of lens proteins due to hyperglycemia was prevented by turmeric and curcumin. Dietary curcumin (0.002%) was effective against the onset and maturation of galactose-induced cataract in rats via exerting antioxidant and antiglycating effects, as it inhibited lipid peroxidation and protein aggregation (Suryanarayana et al. 2003).

NEUROPROTECTIVE POTENTIAL

Herbs and spices, by contributing antioxidants, may influence age-related cognitive decline (Rahman 2003). Free radical–induced neuronal damage is implicated in cerebral ischemia reperfusion (IR) injury, and antioxidants are reported to have neuroprotective activity. The neuroprotective potential of curcumin (300 mg/kg) investigated in cerebral ischemia reperfusion injury observed in cerebral ischemia is mediated through its antioxidant activity by preventing the elevation in lipid peroxidation (Thiyagarajan and Sharma 2004). The protective effect of curcumin against lead-induced neurotoxicity has been evidenced in rats, which was accompanied by a reversal of the decrease in glutathione levels, superoxide dismutase, and catalase activities in the brain regions (Shukla et al. 2003).

ANTI-INFLAMMATORY EFFECT

Lipid peroxides play a crucial role in arthritis and other inflammatory diseases. Herbs and spices are useful in the treatment of symptomatic osteoarthritis owing to their ability to reduce inflammation (Grzanna et al. 2005). Turmeric is the earliest anti-inflammatory drug known in the indigenous system of medicine in India. Turmeric extract, curcuminoids, and volatile oil of turmeric have been found to be effective as anti-inflammatory agents in several studies involving mice, rats, and rabbits. The efficacy of curcuminoids was also established in experimental inflammation in mice and rats (Srimal 1997). Both *in vitro* and *in vivo* animal studies have documented the anti-inflammatory potential of the spice principles curcumin (of turmeric), capsaicin (of red pepper), and eugenol (of clove). Animal studies have revealed that curcumin and capsaicin also lower the incidence and severity of arthritis and also delay the onset of adjuvant-induced arthritis.

The anti-inflammatory effect of curcumin (400 mg) in patients undergoing surgery for hernia/hydrocele was found to be comparable to that of phenylbutazone (100 mg) (Satoskar et al. 1986). In rheumatoid arthritis patients, administration of curcumin produced significant improvement similar to phenylbutazone (Deodhar et al. 1980). Capsaicin has received considerable attention as a pain reliever. In patients with osteoarthritis and rheumatoid arthritis, topical application of creams containing capsaicin was an effective alternative to analgesics employed in systemic medications, which are often associated with potential adverse effects (McCarthy and McCarthy 1991). There is also evidence for the benefit of ginger in ameliorating arthritic knee pain, although the effectiveness is lesser than that of ibuprofen. Ginger contains pungent ingredients such as 6-gingerol and 6-paradol, which possess anti-inflammatory properties (Surh 1999). Human trial has proven the efficacy of ginger extract in ameliorating arthritic knee pain. Ginger doses of 0.5–1.0 g/day have been found to be efficacious in osteoarthritis and rheumatoid arthritis.

Natural anti-inflammatory compounds of spices (curcumin, capsaicin, gingerol) appear to operate by inhibiting one or more of the steps linking pro-inflammatory stimuli with COX activation, such as the blocking by curcumin of NF-κB translocation into the nucleus. It has been shown recently that natural anti-inflammatory compounds such curcumin were as effective as indomethacin (a nonsteroidal anti-inflammatory drug). The presence of eugenol in basil's (Ocimum basilicum) volatile oils, which is known to inhibit the activity of COX-2, makes basil an anti-inflammatory herb that can provide healing benefits along with symptomatic relief for individuals with inflammatory problems like rheumatoid arthritis or inflammatory bowel conditions.

HEPATOPROTECTIVE AND RENAL-PROTECTIVE EFFECTS

Oral (30 mg/kg for 10 days) dietary administration of curcumin to Wistar rats reduced the iron-induced hepatic damage by lowering lipid peroxidation (Reddy and Lokesh 1996). Increasing evidence demonstrates that oxidative stress plays an important etiologic role in the development of alcoholic liver disease. The protective role of curcumin on alcohol- and thermally oxidized sunflower oil (δPUFA)–induced oxidative stress was observed in Wistar rats; curcumin exerts its protective effect by decreasing the lipid peroxidation and improving antioxidant status (Rukkumani et al. 2004).

Eugenol (5 or 25 mg/kg) has been shown to have a protective effect against carbon tetrachloride–induced hepatotoxicity (Nagababu et al. 1995). Oral administration of eugenol (100 mg/kg for 10 days) lowered the liver and serum lipid peroxide levels, serum marker enzymes of hepatic damage, enhanced by intraperitoneal injection of iron, indicating that eugenol reduces the iron-induced hepatic damage by lowering lipid peroxidation (Reddy and Lokesh 1996). Furthermore, the inactivation of the drug-metabolizing system by carbon tetrachloride was countered by eugenol, suggesting that eugenol might act as an antioxidant and inducer of phase II and phase I enzymes (Kumaravelu et al. 1995). The beneficial effect of curcumin in preventing the acute renal failure and related oxidative stress caused by chronic administration of cyclosporine has been demonstrated in rats (Tirkey et al. 2005).

OTHER NUTRACEUTICAL PROPERTIES OF HERBS AND SPICES

Among the other nutraceutical properties of spices, which are independent of their antioxidant influence, are anticholelithogenic effect, digestive stimulant action, and antimicrobial activity. A persistent high-cholesterol diet leads to cholesterol saturation in bile, resulting in the formation of cholesterol gallstones in the gallbladder. The antilithogenic potential of hypocholesterolemic spices—red pepper, turmeric, garlic, onion, and fenugreek seeds—has been evidenced in animal studies (Srinivasan 2013). The antilithogenicity of these spices is considered to be due to lowering of cholesterol concentration and enhancing the bile acid concentration, both of which contribute to lowering of cholesterol saturation index and hence its crystallization. Several spices such as cumin, coriander, ajowan, fennel, mint, and garlic are common remedies used in traditional medicine to cure digestive disorders. Spices exert digestive stimulatory effects via stimulation of bile acid secretion and stimulation of the production and secretion of digestive enzymes from pancreas (Platel and Srinivasan 2004). Antimicrobial activity has been demonstrated *in vitro* for several herbs and spices and essential oils from basil, thyme, oregano, parsley, cilantro, and cinnamon (Cowan 1999). Beneficial antimicrobial phytochemicals include polyphenols, terpenoids and essential oils, alkaloids, and lectins. Polyphenols are capable of forming an irreversible complex with nucleophilic amino acids in protein, leading to their inactivation and therefore loss of function. Polyphenols have been reported to disrupt microbial membranes and inactivate microbial enzymes.

CONCLUSIONS

Oxidative stress is clearly implicated in a wide range of disease processes, including cardiovascular disease, cancer, inflammatory diseases, neurodegenerative diseases, cataract, etc. Herbs and spices, which are normal ingredients of the human diet, are now known to exert health-beneficial antioxidant effects in mammalian systems and in several model systems through their bioactive compounds. The antioxidant properties of herbs and spices are of particular interest in view of the impact of oxidative modification of LDL in the development of atherosclerosis, and suppression of oxidative stress and inflammation in their cancer-preventive role, since both oxidative stress and inflammation are a risk factor for cancer initiation and promotion. The antioxidant potential of spices has far-reaching health implication. The studies to this effect are exhaustive, and experimental evidences are plenty particularly in the case of curcumin of turmeric and eugenol of clove. All the available information essentially endorses that using antioxidant spices at high levels is beneficial to the markers of health, although it is less clearly evident that these are actually beneficial in preventing or protecting oxidative stress–mediated diseases. By virtue of antioxidant activity, these spice bioactive compounds are extrapolated to be anti-inflammatory, antimutagenic and cancer-preventive, antiatherogenic and cardioprotective, hepatoprotective, neuroprotective, anticataractogenic, etc. What essentially remains is integrating this knowledge to ascertain whether such health beneficial effects can be observed in humans.

Although the effective dose of these dietary spices evidenced in animal studies to produce the desired antioxidant influence far exceeds their normal levels encountered in our daily diet, the effectiveness of lower doses of these spices cannot be ruled out. There is also the possibility of deriving the beneficial effect by chronic consumption of these spices in our daily diet. In view of the antioxidant potential of a number of herbs and spices with far-reaching health implication, these food adjuncts deserve to be considered as natural and necessary components of our daily nutrition. Use of spices and herbs in the diet ensures adequate intake of both essential nutrients and health-promoting bioactives in the food supply. Herbs and spices can add substantial variety to the nutrients and bioactives available in the diet. Although the potential health effects of herbs and spices are reported abundantly in the scientific literature, it should be noted that human data of variable quality are limited; vast research literature from *in vitro* and *in vivo* studies suggests that specific herbs and spices may confer unique health benefits. The use of herbs and spices as source of antioxidants to combat oxidative stress warrants further attention in terms of validating the antioxidant capacity and testing their effects on markers of oxidation in clinical trials that are aiming to establish antioxidants as mediators of disease prevention.

REFERENCES

Anwar, M.M., and Meki, A.R. 2003. Oxidative stress in streptozotocin-induced diabetic rats: Effects of garlic oil and melatonin. *Comp. Biochem. Physiol. Mol. Integr. Physiol.* 135: 539–547.

Babu, P.S., and Srinivasan, K. 1995. Influence of dietary curcumin and cholesterol on the progression of experimentally induced diabetes in albino rat. *Mol. Cell. Biochem.* 152: 13–21.

Baghurst, K. 2006. Herbs and spices: An integral part of the daily diet. Position paper, National Centre of Excellence in Functional Foods, Australia.

Balasenthil, S., Ramachandran, C.R., and Nagini, S. 2001. *S*-Allylcysteine, a garlic constituent, inhibits 7,12-dimethylbenz[*a*]anthracene-induced hamster buccal pouch carcinogenesis. *Nutr. Cancer* 40: 165–172.

Bellamy, D., and Pfister, A. 1992. *World Medicine. Plants Patients and People.* Oxford, UK: Blackwell Publishers.

Cao, G., Booth, S.L., Sadowski, J.A., and Prior, R.L. 1998. Increases in human plasma antioxidant capacity after consumption of controlled diets high in fruit and vegetables. *Am. J. Clin. Nutr.* 68: 1081–1087.

Carnesecchi, S., Schneider, Y., Ceraline, J. et al. 2001. Geraniol, a component of plant essential oils, inhibits growth and polyamine biosynthesis in human colon cancer cells. *J. Pharmacol. Exp. Ther.* 298: 197–200.

Chuang, S.E., Kuo, M.L., Hsu, C.H. et al. 2000. Curcumin-containing diet inhibits diethylnitrosamine-induced murine hepatocarcinogenesis. *Carcinogenesis* 21: 331–335.

Cowan, M.M. 1999. Plant products as antimicrobial agents. *Clin. Microbiol. Rev.* 12: 564–582.

Deodhar, S.D., Sethi, R., and Srimal, R.C. 1980. Preliminary studies on anti-rheumatic activity of curcumin. *Indian J. Med. Res.* 71: 632–634.

Durak, I., Aytac, B., Atmaca, Y. et al. 2004. Effects of garlic extract consumption on plasma and erythrocyte antioxidant parameters in atherosclerotic patients. *Life Sci.* 75: 1959–1966.

Duthrie, G.G., and Brown, K.M. 1994. Reducing the risk of cardiovascular disease. In: Goldberg, I. (Ed.), *Functional Foods.* London: Chapman & Hall, 19–38.

Elson, C.E., Underbakke, G.L., Hanson, P., Shrago, E., Wainberg, R.H., and Qureshi, A.A. 1989. Impact of lemongrass oil, an essential oil, on serum cholesterol. *Lipids* 24: 677–679.

Genet, S., Kale, R.K., and Baquer, N.Z. 2002. Alterations in antioxidant enzymes and oxidative damage in experimental diabetic rat tissues: Effect of vanadate and fenugreek (*Trigonella foenum-graecum*). *Mol. Cell. Biochem.* 236: 7–12.

Govindarajan, R., Vijayakumar, M., and Pushpangadan, P. 2005. Antioxidant approach to disease management and the role of 'Rasayana' herbs of Ayurveda. *J. Ethnopharmacol.* 99: 165–178.

Grzanna, R., Lindmark, L., and Frondoza, C.G. 2005. Ginger—A herbal medicinal product with broad anti-inflammatory actions. *J. Med. Food* 8: 125–132.

Gujaral, S., Bhumra, N., and Swaroop, M. 1978. Effect of ginger oleoresin on serum and hepatic cholesterol levels in cholesterol fed rats. *Nutr. Rep. Int.* 17: 183.

Halvorsen, B.L., Carlsen, M.H., Phillips, K.M. et al. 2006. Content of redox-active compounds in foods consumed in the United States. *Am. J. Clin. Nutr.* 84: 95–135.

Helen, A., Rajasree, C.R., Krishnakumar, K., Augusti, K.T., and Vijayammal, P.L. 1999. Antioxidant role of oils isolated from garlic (*Allium sativum* Linn) and onion (*Allium cepa* Linn) on nicotine-induced lipid peroxidation. *Vet. Hum. Toxicol.* 41: 316–319.

Hertog, M.G., Feskens, E.J., Hollman, P.C., Katan, M.B., and Kromhout, D. 1993. Dietary antioxidant flavonoids and risk of coronary heart disease: The Zutphen Elderly Study. *Lancet* 342: 1007–1011.

Huang, M.T., Ho, C.T., Wang, Z.Y. et al. 1994. Inhibition of skin tumorigenesis by rosemary and its constituents carnosol and ursolic acid. *Cancer Res.* 54: 701–708.

Ippoushi, K., Azuma, K., Ito, H., Horie, H., and Higashio, H. 2003. [6]-Gingerol inhibits nitric oxide synthesis in activated J774.1 mouse macrophages and prevents peroxynitrite-induced oxidation and nitration reactions. *Life Sci.* 73: 3427–3437.

Khajuria, A., Zutshi, U., and Bedi, K.L. 1998. Permeability characteristics of piperine on oral absorption—An active alkaloid from peppers and a bioavailability enhancer. *Indian J. Exp. Biol.* 36: 46–50.

Kim, S.S., Oh, O.J., Min, H.Y. et al. 2003. Eugenol suppresses cyclooxygenase-2 expression in lipopolysaccharide-stimulated mouse macrophage RAW264.7 cells. *Life Sci.* 73: 337–348.

Kumaravelu, P., Dakshinamoorthy, D.P., Subramaniam, S., Devaraj, H., and Devaraj, N.S. 1995. Effect of eugenol on drug-metabolizing enzymes of carbon tetrachloride-intoxicated rat liver. *Biochem. Pharmacol.* 49: 1703–1707.

Lantry, L.E., Zhang, Z., Gao, F. et al. 1997. Chemopreventive effect of perillyl alcohol on 4-(methylnitrosamino)-1-(3-pyridyl)-1-butanone induced tumorigenesis in (C3H/HeJ X A/J)F1 mouse lung. *J. Cell. Biochem. Suppl.* 27: 20–25.

Lau, B.H. 2001. Suppression of LDL oxidation by garlic. *J. Nutr.* 131: 985S–988S.

Mahesh, T., Balasubashini, M.S., and Menon, V.P. 2005. Effect of photo-irradiated curcumin treatment against oxidative stress in streptozotocin-induced diabetic rats. *J. Med. Food* 8: 251–255.

Manikandan, P., Sumitra, M., Aishwarya, S., Manohar, B.M., Lokanadam, B., and Puvanakrishnan, R. 2004. Curcumin modulates free radical quenching in myocardial ischaemia in rats. *Int. J. Biochem. Cell. Biol.* 36: 1967–1980.

Manjunatha, H., and Srinivasan, K. 2006. Protective effect of dietary curcumin and capsaicin on induced oxidation of low-density lipoprotein, iron-induced hepatotoxicity and carrageenan-induced inflammation in rats. *FEBS J.* 273: 4528–4537.

McCarthy, G.M., and McCarthy, D.J. 1991. Effect of topical capsaicin in the therapy of painful osteoarthritis of the hand. *J. Rheumatol.* 19: 604–607.

Miquel, J., Bernd, A., Sempere, J.M., Diaz-Alperi, J., and Ramirez, A. 2002. The curcuma antioxidants: Pharmacological effects and prospects for future clinical use (A review). *Arch. Gerontol. Geriatr.* 34: 37–46.

Mittal, R., and Gupta, R.L. 2000. *In vitro* antioxidant activity of piperine. *Exp. Clin. Pharmacol.* 22: 271–274.

Nagababu, E., Sesikeran, B., and Lakshmaiah, N. 1995. The protective effects of eugenol on carbon tetrachloride induced hepatotoxicity in rats. *Free Radic. Res.* 23: 617–627.

Nagashima, K. 1989. Inhibitory effect of eugenol on Cu^{++} catalyzed lipid peroxidation in human erythrocyte membrane. *Int. J. Biochem.* 21: 745–749.

Naidu, K.A., and Thippeswamy, N.B. 2002. Inhibition of human low density lipoprotein oxidation by active principles from spices. *Mol. Cell. Biochem.* 229: 19–23.

Nirmala, C., and Puvanakrishnan, R. 1996. Protective role of curcumin against isoproterenol induced myocardial infarction in rats. *Mol. Cell. Biochem.* 159: 85–93.

Padmaja, S., and Raju, T.N. 2004. Antioxidant effect of curcumin in selenium induced cataract of Wistar rats. *Indian J. Exp. Biol.* 42: 601–603.

Pandya, U., Saini, M.K., Jin, G.F., Awasthi, S., Godley, B.F., and Awasthi, Y.C. 2000. Dietary curcumin prevents ocular toxicity of naphthalene in rats. *Toxicol. Lett.* 115: 195–204.

Platel, K., and Srinivasan, K. 2004. Digestive stimulant action of spices: A myth or reality? *Indian J. Med. Res.* 119: 167–179.

Quiles, J.L., Mesa, M.D., Ramirez-Tortosa, C.L. et al. 2002. *Curcuma longa* extract supplementation reduces oxidative stress and attenuates aortic fatty streak development in rabbits. *Arterioscler. Thromb. Vasc. Biol.* 22: 1225–1231.

Rahman, K. 2003. Garlic and aging: New insights into an old remedy. *Ageing Res. Rev.* 2: 39–56.

Ramirez-Tortosa, M.C., Mesa, M.D., Aguilera, M.C. et al. 1999. Oral administration of a turmeric extract inhibits LDL oxidation and has hypocholesterolemic effects in rabbits with experimental atherosclerosis. *Atherosclerosis* 147: 371–378.

Rauscher, F.M., Sanders, R.A., and Watkins, J.B. 2000. Effects of piperine on antioxidant pathways in tissues from normal and streptozotocin-induced diabetic rats. *J. Biochem. Mol. Toxicol.* 14: 329–334.

Ravikumar, P., and Anuradha, C.V. 1999. Effect of fenugreek seeds on blood lipid peroxidation and antioxidants in diabetic rats. *Phytother. Res.* 13: 197–201.

Reddy, A.C.P., and Lokesh, B.R. 1992. Studies on spice principles as antioxidants in the inhibition of lipid peroxidation of rat liver microsomes. *Mol. Cell. Biochem.* 111: 117–124.

Reddy, A.C.P., and Lokesh, B.R. 1994a. Effect of dietary turmeric (*Curcuma longa*) on iron-induced lipid peroxidation in the rat liver. *Food Chem. Toxicol.* 32: 279–283.

Reddy, A.C.P., and Lokesh, B.R. 1994b. Alterations in lipid peroxides in rat liver by dietary n-3 fatty acids: Modulation of antioxidant enzymes by curcumin, eugenol, and vitamin E. *J. Nutr. Biochem.* 5: 181–188.

Reddy, A.C.P., and Lokesh, B.R. 1996. Effect of curcumin and eugenol on iron-induced hepatic toxicity in rats. *Toxicology* 107: 39–45.

Rukkumani, R., Aruna, K., Varma, P.S., Rajasekaran, K.N., and Menon, V.P. 2004. Comparative effects of curcumin and an analog of curcumin on alcohol and PUFA induced oxidative stress. *J. Pharm. Pharm. Sci.* 7: 274–283.

Satoskar, R.R., Shah, S.J., and Shenoy, S.G. 1986. Evaluation of anti-inflammatory property of curcumin (diferuloylmethane) in patients with post-operative inflammation. *Int. J. Clin. Pharmacol. Ther. Toxicol.* 24: 651–654.

Selvendiran, K., Senthilnathan, P., Magesh, V., and Sakthisekaran, D. 2004. Modulatory effect of Piperine on mitochondrial antioxidant system in benzo(α)pyrene-induced experimental lung carcinogenesis. *Phytomedicine* 11: 85–89.

Sengupta, A., Ghosh, S., and Das, S. 2003. Tomato and garlic can modulate azoxymethane-induced colon carcinogenesis in rats. *Eur. J. Cancer Prev.* 12: 195–200.

Shukla, P.K., Khanna, V.K., Khan, M.Y., and Srimal, R.C. 2003. Protective effect of curcumin against lead neurotoxicity in rat. *Hum. Exp. Toxicol.* 22: 653–658.

Sinha, R., Anderson, D., McDonald, S., and Greenwald, P. 2003. Cancer risk and diet in India. *J. Postgrad. Med.* 49: 222–228.

Soni, K.B., and Kuttan, R. 1992. Effect of oral curcumin administration on serum peroxides and cholesterol levels in human volunteers. *Indian J. Physiol. Pharmacol.* 36: 273–275.

Srimal, R.C. 1997. Turmeric: A brief review of medicinal properties. *Fitoterapia* LXVIII: 483–490.

Srinivasan, K. 2013. Dietary spices as beneficial modulators of lipid profile in conditions of metabolic disorders and diseases. *Food Funct.* 4: 503–521.

Srinivasan, K. 2014. Antioxidant potential of spices and their active constituents. *Crit. Rev. Food Sci. Nutr.* 54: 352–372.

Steiner, M., Khan, A.H., Holbert, D., and Lin, R.I. 1996. A double-blind crossover study in moderately hypercholesterolemic men that compared the effect of aged garlic extract and placebo administration on blood lipids. *Am. J. Clin. Nutr.* 64: 866–870.

Stoilova, I., Krastanov, A., Stoyanova, A., Denev, P., and Gargovaa, S. 2007. Antioxidant activity of a ginger extract (*Zingiber officinale*). *Food Chem.* 102: 764–770.

Subramanian, M., Sreejayan, N., Rao, M.N., Devasagayam, T.P., and Singh, B.B. 1994. Diminution of singlet oxygen-induced DNA damage by curcumin and related antioxidants. *Mutat. Res.* 311: 249–255.

Sukumaran, K., Unnikrishnan, M.C., and Kuttan, R. 1994. Inhibition of tumour promotion in mice by eugenol. *Indian J. Physiol. Pharmacol.* 38: 306–308.

Surh, Y. 1999. Molecular mechanisms of chemopreventive effects of selected dietary and medicinal phenolic substances. *Mutat. Res.* 428: 305–327.

Surh, Y.J. 2002. Anti-tumor promoting potential of selected spice ingredients with antioxidative and anti-inflammatory activities: A short review. *Food Chem. Toxicol.* 40: 1091–1097.

Suryanarayana, P., Krishnaswamy, K., and Reddy, G.B. 2003. Effect of curcumin on galactose-induced cataractogenesis in rats. *Mol. Vis.* 9: 223–230.

Suryanarayana, P., Saraswat, M., Mrudula, T., Krishna, T.P., Krishnaswamy, K., and Reddy, G.B. 2005. Curcumin and turmeric delay streptozotocin-induced diabetic cataract in rats. *Invest. Ophthalmol. Vis. Sci.* 46: 2092–2099.

Tapsell, L.C., Hemphill, I., Cobiac, L. et al. 2006. Health benefits of herbs and spices: The past, the present, the future. *Med. J. Aust.* 185 (Suppl): S4–24.

Thiyagarajan, M., and Sharma, S.S. 2004. Neuroprotective effect of curcumin in middle cerebral artery occlusion induced focal cerebral ischemia in rats. *Life Sci.* 74: 969–985.

Tirkey, N., Kaur, G., Vij, G., and Chopra, K. 2005. Curcumin, a diferuloylmethane, attenuates cyclosporine-induced renal dysfunction and oxidative stress in rat kidneys. *BMC Pharmacol.* 5: 15.

Volate, S.R., Davenport, D.M., Muga, S.J., and Wargovich, M.J. 2005. Modulation of aberrant crypt foci and apoptosis by dietary herbal supplements (quercetin, curcumin, silymarin, ginseng and rutin). *Carcinogenesis* 26: 1450–1456.

Wargovich, M.J., Woods, C., Hollis, D.M., and Zander, M.E. 2001. Herbals, cancer prevention and health. *J. Nutr.* 131 (11 Suppl): 3034S–3036S.

Yu, T.W., Xu, M., and Dashwood, R.H. 2004. Antimutagenic activity of spearmint. *Environ. Mol. Mutagen* 44: 387–393.

Zheng, G., Kenney, P.M., and Lam, L.K. 1992. Myristicin: A potential cancer chemopreventive agent from parsley leaf oil. *J. Agric. Food Chem.* 40: 107–110.

Index

Page numbers followed by f and t indicate figures and tables, respectively.

A

Abacanir, 273t
Academy of Nutrition and Dietetics, 77
1-Acetoxy-pinoresinol, 39, 40
Achillea millefolium, 37
Achillea spp., 30, 37
Acute effects of smoking (ACS), 88–89
Acyclic polysulfides, 35
Acyl-CoA oxidase, 7
Adefovir, 273t
Adenomatous polyposis coli (Apc) gene, 186
Adequate intake (AI) recommendations, for
    breast cancer, 189, 189t
Adipokincs, 234
Adulthood, dietary antioxidants in, 71–76
    bioavailability of natural antioxidants and
        effect on biomarkers, 73–75, 74t
    disease prevention, 75
    needs and importance, 71–73
    supplements and health, 75–76, 76t
Age-related macular degeneration (AMD), 78
Aging, OS theory, 283
Aglycones, 24, 26, 27, 34, 40
Akinesia, 203
Alcohols
    extraction of gluten, 216
    heavy drinking, 168
    moderate consumption, 168
    OS and, 48
α-Lipoic acid (ALA), in obesity, 241
Alkoxyls, 86
Allergies, antioxidants in, 59
Allicin, 35
    S-allyl cysteine and, 283f
Alliin, 35
Allium cepa, antioxidant effects, 284, 286t–287t,
    288
Allium sativum, 38, 283f
    antioxidant effects, 284, 286t–287t, 288
Allium species, 30
Allopurinol, 109
S-Allylcysteine, 292
S-Allyl-l-cysteine sulfoxide, 35
Almonds, 179
Alpha-tocopherol beta-carotene cancer (ATBC),
    99, 139, 174

Alzheimer's disease (AD), 77–79, 204–205
Amelioration, of OS in diabetes, 293
American Heart Association (AHA), 117, 242
American Institute for Cancer Research, 180
American Psychiatric Association (APA), 61
5-Aminosalicylic acid, 225
Amyloid β, 78–79
Anemia, 58
Anorexia, 267
Anthocyanidines, 27, 94
Anthocyanins, 27, 31, 33, 34, 35, 36, 73
    blueberries and, 239
Antiatherogenic effect, of herbs and spices,
    290–291
Anticataractogenesis, 294
Anticlotting properties, of garlic, 290
Anti-inflammatory effect, spices and herbs,
    294–295
Anti-inflammatory properties, of antioxidants,
    257–258
Antilipogenic effects, of EGCG, 238
Antilithogenicity, of spices, 296
Antimitogenic effects, of EGCG, 238
Antioxidant(s)
    activity, substances and compounds with,
        18t–19t
    anti-inflammatory properties, 257–258
    in asthma and allergies, 59
    behavioral alterations, 60–62
    brain development and, 60–61
    cancer chemopreventive effects, 291–293
    celiac disease and, 217, 218–220. *See also*
        Celiac disease
    CHD and stroke, 120–143. *See also* Coronary
        heart disease (CHD); Stroke(s)
    in children's growth and development, 53–64.
        See also Children's growth and
        development
    cognitive function, 60–62
    defective, defense in obesity, 235–236, 236f
    in deficiency diseases treatment, 58–59
    defined, 24, 176
    diabetes and, 152–156. *See also* Diabetes
    dietary
        in adulthood, 71–76. *See also* Adulthood,
        dietary antioxidants in
        in cancer, 174

defined, 167
in elderly, 76–79. *See also* Elderly,
    dietary antioxidants in
food sources and, 23–40. *See also*
    Dietary antioxidants
intake, IBD risks and, 223–224
smoking and, 89–91, 90t, 91f, 95
Down syndrome and, 63, 64f
endogenous, 89, 90t, 103–104, 106–109
    defined, 167
    GSH, 106–107
    lipoic acid, 107–109
exogenous, 89, 90t, 103–104, 109–111
    in cancer, 174
    clinical and experimental evidence in
        obesity, 236–242
    defined, 167
    flavonoids, 110–111
    vitamins C and E, 109–110
general health and, 104
growth and, 56–58, 56t
HIV/AIDS and, 268–271. *See also* Human
        immunodeficiency virus/acquired
        immunodeficiency syndrome
        (HIV/AIDS)
    β-carotene, 269
    factors affecting level in patients, 272–273
    NAC, 271
    polyphenols, 271
    selenium, 270
    supplementation, adverse effects, 273–274
    vitamin A, 268–269
    vitamin C, 269
    vitamin E, 269–270
    zinc, 270–271
hypothesis, CHD and stroke, 119–120, 120f
IBDs and. *See* Inflammatory bowel diseases
        (IBDs)
intake, smoking and, 89–99. *See also*
        Smoking
    dietary antioxidants, interaction, 95
    minerals and trace elements, 94–95.
        See also Minerals; Trace elements
    natural antioxidants, case, 95–98.
        See also Natural antioxidants
    in supplementation studies, 98–99.
        See also Supplementation, studies
    vitamins, 91–94. *See also* Vitamins,
        smoking and
modulation of immune response by, 249–258.
        See also Modulation of immune
        response
natural. *See* Natural antioxidants
in neurodegeneration, 199–207. *See also*
        Neurodegeneration
obesity and, 59–60
    inflammation, 233–243. *See also* Obesity

in pregnancy, 47–51. *See also* Pregnancy
supplementation in cancers, 174–177, 178t
    dilemma of, 177, 178–179
Antioxidant capacity (AC), 176
Antioxidant effects, of herbs and spices, 283–289
    clove (*Eugenia caryophyllus*) and eugenol,
        284, 287t, 289
    garlic (*Allium sativum*) and onion
        (*Allium cepa*), 284, 286t–287t, 288
    ginger (*Zingiber officinale*), 284, 288, 289
    red pepper (*Capsicum annuum*) and black
        pepper (*Piper nigrum*), 284, 288t
    turmeric (*Curcuma longa*) and curcumin,
        284, 285t–286t, 289f
Antioxidant level, factors affecting in HIV/AIDS
        patients, 272–273
    combination therapy (HAARTS), 272, 273t
    medication intake, 272
    opportunistic conditions, 272
    socioeconomic status, 273
Antioxidative stress, 254
Anxiety, 62
Apigenin, 36, 37, 39, 40
Apigenin-acetyl-apiosylglucoside, 35
Apigenin-7-apiosylglucoside, 35
Apiin, 35
Apocarotenoids, 28
ApoE4 gene, 204
Apples, 31, 32t, 33, 177
Apricots, 31, 32t, 179
    carotenoids in, 28
Aqueous cigarette tar (ACT), 84, 86
Arbutus unedo, 33
L-arginine, 251
Arginine, NO from, 13–14
Aromatic plants, 30
Artemisia dracunculus, 37
Arteriosclerosis, 77–78
Arthritis, 294
Artichoke, 27, 32t, 36
Arugula, 181
Ascorbate. *See* Vitamin C
Ascorbic acids. *See* Vitamin C
L-ascorbic acids, 31
Asthma, antioxidants in, 59
Atherogenesis, 283–284
Atherosclerosis, 117, 119, 129, 235, 283–284,
        290
Athletes, antioxidant supplementation for,
        104–105, 109–110
Atrophy, of gray and white matter, 202–203
Attention-deficit hyperactivity disorder (ADHD),
        60, 61–62
Autism spectrum disorders (ASD), 62–63
Autoimmune thyroid diseases (AITDs), 219
Azoxymethane-induced colon carcinogenesis,
        292

B

Bananas, 31
Barley, 216
Basil, 30, 32t, 37, 177, 281, 290, 291, 292t, 295
Basilici herba, 39
Beans, 26, 182, 183
Beef, 179
Behavioral alterations, antioxidants and, 60–62
Benzoic acids, 24, 31, 35
Berries, 31, 32t, 141, 177
    color, 27
Beverages, antioxidant effect, 73
Bioavailability, natural antioxidants, 73–75, 74t
BioCycle Study, 154
Biomarkers
    natural antioxidants bioavailability on, 73–75, 74t
    of OS, 235
Bisabolol oxides, 37
Blackberries, 31, 32t, 177
    color, 27
Blackcurrants, 177
Black grapes, 27, 34
Black pepper, 38
    antioxidant effects, 284, 288t
Black tea, 36
Blackthorn, 32t, 33
Blood antioxidant levels, IBD risks and, 224–225
Blueberries, 177
    anthocyanins and, 239
    color, 27
Body mass index (BMI), 235, 238
Bok choy, 180, 181
Borneol, 30, 37, 284
Bradykinesia, 203
Brain
    development, antioxidants and, 60–61
    Trxs family proteins in, 200–202, 202f
Brassicaceae, 181
Brazilian children, 57
Breast cancer, 188–189
    fiber-rich foods, 188–189, 189t
    folic acid in, 168
    intake recommendations, 189, 189t
    selenium and, 172
    soy in, 183
    vitamin C and, 173–174
Breast-feeding, 57
Broccoli, 179, 180, 181
Bronchoalveolar lavage fluid (BALF), 88
Brussels, 181, 182
Butadiene, 87
Butylated hydroxy toluene (BHT), 37

C

Cabbage, 27, 32t, 35, 180, 181, 182
Caffeic acids, 24, 31, 36, 37–38, 39
Caffeoylquinic acids, 33, 36, 37
Caffeoyltartaric acids, 35
Caftaric acids, 37
Cambridge Heart Antioxidant Study (CHAOS), 99
Camellia sinensis, 27
Camphene, 37
Camphor, 30, 37
Cancers, 75, 166–192
    antioxidant(s), 166–179
        flavonoids on, 97
        folic acid, 167–169, 169t
        food sources, 179
        selenium and, 170–172, 171t
        supplementation, 174–177, 178t
        taking supplements, dilemma of, 177, 178–179
        vitamin C, 172–174, 173t
    breast, 168, 172, 173–174, 188–189
        fiber-rich foods, 188–189, 189t
        intake recommendations, 189, 189t
        soy in, 183
    colon, 167, 170, 291
    colorectal, 167, 187, 188
    forestomach, 291
    FRs in development, 166
    gastric, 174
    intestinal, 225
    liver, 172, 291
    lung, 175, 190
        rodent model, 291
        vitamin C, 173
        vitamin E, 99
    oral, 291
    overview, 166
    pancreatic, 187
    prevention, 174–177, 178t, 179–192
        carotenoids, 184–187. See also
            Carotenoids, in cancer prevention
        colorectal cancer and fiber, 188
        cruciferous vegetables, 181–182
        curcumin, 186, 187
        flavonoids and, 190–192, 190t, 191t
        fruits and vegetables, 179–181
        iodine and thyroid function, 182
        legumes, 182–183
        soy, 183–184
        whole grains, 184
    preventive property, spices and herbs, 291–293, 292t
    prostate, 180–181, 190
        legumes in, 182–183
        selenium and, 99, 170, 172, 175
        soy in, 183

skin, 291
    selenium and, 99, 172
    stomach, 174
Cantaloupe, 179
Capsaicin, 283f, 289, 290, 291
    anti-inflammatory effect, 294, 295
    of red pepper, 284, 288t
Capsicum annuum, 283f
    antioxidant effects, 284, 288t
Caraway, 38
Cardamom, 38, 177
Cardioprotective effect, of herbs and spices,
        290–291
Cardiovascular disease (CVD), 98, 117–118, 184,
        234
    antioxidant(s)
        carotenoids, 130–139, 131t–138t
        lycopene, 142–143
        outcomes risk, RCTs of supplemental
            intake and, 122t–128t
        polyphenols, 140–141
        resveratrol, 141–142
        selenium, 139–140
        vitamin C, 129–130
        vitamin E, 120–129, 122t–128t
Carnosic acid, 37
Carnosol, 37, 39, 291
α-carotene, in cancer prevention, 185, 185t
β-carotene, 30, 31, 72, 76, 96–97, 98
    basil, 290
    cancer, 185, 186t
    CHD and strokes, 130, 139
    diabetes, 154
    food sources, 179
    HIV/AIDS and, 269
Carotene and retinol efficacy trial (CARET),
        175
Carotenoids, 17, 28–30, 29f, 57, 72, 78
    in cancer prevention, 184–187
        β-carotene, 185, 186t
        β-cryptoxanthin, 185
        α-carotene, 185, 185t
        curcumin, 186, 187
        food sources, 184–185
        lutein and zeaxanthin, 186, 187t
        lycopene, 185, 186
    CHD and strokes, 130–139, 131t–138t
    diabetes, 154
    fruits, 30–31
    HIV/AIDS and, 269
    non-provitamin A, smoking and
        dietary antioxidants, 92–93
        natural antioxidants, 96–97
        supplementation studies, 99
Carrots, 28, 179, 185
Carvacrol, 24, 25f, 30, 37, 38, 284
Carvum carvi, 38

Caryophyllus aromaticus, 38
Case–control studies, cancers and, 170, 172,
        179–180, 183, 184, 188
Catalase, 16
Cataract, 77–78
Cataractogenesis, 294
Catechins, 27, 38–39, 62, 75
    GTC, 237–239, 237t
Cauliflower, 181
C–C chemokine receptor 5 (CCR5), 265, 266
CD4 cells, HIV and, 265–266, 265t
Celiac disease, 216–220
    defined, 216
    OS and, 217, 218f
    overview, 216
    potential beneficial effect of dietary
        antioxidant, 220, 220f
    risk, antioxidants and, 217, 218–219
        selenium in, 218–219
        vitamin E in, 218
    treatment, antioxidants and, 219–220
        vitamin C in, 219–220
Cell signaling, hydrogen peroxide in, 11
Cell signaling theory, 199
Cellular pathway messaging, 78
Cellular ROS and RNS, production, 251–252
Central nervous system (CNS) diseases
    signaling pathways, Trxs protein family in,
        205–206
Cereals, 179
Cerebral ischemia, 206–207
Cerebrovascular disease, 117
c-foc expression, 75
Chain reactions, 10
Chalcones, 25f, 26, 27, 33, 34
Chamazulene, 30
Chamomile, 30, 33t, 36, 38
Chamomillae flos, 39
CHD. See Coronary heart disease (CHD)
Chemistry basics, oxygen, 4–7, 5f, 6t
Cherries, 31, 32t, 177
    color, 27
Children's growth and development, antioxidants
        in, 53–64
    ASD, 62–63
    asthma and allergies, 59
    behavioral alterations, 60–62
    brain development, 60–61
    cognitive function, 60–62
    deficiency diseases treatment, 58–59
    Down syndrome, 63, 64f
    growth and, 56–58, 56t
    micronutrients and early development, 53–54,
        55f
    obesity and, 59–60
    OS and health, 54, 56
    overview, 53–56, 55f

Chili powder, 177
Chinese cabbage, 181
Chinese green tea, 27
Chlorogenic acids, 24, 31, 36, 37, 39
Cider apples, 32t, 33
Cigarette smoke. *See* Smoking
Cinnamaldehyde, 30
Cinnamic acids, 24, 31, 35, 38, 39
Cinnamomum zeylanicum, 38
Cinnamon, 38, 177, 281
    EO compound, 30
Cisplatin, 177
Cistus ladanifer, 28
Cistus monspeliensis, 28
Cistus salvifolius, 28
Cistus species, 27, 28
Citrulline, 13–14
Citrus fruits, 31, 32t, 33–34, 72, 292t
    carotenoids, 28
c-jun expression, 75
Classification, natural antioxidants, 24–30
    carotenoids, 28–30, 29f
    EOs, 29f, 30
    phenols and polyphenols, 24–28
        flavonoids, 25f, 26–27, 32t, 33–34, 36
        molecular structures, 25f
        others, 28
        phenolic acids, 24, 25f
        simple, 24, 25t
Clinical evidence, on exogenous antioxidants in
        obesity, 236–242
    ALA, 241
    anthocyanins and blueberries, 239
    CoQ, 241
    curcumin, 237t, 239–240
    fruits, legumes, and nuts, 241–242
    GTCs, 237–239, 237t
    resveratrol, 237t, 240–241
Cloves, 30, 38, 177
    anti-inflammatory effect, 294
    antioxidant effects, 284, 287t, 289
Coenzyme Q (CoQ), 241
Cognitive function, antioxidants and, 60–62
Cohort studies, cancers and, 180, 184, 188, 190
Colitis, development, 222
Collard greens, 179, 181
Colon cancer, 291
    folic acid in, 167
    polyamine biosynthesis in, 291
    selenium and, 170, 172
Colorectal cancer, 187, 188
    fiber and, 188
    folic acid in, 167
Combination therapy (HAARTS), in HIV/AIDS
        patients, 272, 273t
Combined antioxidant supplementation studies,
    99

Condensed tannins, 27
Congenital heart disease, 117
Consumption, dietary antioxidant
    disease prevention in elderly, 77–79
Copper, smoking and
    dietary antioxidants, 94
    natural antioxidants, 97–98
Coriander, 177
Corn, 179
Coronary heart disease (CHD), 117–143
    antioxidant(s), 120–143
        carotenoids, 130–139, 131t–138t
        hypothesis, 119–120, 120f
        lycopene, 142–143
        polyphenols, 140–141
        resveratrol, 141–142
        selenium, 139–140
        vitamin C, 129–130
        vitamin E, 120–129, 122t–128t
    overview, 117–118
    risk factors associated with, 118
    vitamin E on, 99
3-*p*-Coumaroylquinic acid, 31
COX-2 (cyclooxygenase 2), 217, 218, 282
COX-2 gene, 219
Cranberries, 177
Cretan marjoram, 38
Crixivan, 273t
Crocetins, 28
Crocins, 28, 30
Crocus sativus, 28
Crohn's disease (CD), 221, 223–224, 225
Cruciferous vegetables, 181–182
    intake recommendations, 182
    iodine and thyroid function, 182
Cryptochlorogenics, 36, 37
Cryptoxanthin, 31
β-cryptoxanthin, in cancer prevention, 185
Cumin, 177
Curcuma longa, 186, 225, 283f
    antioxidant effects, 284, 285t–286t, 289f
Curcuminoids, 290, 294
Curcumins, 29, 37, 225, 283f, 290, 291, 293, 294
    anti-inflammatory effect, 294–295
    antimutagenic property, 292
    antioxidant effects, 284, 285t–286t, 289f
    in cancer prevention, 186, 187
    cancer-preventive property, 291–292
    hepatoprotective and renal -protective effects,
        295
    in obesity, 237t, 239–240
Curry powder, 177
Cyanidin 3-*O*-glucoside, 31, 33
Cyanidin 3-*O*-rutinoside, 31, 33
Cyanidins, 27, 31, 35, 36
Cyclooxygenase 2 (COX-2), 217, 218, 282
Cyclosporine, 295

Cymbopogon citrates, 290
Cymbopogon citratus, 291, 292t
Cynara cardunculus, 36
Cynarin, 36
Cynaroside, 36
Cysteine, 58
Cysteinylation, 200
Cysteinyl thiols, 200
Cyt P450, 9

D

Daidzein, 26–27
Damaging effects of ROS, common targets, 19–20
Dates, 177
Deeply pigmented fruits, 177
Deep vein thrombosis, 117
Defective antioxidant defense, in obesity,
        235–236, 236f
Deficiency diseases treatment, antioxidants in,
        58–59
Delphinidins, 27, 35, 36
Dementia, 204–205
Depletion, GSH, 87–88
Depression, 62
Development
    antioxidants in children, 53–64
        ASD, 62–63
        asthma and allergies, 59
        behavioral alterations, 60–62
        brain development, 60–61
        cognitive function, 60–62
        deficiency diseases treatment, 58–59
        Down syndrome, 63, 64f
        growth and, 56–58, 56t
        micronutrients and early development,
            53–54, 55f
        obesity and, 59–60
        OS and health, 54, 56
        overview, 53–56, 55f
    cancer, FRs in, 166
Diabetes, 151–157
    amelioration of OS in, 293
    antioxidants and, 152–156
        carotenoids, 154
        lycopene, 154
        polyphenols, 155–156, 156f
        selenium, 155
        serum retinol, 154
        vitamin C, 153
        vitamin E, 153
    diet *vs.* pills, 157
    overview, 151–152
    serum retinol, 154
Diabetes mellitus, 151–152, 183, 216
    gestational, 50–51
    OS in, 293

Diallyl disulfides, 284, 288
Diallyl sulfides, 30, 284, 288, 292
Diallyl thiosulfinate, 35
Diarrhea, 265, 267, 270, 273t
Dicaffeoylquinin acids, 36, 37
Didanosin, 273t
Dielectric constant, 9
Diels–Alder reactions, 15
Dietary antioxidants
    in adulthood, 71–76
        bioavailability of natural antioxidants and
            effect on biomarkers, 73–75, 74t
        disease prevention, 75
        needs and importance, 71–73
        supplements and health, 75–76, 76t
    in cancer, 174
    defined, 167
    in elderly, 76–79
        consumption and disease prevention,
            77–79
        needs and importance, 76–77
    intake, IBD risks and, 223–224
    smoking and, 89–91, 90t, 91f
Dietary antioxidants, food sources and, 23–40
    natural, classification, 24–30
        carotenoids, 28–30, 29f
        EOs, 29f, 30
        phenols and polyphenols, 24–28. *See also*
            Phenols and polyphenols
    natural, distribution, 30–40
        fruits, 30–34, 32t–33t
        grapes and wine, 32t, 34–35
        herbs, 33t, 36–39
        olives and olive oil, 39–40
        vegetables, 32t, 35–36
    overview, 23–24
Dietary folate equivalents (DFEs), 168
Dietary Guidelines for Americans, 168, 181,
        184
Dietary intakes, for vitamins and minerals,
        56–58, 56t
Dietary reference intakes (DRIs), 77, 105
5-Diethoxyphosphoryl-5-methyl-1-pyrroline-*N*-
        oxide (DEPMPO), 86
Diet(s)
    Mediterranean, 77
    pills *vs.*, 157
Diglycoside isolariciresinols, 28
Dihydrochalcones, 33
Dihydroflavonols, 26
2,3-Dihydroxybenzoic acid, 39
3,4-Dihydroxyphenylacetic acid, 24
Dill, 32t, 35
Dill weed, 177
Diosmetin-acetyl-apioglucoside, 35
Diosmetin-apiosylglucoside, 35
Diphenylheptanoid compound, 29

2,2-Diphenyl-1-picrylhydrazyl (DPPH) test, 30, 37
Disease prevention, dietary antioxidants and
    in adulthood, 75
    in elderly, 77–79
Distribution, natural antioxidants, 30–40
    fruits, 30–34, 32t–33t
    grapes and wine, 32t, 34–35
    herbs, 33t, 36–39
    olives and olive oil, 39–40
    vegetables, 32t, 35–36
Diterpene, 291
Dittany, 30
Dog roses, 32t, 33
Down syndrome, antioxidants and, 63, 64f
Doxorubicin, 177
Dried fruits, 177
Dry beans, in cancer prevention, 182

E

Early development, micronutrients and, 53–54,
        55f
Ebselen, 206
Eclampsia, 49
Efavirenz, 272
Eggplant, 27, 32t, 35
Egg yolks, 179
Elderly, dietary antioxidants in, 76–79
    consumption and disease prevention, 77–79
    needs and importance, 76–77
Electron paramagnetic resonance (EPR)
        spectroscopy, 86
Elettaria cardamomum, 38
Ellagic acids, 31
Ellagitannins, 28
Endogenous antioxidants, 89, 90t, 103–104,
        106–109
    defined, 167
    GSH, 106–107
    lipoic acid, 107–109
Endometrium, of women, 48
Endoplasmic reticulum (ER), ROS production
        in, 8, 9
Endothelial isoform of NOS (eNOS), 14, 251–252
Eosinophils, activation, 268
Epicatechin-3-gallate (ECG), 237
Epicatechins (EC), 27, 38–39, 237
Epidemiology, HIV/AIDS, 263–264
Epididymis, 47
Epigallocatechin (EGC), 237
Epigallocatechin-3-gallate (EGCG), 237, 238
Epigallocatechins, 27
Ericaceae family, 27
Eriodictyol glycosides, 36
Eriodictyol-7-O-glucoside, 38
Eriodictyol-7-O-rutinoside, 26
Escherichia coli, 200

Essential oils (EOs), 29f, 30, 35, 36–37, 177, 292t
Eucalyptol, 30, 37
Eugenia caryophyllus, 283f
    antioxidant effects, 284, 287t, 289
Eugenol, 24, 25f, 30, 283f, 292t
    anti-inflammatory effect, 294
    antioxidant effects, 284, 287t, 289
    hepatoprotective and renal -protective effects,
        295
    in tumors, 293
European Food Safety Authority (EFSA), 73,
        75, 176
European Union (EU), 118
Evidence, clinical and experimental
    on exogenous antioxidants in obesity, 236–242
        ALA, 241
        anthocyanins and blueberries, 239
        CoQ, 241
        curcumin, 237t, 239–240
        fruits, legumes, and nuts, 241–242
        GTCs, 237–239, 237t
        resveratrol, 237t, 240–241
Exercise, physical, 103–111
    antioxidants
        endogenous, 106–109. See also
            Endogenous antioxidants
        exogenous, 109–111. See also Exogenous
            antioxidants
        general health and, 104
        supplementation for physically active
            individuals, 104–105
    overview, 103–104
Exhaled nitric oxide (eNO), 88
Exogenous antioxidants, 89, 90t, 103–104,
        109–111
    in cancer, 174
    clinical and experimental evidence in obesity,
        236–242
        ALA, 241
        anthocyanins and blueberries, 239
        CoQ, 241
        curcumin, 237t, 239–240
        fruits, legumes, and nuts, 241–242
        GTCs, 237–239, 237t
        resveratrol, 237t, 240–241
    defined, 167
    flavonoids, 110–111
    vitamins C and E, 109–110
Experimental evidence, on exogenous
        antioxidants in obesity, 236–242
        ALA, 241
        anthocyanins and blueberries, 239
        CoQ, 241
        curcumin, 237t, 239–240
        fruits, legumes, and nuts, 241–242
        GTCs, 237–239, 237t
        resveratrol, 237t, 240–241

F

Familial AD (fAD), 204
Farnesene, 30
Fennel seed, 38
Fenton reaction, 12
Fenugreek seeds, 293
Ferric reducing antioxidant power (FRAP)
        values, 31
Ferritin, 13
Fertility, OS in, 47–48
Ferulic acids, 24, 31, 39
Fibers
    breast cancer, 188–189, 189t
    colorectal cancer and, 188
Figs, 31, 177
Fish, 179
F2-isoprostane levels, 88
Flavanols, 25f, 26, 27, 33, 35, 38, 155
Flavan-3-ols, 27, 33, 34
Flavanones, 25f, 26, 27, 33–34, 36, 97, 155
Flavanonols, 25f, 26
Flavones, 25f, 26, 33, 34, 35, 36, 37, 97, 155, 190
Flavonoids, 25f, 26–27, 32t, 33, 36, 73, 75, 78,
        155
    in cancer prevention, 190–192, 190t, 191t
        292t
        food sources, 190–192, 190t, 191t
    exogenous antioxidants, 110–111
    polymethoxylated, 34
    smoking and
        dietary antioxidants, 93–94
        natural antioxidants, 97
    of tea, 290
    in thyme, 284
Flavonols, 25f, 26, 33, 34, 35, 36, 37, 97, 155,
        190
Flax seeds, 28, 32t
Foeniculum vulgare, 38
Folic acid, cancer and, 167–169, 169t
Food and Nutrition Board (FNB), 168
Food sources, dietary antioxidants and, 23–40
    in cancer, 179
        β-carotene, 179
        carotenoids, 184, 185
        lutein, 179
        lycopene, 179
        selenium, 179
        vitamin A, 179
        vitamin C, 179
    flavonoids, 190–192, 190t, 191t
    of folate and folic acid, 169t
    natural antioxidants, classification, 24–30
        carotenoids, 28–30, 29f
        EOs, 29f, 30
        phenols and polyphenols, 24–28. *See also*
            Phenols and polyphenols

natural antioxidants, distribution, 30–40
    fruits, 30–34, 32t–33t
    grapes and wine, 32t, 34–35
    herbs, 33t, 36–39
    olives and olive oil, 39–40
    vegetables, 32t, 35–36
    overview, 23–24
    of selenium, 171t
    of vitamin C, 173t
Forestomach cancer, 291
Framingham offspring cohort, 235
Free radicals (FRs), 4, 84, 87, 93
    in cancer development, 166
    in cigarette tar, 85–86
    defined, 166, 250
Fruits
    cancer prevention, 179–181
        intake recommendations, 181
    deeply pigmented, 177
    dried, 177
    natural antioxidants distribution in, 30–34,
        32t–33t
    obesity, 241–242
Functional foods, 281

G

Gallic acids, 24, 31, 34, 36, 37
Gallocatechins, 27
Garlic, 30, 32t, 35, 38, 177, 180, 181, 291, 293
    antiatherogenic and cardioprotective effect, 290
    antioxidant effects, 284, 286t–287t, 288
    diallyl sulfide, 292
    S-allylcysteine of, 292
Gas phase, radicals in, 87–88
    GSH depletion, 87–88
    oxidative radicals, 87
    peroxynitrite, 87
Gastric cancer, 174
Gastrointestinal disorders, 215–228
    celiac disease, 216–220
        defined, 216
        OS and, 217, 218f
        overview, 216
        potential beneficial effect of dietary
            antioxidant, 220, 220f
        risk, antioxidants and, 217, 218–219
        treatment, antioxidants and, 219–220
        vitamin C in, 219–220
    IBDs, 221–229. *See also* Inflammatory bowel
        diseases (IBDs)
        OS and, 222–223
        overview, 221
        risks, antioxidant and, 223–225
        treatment, antioxidant and, 225–228,
            226t–227t
Gastrointestinal tract, cancers of, 187

General health, antioxidants and, 104
Genistein, 26–27, 39
Gentisic acids, 31
Geranial, 30
Geraniol, 284, 291
Gestational diabetes mellitus, 50–51
Gingerol, 283f, 284, 288, 289, 291
Gingers, 38, 177, 281, 291
  antioxidant effects, 284, 288, 289
  in arthritic knee pain, 295
  6-gingerol and 6-paradol in, 292
Ginkgo biloba, 281
Ginseng, 281, 292t
GISSI (Gruppo Italiano per lo Studio della
        Sopravvivenza nell'Infarto
        Miocardico), 99
Glaucoma therapy, 207
Glaxo Wellcome, 273t
Gliadin, 216
Glucagon-like polypeptide-1 (GLP-1), 156
Glucose transporter-4 (GLUT4) translocation, 238
β-glucosides, 26–27
Glucosinolates, 181, 182
γ-Glutamylcysteine synthetase (γ-GCS), 200
L-γ-glutamyl-L-cysteinylglycine, 106–107
Glutaredoxins (Grxs), 200, 201, 205–206
Glutathione (GSH), 9, 15, 16, 17, 48, 50, 62,
        200–201, 252, 271
  in CNS pathologies, 206
  depletion, 87–88
  endogenous antioxidant, 106–107
Glutathione peroxidases (GSH-Px), 16, 17, 54, 58,
        63, 94–95, 106, 155, 200, 252, 270
Glutathione reductase (GR), 200–201
Glutathionylation, 200
Gluten, alcohol extraction, 216
Gluten-free diet (GFD), 216
Glutenins, 216
Gluten-sensitive enteropathy, 216
Glycosides, 26, 27, 31, 33–34, 35, 36, 39
Goitrin, 182
Gooseberries, 31, 32t
G proteins, 12
Grapes, 31, 32t, 34, 177, 179
  anthocyanin, 27, 34
  color, 27, 34
  fruit bark, 26
  natural antioxidants distribution in, 32t, 34–35
Green tea, 27, 36
  green tea catechin (GTC), 237–239, 237t
Ground-state oxygen, 4, 6
Growth, antioxidants in children, 53–64
  ASD, 62–63
  asthma and allergies, 59
  behavioral alterations, 60–62
  brain development, 60–61
  cognitive function, 60–62

deficiency diseases treatment, 58–59
  Down syndrome, 63, 64f
  growth and, 56–58, 56t
  micronutrients and early development, 53–54,
        55f
  obesity and, 59–60
  OS and health, 54, 56
  overview, 53–56, 55f
Gruppo Italiano per lo Studio della
        Sopravvivenza nell'Infarto
        Miocardico (GISSI), 99
GTP-cyclohydrolase (GCH1), 255
Guava, 177, 179

H

Halimioides, 28
Head, artichoke, 27, 32t, 36
Health
  adult, antioxidant supplements and, 75–76, 76t
  general, antioxidants and, 104
  pediatric, OS and, 54, 56
Health Professionals Study, 180–181
Heart Outcomes Prevention Evaluation (HOPE)
        study, 99, 175
Heat shock proteins (HSPs), 107
Heavy drinking, defined, 168
HELENA study, 58
Helicobacter pylori, 174
HELLP syndrome, 49
Heme oxygenase-1 (HO-1), 204
Hemorrhagic stroke, 118, 129
Hepatoprotective effects, spices and herbs, 295
Herbs, 177, 281–296
  amelioration of OS in diabetes, 293
  antiatherogenic and cardioprotective effect,
        290–291
  anticataractogenesis, 294
  anti-inflammatory effect, 294–295
  antioxidant effects, 283–289
    clove (*Eugenia caryophyllus*) and
          eugenol, 284, 287t, 289
    garlic (*Allium sativum*) and onion
          (*Allium cepa*), 284, 286t–287t, 288
    ginger (*Zingiber officinale*), 284, 288, 289
    red pepper (*Capsicum annuum*) and black
          pepper (*Piper nigrum*), 284, 288t
    turmeric (*Curcuma longa*) and curcumin,
          284, 285t–286t, 289f
  cancer-preventive property, 291–293, 292t
  hepatoprotective and renal-protective effects,
        295
  natural antioxidants distribution, 33t, 36–39
  neuroprotective potential, 294
  other nutraceutical properties, 296
  overview, 281–283, 283f
Hernia, 295

Hesperetin, 26, 38
Hesperidin, 26, 34
Hespiridin, 38
High-density lipoprotein (HDL), 142, 238, 290–291
High-fat diet (HFD), 238, 240
Highly active antiretroviral therapy (HAART), 272, 273t
Hipovitaminosis A, 57
HIV/AIDS. *See* Human immunodeficiency virus/ acquired immunodeficiency syndrome (HIV/AIDS)
Homeostasis, redox, 250–251
Homeostasis model assessment of insulin resistance (HOMA-IR), 154
Homovanillic acid, 39
Homovanillyl alcohol, 40
HOPE (Heart Outcomes Prevention Evaluation) study, 99, 175
Hordein, 216
Horseradish, 181
Human immunodeficiency virus/acquired immunodeficiency syndrome (HIV/AIDS), 263–274
    antioxidants and, 268–271
        β-carotene, 269
        NAC, 271
        polyphenols, 271
        selenium, 270
        supplementation, adverse effects, 273–274
        vitamin A, 268–269
        vitamin C, 269
        vitamin E, 269–270
        zinc, 270–271
    epidemiology, 263–264
    factors affecting antioxidant level in patients, 272–273
        combination therapy (HAARTS), 272, 273t
        medication intake, 272
        opportunistic conditions, 272
        socioeconomic status, 273
    HIV-1 *vs.* HIV-2, 264, 264t
    infections, types, 264, 264t
    malnutrition and, 266–267
    nutrition and, 267
    OS and, 267–268
    overview, 263–265
    pathomechanism, 265–266
        CD4 cells and, 265–266, 265t
        viral load, 266
    prevention, 274
    transmission, 264, 265
Human leukocyte antigen (HLA), 216
Humans
    smoking on OS in, 88–89
    sperms, OS and, 47
Hund's rule, 5
Hydrocele, 295

Hydrogen peroxide, 10–12, 86
Hydrolyzable tannins, 28
p-Hydroxybenzoic acids, 24, 31, 39
Hydroxycinnamic acids, 33
Hydroxyl radicals, 12–13
Hydroxytyrosol, 24, 25f, 39–40
Hypercholesterolemia, 290
Hyperglycemia, 152
Hyperici herba, 39
Hypochlorous acid (HOCl), 14–15
Hypothyroidism, 182
Hypoxia-ischemia (HI), 202–203
Hyssop, 37
Hyssopus officinalis, 37

I

IBDs. *See* Inflammatory bowel diseases (IBDs)
Ibuprofen, 295
IFN-γ (interferon-γ), 217, 218, 219, 220, 255
IL (Interleukin), 217, 218, 219, 220
IL-6 (interleukin-6), 107, 220
Imatinib, 177
Immune response, modulation, 249–258
    anti-inflammatory properties of antioxidants, 257–258
    antioxidant systems, 252–254
    overview, 249
    small redox molecules and redox homeostasis, 250–251
    Th1-type immune response, 254–256, 255f
    in vitro, monitoring, 256–257, 257f
Indinavir, 273t
Indole glucosinolates, 182
Indoles, 181
Indomethacin, 291
Indonesian children, 57
Inducible isoform of NOS (iNOS), 14, 217, 219, 251–252
Inflammation
    anti-inflammatory effect, spices and herbs, 294–295
    anti-inflammatory properties, of antioxidants, 257–258
    obesity and
        antioxidants in, 233–243. *See also* Obesity condition, 234
Inflammatory bowel diseases (IBDs), 221–229
    OS and, 222–223
    overview, 221
    risks, antioxidant and, 223–225
        blood antioxidant levels and, 224–225
        dietary antioxidant intake, 223–224
        treatment, antioxidant and, 225–228, 226t–227t
iNOS (inducible isoform of NOS), 14, 217, 219, 251–252

iNOS gene, 219
Intakes
    dietary
        antioxidants, IBD risks and, 223–224
        for vitamins and minerals, 56–58, 56t
    DRIs, 77, 105
    medication, HIV/AIDS patients and, 272
    recommendations
        breast cancer, 189, 189t
        cruciferous vegetables, 182
        fruits and vegetables, 181
        soy, 183, 184
        whole grains, 184
Interferon-γ (IFN-γ), 217, 218, 219, 220, 255
Interleukin (IL), 217, 218, 219, 220
Interleukin-6 (IL-6), 107
Intestinal cancer, 225
Intrauterine growth restriction (IUGR), 49
Invirase, 273t
In vitro immune response, monitoring, 256–257,
        257f
In vitro systems, antioxidant effects
    curcumin in, 284, 285t–286t, 289f
    eugenol, 284, 287t, 289
In vivo systems, antioxidant effects
    curcumin in, 284, 285t–286t, 289f
    eugenol, 284, 287t, 289
Iodine function, cruciferous vegetables and,
        182
    intake recommendations, 182
Iraqi children, 59
Iron
    smoking and
        dietary antioxidants, 95
        natural antioxidants, 98
    supplementation, 57–58, 59
Ischemia, defined, 118
Ischemia–reperfusion injury, 201
Ischemic stroke, 118, 129
Isoflavones, 25f, 26–27, 97, 155
Isophorone, 30
Isoprene, 87
Isorhamnetin, 35, 37
Isothiocyanates, 181

J

Juniper berry, 38
Juniperus communis, 38

K

Kaempferol, 26, 35, 38
Kale, 179, 181, 186
Kidney stones, 273t
Kinase-driven pathways, on hydrogen peroxide,
        11

Kiwi fruit, 72
Kohlrabi, 181
Kwashiorkor, 58

L

Lamivudin, 272
Lariciresinols, 28
Laurels, 38
Lauri folium, 39
Laurus nobilis, 38
Lavender, 291
Leafy greens, 180
Legumes, 181
    in cancer prevention, 182–183
        dry beans, peas, and lentils, 182
        prostate cancer, 182–183
    in obesity, 241–242
Leguminosae family, 26
Lemon balm, 26, 33t, 37, 38
Lemon bark, 26
Lemongrass, 30, 290, 291, 292t
Lemon peel, 34
Lentils, in cancer prevention, 182, 183, 184
Lettuce, 180
Leucocistus, 28
Lewy bodies, 203, 204
Lewy neurites, 203
Lignans, 28
    in whole grains, 184
Ligstroside, 39, 40
Limonene, 30, 292t
Lind's study, 57–58
Linoleic acid, 223
Lipid peroxidation, 152, 295
Lipid peroxides, 294
Lipid theory, 283
Lipoic acid, 107–109
Lipophilic antioxidant, 72
Lipoprotein oxidation, singlet oxygen in, 15
Lipoyllysine, 108
Liver cancer, 172, 291
Low-density lipoprotein (LDL), 72, 92, 98, 109,
        119, 142, 235, 238, 290–291
Lung cancer, 175, 190
    rodent model, 291
    vitamin C and, 173
    vitamin E on, 99
Lutein, 31, 72, 78, 139, 179
    in cancer prevention, 186, 187t
Luteolin, 26, 36, 37, 39, 40, 62
Luteolin-7-*O*-glucoside, 36
Lycopene, 31, 72, 97, 99
    cancer prevention, 180–181, 184, 185, 186
    CHD and strokes, 142–143
    diabetes, 154
    food sources, 179

M

Mace, 38, 281
Magnesium, supplementation in diabetes, 157
Mainstream (inhaled) smoking, 84–85
Majoranae folium, 39
Male subfertility, 47–48
Malnutrition
    children, 53–54
    HIV/AIDS and, 266–267
Malondialdehyde (MDA), 48, 49, 50
Malvidin, 27
Malvidin glycoside, 34
Mandarin peel, 32t, 34
Mangoes, 177, 179
Marjoram, 30, 33t, 38, 177
Matricaria chamomilla, 38
M-coumaric acid, 38
Medication intake, 272
Mediterranean diet, 77
Melissa folium, 39
Melissa officinalis, 26, 37
Melons, carotenoids in, 28, 31
Mental development, antioxidants and, 60–61
Mentha piperita, 39
Mentha pulegium, 38
Mentha spicata, 292t
Mesalazine, 225
Metallothionein, 13
Methanols, 37
Methotrexate, 177
Methyl allyl sulfides, 30
Methylphenidate, 61
1-Methyl-4-phenylpyridinium (MPP+), 205
1-Methyl-4-phenyl-1,2,3,6-tetrahydropyridine
        (MPTP), 205
Micronutrients
    deficiency, 266–267, 273
    early development and, 53–54, 55f
    examples, 267
Milk, 179
Minerals
    child growth and development, 54, 56, 56t,
        57–58, 59–62
    smoking and, 94–95
        copper, 94
Mint, 291, 292t
Miscarriage, OS and, 48
Mitochondria, ROS production in, 7
Mitogen-activated protein kinases (MAPKs),
        109
Mn-superoxide dismutase (Mn-SOD), 109
Moderate alcohol consumption, defined, 168
Modulation of immune response, 249–258
    anti-inflammatory properties of antioxidants,
        257–258
    antioxidant systems, 252–254

    overview, 249
    small redox molecules and redox
        homeostasis, 250–251
    Th1-type immune response, 254–256, 255f
    in vitro, monitoring, 256–257, 257f
Monitoring, immune response *in vitro*, 256–257,
        257f
Monoglycoside 7-hydroxymatairesinols, 28
Monoterpene alcohol, 291
Monoterpenes, 30
Morbidity, in mother and fetus, 47, 48–50
Morellos, 31
    color, 27
Mortality
    mother and fetus, OS and, 47, 48–50
    underweight children, 53–54
Mother-to-child transmission (MTCT), 264, 265
Mountain tea, 33t, 36, 38
Mouse models
    anthocyanins administration in, 239
    carcinogenesis in, 291–293
    celiac disease, 219
    cognitive tests in, 78
    diet-induced obesity in, 238
    GSH deficiency and, 106–107
    IBD, 228
    lung cancer, 291
    signaling pathways in CNS diseases, 205–206
    tumor promotion, 291
Mouth sores, 267
Mozzarella cheese, 179
mTOR (target of rapamycin), 271
Muscle damage, vitamins C and E, 109–110
Mustard seed, 177, 181
Myeloperoxidase, 14–15
Myocardial infarction, vitamin E on, 99
Myricetin, 26, 36, 190
Myristica fragrans, 38
Myristicin, 30, 35, 291, 292t
Myrosinase, 181

N

N-acetyl cysteine (NAC), 106, 177
    HIV/AIDS and, 271
NADPH oxidases (NOX), 251
Naphthalene, 294
Naringenin, 26, 36, 38, 39
Naringin, 26, 34, 38
National Cancer Institute, 172, 174, 180, 181, 182
National Health and Nutrition Examination
        Surveys (NHANES), 72, 105, 154
National Institutes of Health (NIH), 118, 187
Natural antioxidants
    bioavailability and effect on biomarkers,
        73–75, 74t
    classification, 24–30

carotenoids, 28–30, 29f
EOs, 29f, 30
phenols and polyphenols, 24–28. *See also*
Phenols and polyphenols
distribution, 30–40
fruits, 30–34, 32t–33t
grapes and wine, 32t, 34–35
herbs, 33t, 36–39
olives and olive oil, 39–40
vegetables, 32t, 35–36
smoking and, 95–98
copper, 97–98
flavonoids, 97
iron, 98
selenium, 98
vitamin A and non–provitamin A
carotenoids, 96–97
vitamin C, 95–96
vitamin E, 96
zinc, 97
Natural killer cells, 48
Nausea, 272, 273t
Needs and importance, of dietary antioxidants
in adulthood, 71–73
in elderly, 76–77
Nelfinavir, 273t
Neochlorogenic acids, 31, 36, 37
Neohesperidin, 34
Neonatal stroke, 202
Neopterin, 255–256, 257
Neoxanthine, 31
Neral, 30
Neurodegeneration, 199–207
pathologies in, 202–205
AD, 204–205
PA, 202–203
PD, 203–204
pharmacological approaches, 206–207
redox control and ROS and RNS, 199–200
signaling pathways in CNS diseases, Trxs
protein family in, 205–206
Trxs family proteins in brain, 200–202, 202f
Neuronal isoform of NOS (nNOS), 14, 251–252
Neuroprotective potential, 294
Nevirapine, 272
Nicotinamide adenine dinucleotide phosphate
(NADPH) oxidase, 11–12, 17
Nicotine, in cigarettes, 96
NIH (National Institutes of Health), 118, 187
Nipradilol, 207
Nitric oxide (NO), 13–14, 85, 86, 87, 217
Nitrosoperoxycarbonate, 14
Nitroso thiols, 200
N-methyl-D-aspartate (NMDA), 203
Noncommunicable diseases (NCDs), 117
Nonpolar solvents, 9
Non–provitamin A carotenoids, smoking and

dietary antioxidants, 92–93
natural antioxidants, 96–97
supplementation studies, 99
Norepinephrine, 238
Norvir, 273t
NO synthetase (NOS), 13–14, 251–252
Nuclear factor kappa B (NF-κB), 109, 217, 223,
254–255, 257, 267–268
Nuclear magnetic resonance analysis, of phenols,
40
Nurses' Health Study, 72, 130, 173, 180
Nutmeg, 38
Nutraceutical properties, of spices and herbs, 296
Nutrition
in cancer care, 191–192
HIV and, 267
Nutritional Prevention of Cancer Trial, 99
Nuts, 179
in obesity, 241–242

O

Obesity, 59–60, 233–243
clinical and experimental evidence on
exogenous antioxidants in, 236–242
ALA, 241
anthocyanins and blueberries, 239
CoQ, 241
curcumin, 237t, 239–240
fruits, legumes, and nuts, 241–242
green tea catechins, 237–239, 237t
resveratrol, 237t, 240–241
defective antioxidant defense in, 235–236,
236f
as inflammatory condition, 234
OS and, 48, 234–235
overview, 233–234
pediatric, 54
recommendations, 243
safety concerns and open questions, 242–243
Ocimum basilicum, 37, 290, 292t, 295
Old age. *See* Elderly
Oleuropein, 24, 39–40
Olives and olive oils, 24, 32t
natural antioxidants distribution, 39–40
Onions, 32t, 35, 177, 180, 181
antioxidant effects, 284, 286t–287t, 288
red, 27, 32t
Oocyte, OS and, 48
Opportunistic conditions, 272
Oral cancer, 291
Oranges, 31, 34, 177, 179
Oregano, 26, 30, 33t, 37, 38–39, 177, 292t
Organosulfur compounds, 30
Origanum majorana, 38
Origanum microphyllum, 38
Origanum species, 24, 37

Origanum vulgare, 26, 37, 38
OS. *See* Oxidative stress (OS)
Osteoarthritis, 295
Outcomes, CVD
    risk of
        observational studies on antioxidant
            intake and, 131t–138t
        RCTs of supplemental antioxidant intake
            and, 122t–128t
Overweight children, 54, 59–60
Oxidative burst reaction, 11
Oxidative radicals, 87
Oxidative stress (OS), 16–17, 203
    in cataractogenesis, 294
    children's health and, 54, 56
    in chronic diabetic complications, 152
    defined, 84, 119, 215
    in diabetes, amelioration, 293
    gastrointestinal disorders, 215–228
        celiac disease and, 217, 218f. *See also*
            Celiac disease
        IBDs, 222–223. *See also* Inflammatory
            bowel diseases (IBDs)
    HIV/AIDS and, 267–268
    obesity and, 48, 234–235
    in pregnancy, 47–51
        fertility, 47–48
        gestational diabetes mellitus, 50–51
        IUGR, 49
        miscarriage, 48
        overview, 47
        PPROM, 50
        preeclampsia, 48–49
        preterm labor, 49–50
    smoking and, 84–99
        antioxidant intake, interrelationship,
            89–99
        chemistry, interrelationship, 85–88.
            See also Smoking
        effects in humans, 88–89
        overview, 84–85
Oxygen
    chemistry basics, 4–7, 5f, 6t
    derived ROS, types, 10–19
        HOCl and myeloperoxidase, 14–15
        hydrogen peroxide, 10–12
        hydroxyl radicals, 12–13
        OS, 16–17
        ozone, 15–16
        peroxynitrite, 13–14
        singlet oxygen, 15
        substances and compounds with
            antioxidant activity, 18t–19t
    ground-state, 4, 6
    singlet, 4, 5, 15
    in triplet state, 4, 5f

Oxygen radical absorbance capacity (ORAC),
    176, 177, 178t
Ozone, 15–16

P

Pancreatic cancer, 187
Papaya, 179
Paprika, 177
PARK2 gene, 204
Parkin, 204
Parkinson disease (PD), 77–78, 203–204
Parsley, 32t, 35, 291, 292t
    EO compound, 30
Passive smoking, 84–85
Pathologies, in neurodegeneration, 202–205
    AD, 204–205
    PA, 202–203
    PD, 203–204
Pathomechanism, HIV/AIDS, 265–266
    CD4 cells and, 265–266, 265t
    viral load, 266
p-benzoquinone (*p*-BQ), 98
p-coumaric acids, 24, 31, 37, 39, 40
p-coumaroyltartaric acid, 35
p-cymene, 30, 37
Peaches, 31, 32t, 141, 177
    carotenoids in, 28, 31
Pears, 31, 32t, 177
Peas, in cancer prevention, 182, 183, 184
Pelargonidins, 27, 35
Pelargonin, 31
Pennyroyal, 30, 33t, 38–39
Peonidin-3-arabinoside, 27
Peonidin 3-*O*-rutinoside, 33
Peonidins, 27, 35, 36
Pepper, 177
Peppermint, 177
Perillyl alcohol, 291
Perinatal asphyxia (PA), 202–203
Peripheral arterial disease (PAD), 117
Peripheral blood mononuclear cells (PBMCs),
    256–257, 257f
Peroxidases, 16
Peroxiredoxins (Prxs), 16–17, 200, 201, 206
Peroxisomes, ROS production in, 7
Peroxyls, 86
Peroxynitrite, 13–14, 87, 201
Perrone's study, 57–58
Petroselinum crispum, 292t
Petunidin, 27, 31
Petunidin glycoside, 34
Phagocytic processes by cells, hydrogen peroxide
    in, 11
Pharmacological approaches, neurodegeneration,
    206–207

α-Phellandrene, 35
β-Phellandrene, 30, 35
Phenolic acids, 24, 25f, 32t–33t, 62
    fruits, 31–33
    grapes, 34
    herbs, 36–37
    olives and olive oil, 39–40
    vegetables, 35–36
Phenolic terpenes, 37
Phenols and polyphenols, 24–28, 32t–33t
    allergies in children, 59
    flavonoids, 25f, 26–27, 32t, 33–34, 36, 73, 75
    in fruits, 31–33
    in grapes, 34
    herbs, 36–37
    molecular structures, 25f
    olives and olive oil, 39–40
    others, 28
    phenolic acids, 24, 25f, 31–33, 32t–33t
    simple, 24, 25f
    in vegetables, 35–36
Phenylbutazone, 295
Phenylpropanoids, 24, 30
Phloretin, 27
Photolysis, 12
Photosynthesis, singlet oxygen in, 15
Physical exercise, 103–111
    antioxidants
        endogenous, 106–109. See also
            Endogenous antioxidants
        exogenous, 109–111. See also Exogenous
            antioxidants
        general health and, 104
        supplementation for physically active
            individuals, 104–105
    overview, 103–104
Physically active individuals, antioxidant
    supplementation for, 104–105
Physicians' Health Study II (PHS II), 175–176
Phytoene, 31
Phytoestrogens, 28
Phytofluene, 31
Phytohemagglutinin (PHA), 256
Pills, diet vs., 157
Pineapples, 31
α-Pinene, 30, 37
Pinoresinols, 28, 39, 40
Piperine, 283f, 293
    of black pepper, 284, 288t
Piper nigrum, 38, 283f
    antioxidant effects, 284, 288t
Pleiotropic effect, 141
Plums, 31, 177
Poliomintha longiflora, 292t
Polygonum cuspidatum, 141
Polymethoxylated flavonoids, 34

Polyphenols, 24–28, 32t–33t, 73, 78
    allergies in children, 59
    in CHD and strokes, 140–141
    diabetes, 155–156, 156f
    dietary, antiobesity effects, 237t
    flavonoids, 25f, 26–27, 32t, 33–34, 36, 73, 75
    in fruits, 31–33
    in grapes, 34
    herbs, 36–37
    HIV/AIDS and, 271
    molecular structures, 25f
    olives and olive oil, 39–40
    others, 28
    phenolic acids, 24, 25f, 31–33, 32t–33t
    simple, 24, 25f
    in vegetables, 35–36
Polyunsaturated fatty acids (PUFA), 61
Pomace, 32t
Pomegranate, 177
Poultry, 179
Preeclampsia, OS in, 47, 48–49
Pregnancy, OS in, 47–51
    fertility, 47–48
    gestational diabetes mellitus, 50–51
    IUGR, 49
    miscarriage, 48
    overview, 47
    PPROM, 50
    preeclampsia, 48–49
    preterm labor, 49–50
Preterm labor, 49–50
Preterm premature rupture of membrane
    (PPROM), 50
Prevention
    disease, dietary antioxidants and
        in adulthood, 75
        in elderly, 77–79
    HIV/AIDS, 274
Prevention, cancer, 174–177, 179–192
    carotenoids, 184–187
        β-carotene, 185, 186t
        β-cryptoxanthin, 185
        α-carotene, 185, 185t
        curcumin, 186, 187
        food sources, 184–185
        lutein and zeaxanthin, 186, 187t
        lycopene, 185, 186
    colorectal cancer and fiber, 188
    cruciferous vegetables, 181–182
        intake recommendations, 182
        iodine and thyroid function, 182
    curcumin, 186, 187
    flavonoids and, 190–192, 190t, 191t
        food sources, 190–192, 190t, 191t
    fruits and vegetables, 179–181
        intake recommendations, 181

legumes, 182–183
    dry beans, peas, and lentils, 182
    soy, 183–184
    spices and herbs, 291–293, 292t
    whole grains, 184
        intake recommendations, 184
Proanthocyanidins, 27
Procyanidins, 62
Production, ROS, 7–10, 8f, 9f
Progoitrin, 181
Progression, HIV, 265t
Prolamins, 216
Prostaglandins, 217
Prostate cancer, 180–181, 190
    legumes in, 182–183
    selenium and, 99, 170, 172, 175
    soy in, 183
Protocatechic acids, 24, 31, 38
Protocatechuic acids, 37
Provitamin A carotenoids, smoking and
    dietary antioxidants, 92–93
    natural antioxidants, 96–97
    supplementation studies, 99
Prunus avium, 31
Prunus spinosa, 33
Psyllium, 188
Pulegone, 30
Pulmonary embolism, 117
Pumpkin, 179
Pycnogenol, 62
Pyruvoyl tetrahydropterin synthase, 255–256

Q

Quercetin 3-glucoside, 34
Quercetin 3-glucuronide, 34
Quercetin 3-O-rutinoside, 33
Quercetin–rhamnoglucoside, 35
Quercetin 3-rutinoside, 34
Quercetins, 26, 35, 36, 37, 38, 39, 62, 73, 93–94,
    110, 283f, 291
Quinic acids, 31
Quinones, in cigarette tar, 86

R

Rac, transcription factor, 12
Radicals
    cigarette tar, 85–87
        FRs, 85–86
        quinones, 86
        trace heavy metals, 86–87
    gas phase, 87–88
        GSH depletion, 87–88
        oxidative radicals, 87
        peroxynitrite, 87

Radish, 27, 32t, 35, 181
Raisins, 177
Randomized controlled trials (RCTs), 119, 120, 177
    for cancer prevention, 174
    meta-analysis of, 139
    selenium supplementation, examination,
        139–140
    of supplemental antioxidant intake and CVD
        outcomes risk, 122t–128t
RAS homolog gene family member A (RhoA)
    gene, 108
Raspberries, 31, 32t, 177
    color, 27
Reactive nitrogen species (RNS), 84, 87
    cellular, production, 251–252
    redox control and, 199–200
    small redox molecules and redox
        homeostasis, 250–251
Reactive oxygen species (ROS), 3–20, 84, 119
    activation, 267
    in cell turnover and replacement, 3
    cellular, production, 251–252
    common targets of damaging effects, 19–20
    defined, 3, 166
    forms of, 3, 4
    generation, 8f, 48, 103, 152
    O_2-derived, types, 10–19
        HOCl and myeloperoxidase, 14–15
        hydrogen peroxide, 10–12
        hydroxyl radicals, 12–13
        OS, 16–17
        ozone, 15–16
        peroxynitrite, 13–14
        singlet oxygen, 15
        substances and compounds with
            antioxidant activity, 18t–19t
    oocyte maturation, ovulation, and
        fertilization, 48
    OS by, 48, 54
    overview, 3–4
    oxygen chemistry basics, 4–7
        generation as by-products and
            intermediates, 5f
        relative rate constants for, 6t
        standard reduction potentials for redox
            couples, 6t
    production, 7–10, 8f, 9f
    redox control and, 199–200
    regulation, 8f
    small redox molecules and redox
        homeostasis, 250–251
Recommendations
    intake
        breast cancer, 189, 189t
        cruciferous vegetables, 182
        fruits and vegetables, 181

soy, 183–184
  whole grains, 184
obesity, 243
Recommended daily allowance (RDA), 72, 104
  for folate, 168, 169t
Red cabbage, 27, 32t, 35
Red currants, 31, 32t
  color, 27
Red grapes, 27, 34
Red onion, 27, 32t
Redox control, ROS and RNS and, 199–200
Redox couples, ROS
  standard reduction potentials for, 6t
Redox homeostasis, 250–251
Redox molecules, small, 250–251
Red pepper
  anti-inflammatory effect, 294
  antioxidant effects, 284, 288t
Red wine, 141, 177
Regulated on activation, normal T-cell expressed
    and secreted (RANTES) protein, 16,
    270
Relative rate constants, for ROS, 6t
Renal-protective effects, spices and herbs, 295
Respiratory burst reaction, 11, 250
Resveratrols, 28, 35, 111, 156, 237t
  CHD and strokes, 141–142
  in obesity, 237t, 240–241
Retinal, 92
Retinoic acid (RA), 72, 92, 219
  in gliadin tolerance, 219
Retinol activity equivalents (RAE), 72
Retinols, 57, 60, 92, 185
  diabetes, 154
Retinyl esters, 92
Retrovir, 273t
Rheumatic heart disease, 117
Rheumatoid arthritis, 295
RhoA (RAS homolog gene family member A)
    gene, 108
Riboflavin, 58
Rice, 179
Risk(s)
  antioxidants and
    celiac disease, 217, 218–219
    IBDs, 223–225. *See also* Inflammatory
      bowel diseases (IBDs)
  CVD outcomes
    observational studies on antioxidant
      intake and, 131t–138t
    RCTs of supplemental antioxidant intake
      and, 122t–128t
  factors associated with stroke and CHD, 118
Ritonavir, 273t
Rormarini folium, 39
ROS. *See* Reactive oxygen species (ROS)

Rosa canina, 26, 33
Rosaceae family, 27
Rosa micrantha, 26, 33
Rosemary, 30, 32t, 37, 291, 292t
Rosemary officinalis, 37, 291, 292t
Roses, 32t, 33
Rosmanol, 39
Rosmarinic acid, 24, 37–38
Rutabaga, 181
Rutin, 38, 62
Rye, 28, 32t, 216

S

Safety concerns, in obesity, 242–243
Safflower, 179
Saffron, 28, 29
Safranal, 30
Sage, 30, 33t, 36, 37, 177, 292t
Salicylic acids, 24, 31
Salvia cryptantha, 37
Salvia multicaulis, 37
Salvianolic acid, 39
Salvia officinalis, 37, 39, 292t
Salvia species, 37
Saquinavir, 273t
Satureja herba, 39
Satureja hortensis, 37
Satureja species, 24, 37
Satureja thymbra, 38
Savory, 30, 33t, 37, 38, 177
Schenck-ene reactions, 15
Secalin, 216
Secoisolariciresinols, 28
Selenium, 54, 56t, 58, 60, 72, 106, 167
  cancer and, 170–172, 171t
  celiac disease, 218–219
  CHD and strokes, 139–140
  diabetes, 155
  food sources, 179
  HIV/AIDS and, 270
  intestinal cancer and, 225
  smoking and
    dietary antioxidants, 94–95
    natural antioxidants, 98
    supplementation studies, 99
Selenium and vitamin E cancer prevention trial
    (SELECT), 175
Selenoenzymes, 172
Selenol, 16
Selenoproteins, 219
Seminal fluid, 47
Serpylli herba, 39
Serratia vaccinii, 239
Serum retinol diabetes, 154
Sesame seeds, 28, 32t

Sesamin, 28
Sesaminols, 28
Sesamolin, 28
Sesamolinols, 28
Sesquiterpenes, 30
Sideritis syriaca, 38
Sidestream smoking, 84
Signaling pathways, in CNS diseases
    Trxs protein family and, 205–206
Silymarin, 291
Simple phenols, 24, 25f
Sinapic acids, 24, 39
Singlet oxygen, 4, 5, 15
Skin cancer, 291
    selenium and, 99, 172
Skin photosensitivity, singlet oxygen in, 15
Small redox molecules, 250–251
Smoking, OS and, 48, 84–99
    antioxidant intake, interrelationship, 89–99
        dietary antioxidants, 89–91, 90t, 91f
        dietary antioxidants, interaction, 95
        minerals and trace elements, 94–95.
            See also Minerals; Trace elements
        natural antioxidants, case, 95–98.
            See also Natural antioxidants
        in supplementation studies, 98–99.
            See also Supplementation, studies
        vitamins, 91–94. *See also* Vitamins,
            smoking and
    chemistry, interrelationship, 85–88
        cigarette tar, radicals in, 85–87. *See also*
            Radicals, cigarette tar
        gas phase, radicals in, 87–88. *See also*
            Radicals, gas phase
    effects in humans, 88–89
    overview, 84–85
S-nitrosylation, 200
Socioeconomic status, HIV/AIDS patients and, 273
Sodium selenite, 172
Solvents, dielectric constant in, 9
Soy, in cancer prevention, 183–184
    intake recommendations, 183–184
Soya, 26
Soya milk, 27
Soybean oils, 179
Spearmint, 291, 292t
Sperms, OS and, 47
Spices, 177, 281–296
    antiatherogenic and cardioprotective effect,
        290–291
    anticataractogenesis, 294
    anti-inflammatory effect, 294–295
    antioxidant effects, 283–289
        clove (*Eugenia caryophyllus*) and
            eugenol, 284, 287t, 289
        garlic (*Allium sativum*) and onion
            (*Allium cepa*), 284, 286t–287t, 288

ginger (*Zingiber officinale*), 284, 288,
        289
    red pepper (*Capsicum annuum*) and black
        pepper (*Piper nigrum*), 284, 288t
    turmeric (*Curcuma longa*) and curcumin,
        284, 285t–286t, 289f
    bioactive compounds, 283f
    cancer-preventive property, 291–293, 292t
    hepatoprotective and renal-protective effects,
        295
    neuroprotective potential, 294
    OS in diabetes, amelioration, 293
    other nutraceutical properties, 296
    overview, 281–283, 283f
Spinach, 32t, 179, 185, 186
Spin trapping, 86
Sporadic PD, 204
Sprouts, 181, 182
Squash, 179, 185
Standard reduction potentials, for ROS redox
        couples, 6t
Stavudine, 272
Stomach cancer, 174
Strawberries, 31, 33, 72, 177
Streptozotocin-induced diabetes, 293, 294
Stroke(s), 117–143
    antioxidant(s), 120–143
        carotenoids, 130–139, 131t–138t
        hypothesis, 119–120, 120f
        lycopene, 142–143
        polyphenols, 140–141
        resveratrol, 141–142
        selenium, 139–140
        vitamin C, 129–130
        vitamin E, 120–129, 122t–128t
    hemorrhagic, 118, 129
    ischemic, 118, 129
    neonatal, 202
    overview, 117–118
    risk factors associated with, 118
    vitamin E on, 99
Stunted children, 57, 58
Subfertility, male, 47–48
Substantia nigra (SNc), 203, 204
Sudanese infants and children, 57
Sulfenic acids, 200
Sulfenylation, 200
Superoxide anion radicals, 6–7, 9
Superoxide dismutase (SOD), 11–12, 63, 86, 109,
        201, 252
Supplementation
    adult health and, 75–76, 76t
    in cancers, 174–177, 178t
        dilemma of, 177, 178–179
    on HIV/AIDS patients
        adverse effects, 273–274
    magnesium, in diabetes, 157

for physically active individuals, 104–105
studies, 98–99
combined antioxidant, 99
non–provitamin A carotenoid, 99
selenium, 99
vitamin C, 98–99
vitamin E, 99
Swallowing problems, 267
Swedish Mammography Cohort, 173
Sweet potatoes, 179
α-Synuclein, 204
Syringaresinols, 28, 40
Syringic acids, 24, 37, 38, 39

T

Table grapes, 34
Table olives, 39
Tannins, 28
Tar, cigarette
radicals in, 85–87
FRs, 85–86
quinones, 86
trace heavy metals, 86–87
Target of rapamycin (mTOR), 271
Tarragon, 33t, 37, 177
Taxifolin, 26, 62
Tea, 27, 33t, 75
black, 36
flavonoids of, 290
green, 27, 36
mountain, 33t, 36, 38
Terpinen-4-ol, 30
α-Terpineols, 30, 37
Tetrachloride–induced hepatotoxicity, 295
Tetraterpenes, 28
Thiobarbituric acid, 272
Thiobarbituric acid reactive substances
(TBARS), 88
Thiocyanate ions, 182
Thiolation, 200
Thiol group, 16
Thioredoxin protein family (Trxs), 200
Thioredoxin reductases (TrxR), 200
Thioredoxins (Trxs), 16–17
protein family
in brain, 200–202, 202f
in signaling pathways in CNS diseases,
205–206
Th1-type immune response, 254–256, 255f
Thyme, 30, 32t, 37, 177, 284, 292t
Thymi herba, 39
Thymol, 24, 25f, 30, 37, 38, 284, 292t
Thymus, 24
Thymus serpyllum, 26
Thymus species, 37
Thymus vulgaris, 284

Thymys serpyllum, 37
Thymys vulgaris, 37, 292t
Thyroid function, cruciferous vegetables and,
182
intake recommendations, 182
Tight junction (Tj), 220
Tiliae officinalis, 39
Timolol, 207
Tocopherols, 24, 29f, 39, 72, 92, 96, 153, 179,
218; *See also* Vitamin E
Toenail selenium concentration, 170, 172
Tomatoes, 97, 179, 180–181, 185, 186
Total particulate matter (TPM), 86
Trace elements, smoking and, 94–95
heavy metals in cigarette tar, 86–87
iron, 95
selenium, 94–95
zinc, 94
Transmission, HIV/AIDS, 264, 265
trans-3,4′,5-trihydroxystilbene, 28
Tricarboxylic acid cycle, 108
Trigonella foenum-graecum, 293
Triplet oxygen, 4, 5f
Triterpene carnosic acid, 39
Triterpenic acid, 39
Trolox, 284
Trolox equivalent antioxidant capacity (TEAC),
88
Tryptophan, Th1-type immune response on,
254–256, 255f, 257
Tumor, in mouse, 291
Tumor necrosis factor-α (TNF-α), 217, 218, 220
Turmeric, 177, 186, 281, 291, 294
antiinflammatory drug, 294
antioxidant effects, 284, 285t–286t, 289f
cancer-preventive property, 291
Turnips, 181, 182
Type 2 diabetes mellitus (T2DM), 233, 234
Tyrosol, 24, 25f, 39, 40

U

Ubiquinol, 62
Ulcerative colitis (UC), 221, 223–224, 225
Uncoupling proteins (UCPs), 7, 9f
Undernourishment, during childhood, 53–54
Underweight children, 54, 57
United Nations Children's Fund (UNICEF),
53
Ursolic acid, 39
U.S. Department of Agriculture, 141
U.S. Preventive Services Task Force, 176

V

Vanillic acids, 24, 31, 37, 38, 39, 40
Vanillin, 39, 40

Vegetables
  in cancer prevention, 179–181
    cruciferous, 181–182
    intake recommendations, 181
  carotenoids in, 28
  natural antioxidants distribution in, 32t,
      35–36
Videx, 273t
Vinblastine, 177
Vinyl dithiins, 30, 35
Viracept, 273t
Viral load, HIV, 266
Virgin olives, 39
Vitamin(s)
  in adulthood, 72, 76
  in child growth and development, 56–62, 56t
  in old Age, 76–77
  smoking and, 91–94
    flavonoids, 93–94
    non–provitamin A carotenoids, 92–93
    vitamin A, 92–93, 94. See also Vitamin A
    vitamin C, 91–92, 94. See also Vitamin C
    vitamin E, 92, 94. See also Vitamin E
  vitamin B, 59
  vitamin D, 76
Vitamin A, 28, 54, 56–57, 56t, 58–59, 60, 72,
      76, 77
  in cancer prevention, 185
  food sources, 179
  HIV/AIDS and, 268–269
  smoking and
    dietary antioxidants, 92–93, 94
    natural antioxidants, 96–97
Vitamin B, 59
Vitamin C, 17, 31, 37, 48, 50, 54, 56t, 58, 59, 60,
      72, 73, 76, 77, 90t
  cancers, 172–174, 173t, 177
  celiac disease, 219–220
  CHD and strokes, 129–130
  diabetes, 153, 157
  DRIs of, 105
  exogenous antioxidant, 109–110
  food sources, 179
  HIV/AIDS and, 269
  smoking and
    dietary antioxidants, 91–92, 94
    natural antioxidants, 95–96
  supplementation studies, 98–99
Vitamin D, 76
Vitamin E, 17, 48, 50, 54, 56t, 58, 59, 60, 61, 72,
      76, 77
  celiac disease, 218
  CHD and stroke, 120–129, 122t–128t
  diabetes, 153, 157
  exogenous antioxidant, 109–110
  food sources, 179

HIV/AIDS and, 269–270
  intake, athletes and, 105
  smoking and, 92, 94
    natural antioxidants, 96
  supplementation studies, 99
Vitis vinifera, 34
Vomiting, 267, 272

W

141 W94, 273t
Wasabi, 181
Watercress, 181
Watermelon, 28, 179
Wheat, 179, 216
Wheat germ, 179
White grapes, 34
White pepper, 38
Whole grains, in cancer prevention, 184
  intake recommendations, 184
Wild roses, 32t, 33
Wild thyme, 26
Wine grapes, 34
Wines, 28, 141
  natural antioxidants distribution in, 34–35
  red, 141, 177
Women's Health Study (WHS), 175
World Cancer Research Fund, 180, 181
World Health Organization (WHO), 56–57, 56t,
      117, 263
ω-3 PUFA, 61

X

Xanthophylls, 186

Z

ζ-carotene, 31
Zeaxanthin, 31, 72
  in cancer prevention, 186, 187t
Zidovudine, 272, 273t
Zinc
  HIV/AIDS and, 270–271
  smoking and
    dietary antioxidants, 94
    natural antioxidants, 97
  supplementation, 54, 56t, 57–58, 59, 60,
      61–62
    for neurodevelopment, 60–61
Zinger officinale, 283f
Zingiber, 290
Zingiberaceae, 186
Zingiber officinale, antioxidant effects, 284, 288,
      289
Zingiber officinalis, 38

Printed in the United States
by Baker & Taylor Publisher Services